Dermatology for the House Officer

Second Edition

D1519609

BOOKS IN THE HOUSE OFFICER SERIES

Dermatology for the House Officer

Second Edition

Peter J. Lynch, M.D.

Professor and Head
Department of Dermatology
University of Minnesota Medical Center
Minneapolis, Minnesota

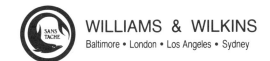

WILLIAMS & WILKINS
Baltimore • London • Los Angeles • Sydney

Editor: Nancy Collins
Associate Editor: Carol Eckhart
Copy Editor: Lindsay Edmunds
Design: JoAnne Janowiak
Illustration Planning: Wayne Hubbel
Production: Raymond E. Reter

Copyright ©, 1987
Williams & Wilkins
428 East Preston Street
Baltimore, MD 21202, U.S.A.

Accurate indications, adverse reactions, and dosage schedules for drugs are provided in this book, but it is possible that they may change. The reader is urged to review the package information data of the manufacturers of the medications mentioned.

Printed in the United States of America

First Edition, 1982

Library of Congress Cataloging in Publication Data
Main entry under title:

Lynch, Peter J., 1936-
  Dermatology for the house officer.
  Bibliography: p.
  Includes index.
  1. Skin—Diseases. I. Title. [DNLM: 1. Skin Diseases. WR 140 L987d]
RL71.L96 1987   616.5   86-13176
ISBN 0-683-05251-9

87 88 89 90   10 9 8 7 6 5 4 3 2

For Barbara, Deborah, and Timothy

There have been many times when the press of professional activity has distracted me from you who are the mainstay of my happiness and peace of mind. Certainly this occurred during preparation of this manuscript. Perhaps public acknowledgment of your forbearance will serve in some small way to thank you for your love and understanding.

Foreword to the First Edition

In his preface, Dr. Lynch writes that this book has three unique features. But it has a fourth: the unique style of the author. No one else has done what he has accomplished with such flare. It is the first book written in a style that makes the study of skin disease both exciting and approachable for the neophyte.

The text is neither all-inclusive nor artificially abbreviated, but contains a wealth of information written in a style that expresses the personal touch and philosophy of the author. Dermatology, like other medical and surgical disciplines, is an art and science of diminishing return: the more one learns the less use he or she has for that information. This truth often discourages the beginner. More than 95% of all skin diseases for which patients approach a physician are included in the 75 conditions that are discussed in this book. But the student need not even learn 75 diseases as distinct entities; the problem-oriented approach permits most of the diseases to be included in one of the ten groups. Once the clinician has grouped an unknown disease, the possibilities are relatively few; usually a maximum of 11 or 12 distinct diseases must be considered. Thus, even the novice can make a correct diagnosis by using the information obtained from observing and palpating skin lesions.

The author states that this book is written for the same purpose that training wheels are put on a bicycle: it is not intended for the developed free-wheeling clinician. But, in reality, it is written for a certain group of experienced dermatologists -- those who wish to teach skin disease to nondermatologists and make it understandable, exciting, and just plain fun.

W. Mitchell Sams, Jr., M.D.

Professor and Chairman
Department of Dermatology
University of Alabama in Birmingham

Preface

I am gratified that the response to this textbook has warranted the publication of a second edition. In preparing this new edition I have retained the philosophy and the format of the original text. The intended audience is still medical students, house officers, and those practicing general medicine. The text continues to be problem oriented in approach and incorporates the use of a clinical algorithm based on lesion morphology (see page 72). This approach was originally chosen, and continues to be used, because it allows for rapid, accurate, on-site diagnosis of otherwise unrecognized skin disease. The text also remains quite brief, and the number of diseases covered has been intentionally restricted. Only 75 entities, those which make up the most common, serious, contagious, and treatable dermatologic problems, are discussed in detail. Fortunately, these 75 diseases encompass more than 95% of all patient encounters for skin problems, thus offering the potential for excellent accuracy and completeness. Further discussion regarding the importance and usefulness of this approach can be found in the preface to the first edition and in Chapter 6.

This second edition also offers much that is new. For each disease the sections on pathophysiology and therapy have been completely rewritten. The recently recognized entities of dysplastic nevus syndrome and acquired immunodeficiency syndrome (AIDS) have been added. References current to mid-1986 have been included, and those prior to 1980 have been deleted. Appendices listing current dermatologic monographs and reference textbooks have been updated. Finally, larger type has been used to enhance readability.

I am once again grateful for the assistance rendered by the editorial staff at Williams & Wilkins and would particularly like to thank my secretary Cynthia Utter for the many hours she has spent typing and proofreading the manuscript. Without her efforts this text would not have been possible.

Peter J. Lynch, M.D.

Contents

Anatomy and Physiology

The skin is an impressively large and heavy organ. It occupies well over a square meter of surface area and accounts for about 20% of total body weight. As the boundary between our body and a hostile world it serves several functions. First, the skin acts as a barrier for fluid movement. Internal fluids are kept within the body and external fluids are withheld from penetration. Second, the skin serves as the major means of temperature control for the body. Conservation of body heat occurs both through vasoconstriction and through the insulating properties of the skin itself. Cooling of the body occurs by way of vasodilation and through evaporation of sweat. Third, the skin offers important protection from ultraviolet light. Both melanin production by melanocytes and keratin production by keratinocytes serve to decrease the amount of damage done to cellular DNA as a result of ultraviolet light penetration. Fourth, the skin operates as the source of sensory input to the body. Sensory nerve endings which terminate in the papillary dermis carry important information to the brain regarding our external environment. Fifth, the skin is an organ of metabolism for some important molecules. This role is exemplified by the ability of epithelial cells to synthesize vitamin D.

The skin is composed of three layers: the epidermis, the dermis, and the fatty layer. Embryologically the epidermis is derived from ectodermal tissue whereas the other two layers are mesodermal structures.

EPIDERMIS (Fig. 1-1)

The epidermis is the outermost layer of the skin and it is the thinnest of the three layers. In practical terms it is no thicker than three or four pages in this book. The epidermis is responsible for the impervious nature of the skin. Fluid movement is restricted by the presence of a barrier zone which occurs at the junction of living and nonliving keratinocytes in the outer third of the epidermis. Penetration of ultraviolet light is greatly reduced by the presence of melanin and keratin within the epidermal cells. The epidermis is composed of four cell types: keratinocytes, melanocytes, Langerhans cells, and Merkel cells.

<u>Keratinocytes</u>. Keratinocytes account for 95% of all of the cells of the epidermis. These cells are mainly responsible for the production of the fibrillar protein known as keratin but to a lesser degree other proteins and sterols are also synthesized. Keratinocytes begin their life as germinative, undifferentiated cells at the dermal-epidermal junction. These cells are known as

basal cells. Cells in the basal layer and in the layer immediately
above it are continuously dividing in such a way that one-half of
the cells remain in place to provide cells for replenishment while
the other half begin a progressive journey to the skin surface where
they will be exfoliated. These basal cells (which already show some
degree of perinuclear keratin formation) are attached to one another
and to the underlying basement membrane in a series of junction
points known as desmosomes. These desmosomal connections are
continuously resorbed and rebuilt as cells move by one another
during their outward journey. By way of these desmosomes and other
connecting points known as gap junctions, a rather constant
200-angstrom distance is kept between adjacent cells. This
intercellular space allows for the diffusion of nutrients to the
cells as they move outward.

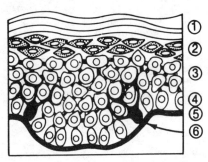

Figure 1-1. The structure of the epidermis. The epidermis is made
up of multiple layers: 1, the stratum corneum; 2, the granular cell
layer; 3, the prickle cell layer; 4, the basal layer; and 5, the
basement membrane layer. 6 points to a dendritic melanocyte found
in the basal layer.

As cells migrate outward from the basal layer the desmosomes, as
a result of histologic fixation artifact, becomes visible as
prickles or spines. Thus the mid layer of the epidermis has become
known as the spinous or prickle cell layer. Cell activity in this
layer is dominated by the production of keratin, the fibrils of
which are now seen to extend to the cytoplasmic wall where they
connect to the membrane at the site of desmosome formation.
In the outermost portion of the spinous layer, the keratinocytes
begin to change in rather noticeable ways. Granules of two types
are now found in the cytoplasm and the shape of the cells becomes
increasingly flattened. The larger of the two types of granules,
the keratohyalin granule, develops within and around the fibrillar
protein contributing in some unknown way to the functional maturity
of keratin. The smaller granules, membrane coating granules or

Odland bodies, attach to the cytoplasmic membrane where their contents convert the already present intercellular material to a "cement" which is impervious to the movement of fluid. At the same time cell membranes become closely opposed with the formation of "tight" junctions. Further out, the flattened keratinocytes die, losing their keratohyalin granules and nuclei and converting the granular layer to the stratum corneum layer. The dead cells in this layer gradually exfoliate at the rate which causes a steady-state equilibrium and thus a constant thickness of the epidermis.

Studies of cell kinetics suggest that, in normal epidermis, mitotically active basal cells have a cell cycle time of 200 to 400 hours and further suggest that a basal cell moves to the stratum corneum in an average time of approximately 2 weeks. The control for these kinetics depends on the presence of a number of molecules such as epidermal growth factor, chalones, prostaglandins, and polyamines. These molecules affect the cell machinery through several mechanisms, including that of the cyclic AMP-cyclic GMP system. Disturbances in epidermal cell kinetics occur in a variety of skin diseases and have been especially well studied in psoriasis.

The keratin produced by these epidermal cells consists of multiple proteins most of which have now been identified in vitro through electrophoretic studies and in vivo through attachment of monoclonal antikeratin antibodies.

Melanocytes. Melanocytes account for about 1% of the cells of the epidermis. These dendritic, pigment producing cells are derived from the neural crest and are first identified in the epidermis in 8-week-old embryos. They are found exclusively in the basal layer where they are interspersed among the basal keratinocytes. Each melanocyte, by way of its dendritic process, is in contact with 30 to 40 nearby keratinocytes. Melanin pigment, which occurs through polymerization of tyrosine-derived indole quinones, develops in membrane-bound organelles known as melanosomes in the cytoplasm of these cells. These pigmented granules then move from the central cytoplasm into the finger-like dendritic processes. From there they are transferred by way of a phagocytic process into the cytoplasm of the multiple keratinocytes which surround each melanocyte.

Variation in normal skin color, including that due to racial differences, is determined not by the number of melanocytes but rather by the number and size of the melanosomes which are produced and transferred to keratinocytes.

Ultraviolet light, primarily that of 290- to 320-nanometer wavelengths (UVB), darkens the skin both through immediate photooxidation of preformed melanin and, more importantly, through new melanin production in the delayed process known as tanning. An increased amount of melanin pigmentation in the epidermis, whether due to natural coloring or to tanning, decreases the amount of ultraviolet light allowed to pass through the epidermis, thus protecting the cellular DNA of deeper structures from ultraviolet light damage. Individuals such as albinos or those of Celtic background with absent or limited ability to produce melanin are at considerably increased risk for the development of skin cancer. The skin darkens in response to other stimuli besides that of ultraviolet light irradiation. Endocrine changes associated with increased elaboration of melanocyte stimulating hormone (MSH) and adrenal corticotropic hormone (ACTH) cause darkening, as does the presence of inflammation through the poorly understood process known as postinflammatory hyperpigmentation.

Nevus cells are pigment producing cells that are almost certainly derived from melanocytes. These rounded-up cells lack dendritic processes and occur in nests or clusters. Pigmented lesions containing such clusters are termed nevi. Lesions containing nests of nevus cells only at the dermal-epidermal junction are known as junctional nevi; lesions containing nests of nevus cells both at the dermal-epidermal junction and within the dermis are known as compound nevi; lesions containing nests of nevus cells only within the dermis are known as intradermal or, more simply, dermal nevi. The nevus cells in the deepest portions of intradermal nevi lack the enzyme(s) necessary to produce melanin from tyrosine. It is not certain whether this simply represents disappearance of the enzyme system due to aging or whether these latter cells might have an embryologic derivation from neural cells other than melanocytes.

Langerhans Cells. Langerhans cells account for 3 to 5% of the cells in the epidermis. They are dendritic cells and thus superficially resemble melanocytes. They do not, however, produce pigment and they possess cell surface markers which identify them as being of monocyte-macrophage lineage. They presumably originate in the bone marrow and from there move in and out of the epidermis as required by their role as processors of antigens which come into contact with the skin. After appropriate processing, Langerhans cells present the altered antigens to immunocompetent helper T cell lymphocytes which in turn trigger the inflammatory reaction of allergic contact dermatitis. Langerhans cells are also found in other benign and malignant inflammatory infiltrates such as occur in lichen planus, mycosis fungoides, and diseases of the histiocytosis X group. Finally, Langerhans cells are unusually susceptible to deactivation or destruction by ultraviolet light irradiation. This property may be important in the induction of immune tolerance and in the pathogenesis of sunlight induced cutaneous malignancy.

Merkel Cells. These are dendritic cells which, like melanocytes, are located in the basal layer of the epidermis. Microscopic studies show that the fine terminal filaments of cutaneous nerves preferentially abut at or near the cytoplasmic membrane of these cells. This observation has led to the suggestion that Merkel cells may play some role in skin sensation. Monoclonal antikeratin antibodies attach to the filaments within the cytoplasm of Merkel cells, suggesting an origin from epithelial, rather than neural, tissues. Merkel cells may undergo uncontrolled proliferation to form rather aggressive, but rarely encountered, cutaneous tumors.

DERMAL-EPIDERMAL JUNCTION

This undulating junction separates the ectodermally derived epidermis from the mesodermally derived dermis (Fig. 1-2). The basement membrane layer or zone presumably serves to attach the epidermis to the dermis and probably also plays a role in supporting the shape of the plasma membrane of the basal cells. From the top downward this basement membrane junction zone is made up of 1) the plasma membrane of the epidermal basal cells together with their hemidesmosomes, 2) an electron lucent layer (lamina lucida), and 3) an electron dense band (the basal lamina) to which are attached connective tissue fibrils (anchoring fibrils) from the underlying dermis. These features can be recognized only on electron microscopy. Fluids and other small- to medium-sized molecules pass easily through these layers but cells and very large molecules can only pass through disrupted areas.

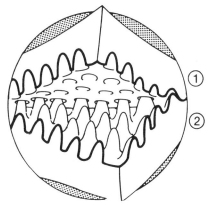

Figure 1-2. This drawing demonstrates the undulating interface between the overlying epidermis and the underlying dermis. The basement membrane layer occurs at this epidermal-dermal junction. 1, the dermis with its irregular surface known as the rete ridges; 2, the dermis with its irregular surface caused by upward projections of the papillary dermis.

The dermal-epidermal junction is important for a number of reasons: 1) it is the site of immunoglobulin and complement deposition in several immunologically mediated diseases such as lupus erythematosus and pemphigoid, 2) it is the site of blister formation for several of the immunobullous diseases, and 3) it appears to be a "resistant factor" in the prevention of dermal invasion during the transformation of in situ to invasive basal and squamous cell carcinoma.

DERMIS

Three somewhat indistinct compartments can be described within the dermis. The uppermost is relatively thin and consists mostly of the loose, areolar connective tissue which lies between the rete ridges of the epidermis. This compartment, known as the papillary dermis, is distinguished by its lighter staining and by the vertical orientation of the connective tissue fibers.

Just below the papillary dermis lies the thicker, major compartment of the dermis known as the reticular dermis. The collagen and elastic fibers found in this section are densely packed and are oriented in a horizontal fashion. It is this tissue that is responsible for the amazing strength and elasticity of the skin.

The lowest of the three compartments consists of the dermal and subdermal fat. Fingers and islands of fat cells are found intermingled with sections of connective tissue at the junction between the two layers but even in the deepest layers of fat, thin septa of connective tissue outline larger globules of fatty tissue. The fatty layer, by way of its cushioning effect, protects the body from mechanical trauma. Fat cells may also be important as storage and metabolic units. The most important cells and structures found in these three compartments are discussed in the following paragraphs.

Fibroblasts. These mesenchymal, spindle shaped cells are responsible for the synthesis of the collagen, reticulin, and elastic fibers of the dermis. The initial construction of all three fibers occurs within the fibroblast but the determination of the final morphologic features occurs in an extracellular location where enzymes clip unnecessary terminal portions from both ends of the fibrillar molecules. Elastic fibers are branched fibers which are folded extensively in their relaxed state. This configuration allows for great distensibility and excellent rebound when the skin has been deformed through stretching. Collagen fibers constitute the bulk of the dermis. They are unbranched, long, thin fibers made up of a triple helix of polypeptide chains. Variation in the amino acids of these polypeptide chains and the way in which these chains are bundled account for the five or more types of collagen known to be present in the human body. Collagen fibers are responsible for the leather-like toughness and flexibility of skin. Reticulin fibers are closely related to collagen fibers but their exact role is not known. All of these dermal fibers lie in a fluid or semisolid matrix of mucopolysaccharides which collectively are known as the ground substance. Presumably ground substance, which is elaborated by fibroblasts, serves as a lubricant which allows for smooth, easy movement of the fibers during bending and twisting of the skin.

Blood Vessels. Small arterial blood vessels (arterioles) occur throughout the mid dermis. They are connected at their proximal end to muscular arteries of the subcutaneous tissue and at their distal end to capillary loops. These capillary loops, together with their associated venules, form a complex network in the papillary dermis where they carry nutrients both to the upper dermis and to the epidermis. The blood vessels of the skin, by virtue of dilation or contraction, also serve an important role in heat discharge and heat conservation. Finally, blood vessels carry leukocytes to the skin where they participate in immunologic reactions and in the defense mechanism of inflammatory response.

Nerves. Both myelinated and nonmyelinated sensory nerves are found within the dermis. The nonmyelinated nerves terminate for the most part as small free twigs at, or just above, the dermal-epidermal junction. Some of the myelinated fibers end in specialized nerve endings. The less well myelinated fibers are primarily responsible for itching and light pain, whereas the myelinated fibers are the principal conveyers of deep pain, pressure, and temperature. Motor nerves to the skin are entirely autonomic in type. They are sympathetic nerves responsible for the function of eccrine sweat glands, for the determination of blood vessel flow rates, and for the contraction of the arrectores pilorum muscles of the hair follicles.

Miscellaneous Cells. Fat cells are found in clusters within the lower portion of the dermis and constitute the majority of the cells between the lower dermis and the fascia of the underlying muscles. Muscle cells as part of the arrectores pilorum muscles are responsible for the tenting of hair follicles ("goose flesh") which occurs under some traumatic environmental conditions. A few other smooth muscle cells are found around the nipples and in the scrotum. Striated muscle is present in the skin only as part of the platysma muscle of the anterior chest. Mast cells are present as scattered isolated cells throughout the superficial dermis. These cells release vasoactive and chemotactic mediators when IgE molecules present on their outer surfaces are bridged by appropriate antigens. These mediators play an important role in all inflammatory diseases of the skin.

ADNEXAL STRUCTURES

Hair Follicles. Hair follicles (Fig. 1-3) are composed primarily of epidermally derived cells. Early in embryogenesis clusters of pluripotential epidermal cells "bud" down from the basal

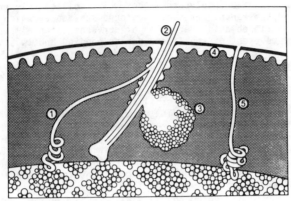

Figure 1-3. The adnexal structures of the skin. 1, an apocrine sweat gland connected by its duct to a hair follicle; 2, a hair shaft lying within a hair follicle; 3, a sebaceous gland attached to a hair follicle; 4, the epidermis, containing the pluripotential cells which form the anlage of hair follicles and eccrine sweat glands; 5, an eccrine sweat gland and duct which opens directly onto the skin surface.

layer and extend into the dermis where they form the hair follicle. A cup shaped indentation at the base of the epidermal bud accepts a specialized dermal papilla with its contribution of blood vessels. The epidermal cells which surround the dermal papilla then differentiate into both matrix cells responsible for the construction of hair keratin and into the cells which make up the inner root sheath of the hair follicle. Hair keratin, because of its greater sulfur content, is "harder" than regular epidermal keratin and thus can form a solid, tough hair shaft. Hair follicles are found everywhere on the skin except on the palms, soles, and mucous membranes. However, ectopic follicles composed mainly of sebaceous glands occasionally do appear on mucosal surfaces as small yellow papules. Such lesions are known as Fordyce spots when they occur on the lips and in the mouth.

The varieties of hair produced by hair follicles differ greatly depending on the type and location of the follicles. Thus thickness, length and curliness are different for scalp hair, eyebrows, eyelashes, vellus hair, beard hair, pubic hair, and trunk hair.

Hair grows in a cyclical fashion. Scalp hair follicles, for example, produce a continuous strand of hair at a rate of about 0.4 mm per day. This continuous growth goes on for several years when, for unknown reasons, the actively growing follicles (anagen phase) rapidly convert to the resting stage (telogen phase). At this point hair protein construction stops and the epidermal bud of the hair follicle retreats toward the basal layer. During this retreat the hair shaft loosens in the follicle and is soon shed as a "club," or telogen, hair. Then, after a resting stage of several months, the epidermal bud spontaneously relengthens and hair construction begins all over again. This cyclical process is carried out in a random, nonsynchronous fashion in each of the 100,000 or so follicles of the scalp. As a part of this cycle, 50 to 100 follicles switch to telogen phase each day. The resultant loss of 50 to 100 hairs per day should be considered as a normal event since it is balanced by the simultaneous reentry into anagen phase of a roughly similar number of previously resting follicles.

When the hair follicle shifts to the growing phase, protein production starts slowly. This results in a hair shaft with a tapered tip. These thin tips are soft and flexible in comparison to sharply edged, nontapered hairs that have been cut during shaving. For this reason shaved hair as it regrows looks and feels coarser than uncut hair. In actuality, shaving has no other effect on shaft diameter or hair growth rates.

Nail Growth. In a manner of speaking the fingernails and toenails can be viewed as arising from a "follicle" analogous to that of the hair follicle (Fig. 1-4). The orientation of this "follicle" of course lies parallel instead of vertical to the surface of the skin. The nail matrix from which the nail plate grows lies deep to the posterior nail fold. The nail plate, which is made of hard keratin very similar to that of the hair shaft, grows outward from the matrix. During this outward growth it rests on and is supported by the nail bed. Epidermal cells from the nail bed contribute only a very thin layer of cells to the ventral surface of the nail plate as it grows outward. Keratin produced from the epidermal cells of the overlying posterior nail fold attaches to the dorsal surface of the nail plate to form the cuticle. Damage to the cuticle such as occurs with "hang nail" formation or overly vigorous manicuring breaks the seal between the cuticle and the nail plate. This creates a blind pocket under the nail fold and allows for the development of paronychial infection.

The lunula of the nail is the crescent shaped area of whiteness found at the proximal end of the nail plate. It is a reflection of the underlying nail matrix as it extends distally from under the posterior nail fold. The lunula is always visible on thumbnails and is usually present on the fingernails. The white or opaque color of the tip of the nail plate where it overhangs the distal end of the nail bed occurs because of light refraction from the ventral surface of the free nail plate.

The nail plate grows at a rate of about 0.1 mm per day. Damage done to the nail matrix will not be visible for several weeks until the damaged nail emerges from underneath the nail fold. The damaged

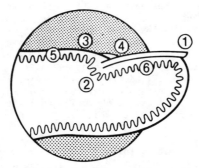

Figure 1-4. The components of a fingernail and its contiguous
structures. The various parts of a nail "follicle": 1, the nail
plate; 2, the nail matrix which consists of specialized epithelial
cells from which grows the nail plate; 3, the posterior nail fold
which overlies both the nail matrix and the proximal portion of the
nail plate; 4, the cuticle which attaches the posterior nail fold to
the nail plate; 5, the surface epithelium which is continuous with
the epithelially derived nail matrix and nail bed; 6, the nail bed
which underlies the nail plate.

portion then takes an additional several months to traverse the
length of the nail bed. Total replacement of a damaged fingernail
requires 3 to 4 months of growth whereas toenails require 6 to 9
months of growth. A certain amount of ridging and splitting of the
nail plate is a consequence of the aging process and is not
medically reversible.

    Sebaceous Glands. Sebaceous glands are formed from epidermally
derived cells which bud outward from the side of the hair follicle
(Fig. 1-3). Sebum, formed from holocrine secretion of the sebaceous
cells within the gland, travels to the surface of the skin via the
lumina of the hair follicle. Essentially all hair follicles have
sebaceous glands but over most of the body the glands are small and
relatively inactive. However, over the face, scalp, and upper trunk
the sebaceous glands are much larger and, under androgenic
stimulation, they are extraordinarily productive. Sebum accounts
for the majority of lipid found on the face and scalp but elsewhere
on the body much of the surface lipid is formed as a by-product of
keratin synthesis by keratinocytes. The lipids produced by
sebaceous cells and by keratinocytes are made up primarily of
glycerides but sterol synthesis in sebum is directed toward squalene
whereas sterol synthesis in keratinocytes is directed toward
cholesterol. Sebum elaboration is a continuous process and the rate
at which it is delivered to the surface of the skin is seemingly
unaffected by temperature, sweating, or sebum removal.

The physiologic role of lipids produced by either sebaceous cells or keratinocytes is uncertain but it is widely believed that surface lipids retard evaporative moisture loss from epidermal cells and thus are important in skin hydration and lubrication.

Eccrine Sweat Glands. Eccrine sweat glands develop from buds of epidermal cells which extend downward onto the dermis from the overlying epithelium (Fig. 1-3). Unlike sebaceous glands, these sweat glands are entirely distinct from the hair follicle and instead open through a coiled duct directly onto the surface of the skin. Sweat glands occur over the entire skin surface. Sweat glands on the palms, soles, axillae, and forehead are under both psychologic and thermal control, whereas those located elsewhere respond entirely to thermal stimuli. Eccrine sweat glands are innervated by sympathetic nerve fibers but, somewhat unexpectedly, physiologic mediation of sweating is due to cholinergic mediators of transmission.

Stimulation of sweating results in the formation of isotonic plasma-like fluid in the secretory portion of the gland. However, as a result of sweat processing in the ductal system, the fluid delivered to the skin surface is usually low in sodium and chloride and high in potassium, urea, ammonia, and some amino acids. Eccrine sweat glands have the potential to deliver astounding amounts of fluid to the skin surface. For short periods more than 1 liter per hour can be elaborated and up to 10 liters can be lost in 1 day. Sweat delivered to the surface of the skin cools the skin through evaporation. As a result blood flowing through the skin is also cooled. Through this process, sweating represents the most important thermoregulatory mechanism available to the body. Unfortunately, little or no significant loss of toxic substances can be accomplished by sweating and thus sweat glands cannot be viewed as miniature kidneys.

Apocrine Sweat Glands. Apocrine sweat glands are epidermally derived structures which, like sebaceous glands, open into the hair follicles (Fig. 1-3). They are phylogenetic remnants from the sexually important scent glands of animals but seem to have no direct usefulness in humans today. Apocrine glands are found primarily in the axillae, perineum, and on the areolae. They occasionally occur ectopically elsewhere. Embryologic derivations of apocrine glands occur in the ear (ceruminous glands) and eyelid (Moll's glands) and form the glandular tissue of the breasts. Apocrine sweat can be produced continuously or can appear in response to psychologic stimuli. Apocrine sweat has no intrinsic odor but odor is quickly produced when the sweat delivered to the surface is acted upon by skin bacteria.

SELECTED READING

Eyre DR: Collagen: Molecular diversity in the body's protein scaffold. Science 207:1315, 1980.

Sandberg LB, Soskel NT, Leslie JG: Elastin structure, biosynthesis, and relation to disease states. N Engl J Med 304:566, 1981.

Adams JS, Clemens TL, Parrish JA, Holick MF: Vitamin-D synthesis and metabolism after ultraviolet irradiation of normal and Vitamin-D-Deficient subjects. N Engl J Med 306:722, 1982.

Lavker RM, Sun T-T: Heterogeneity in epidermal basal keratinocytes: Morphological and functional correlations. Science 215:1239, 1982.

Burgeson RE: Genetic heterogeneity of collagens. J Invest Dermatol 79(Suppl):25s, 1982.

Prockop DJ: How does a skin fibroblast make type I collagen fibers? J Invest Dermatol 79(Suppl):3s, 1982.

Marcelo CL, Tong PSL: Epidermal keratinocyte growth: Changes in protein composition and synthesis of keratins in differentiating cultures. J Invest Dermatol 80:37, 1983.

Weinstein GD, McCullough JL, Ross P: Cell proliferation in normal epidermis. J Invest Dermatol 82:623, 1984.

Bladon PT, Wood EJ, Cunliffe WJ: Intracellular epidermal fibrous proteins. Clin Exp Dermatol 9:18, 1984.

Ogawa H, Yoshiike T: Keratin, keratinization, and biochemical aspects of dyskeratosis. Int J Dermatol 23:507, 1984.

Katz SI: The epidermal basement membrane zone - Structure, ontogeny, and role in disease. J Am Acad Dermatol 11:1025, 1984.

Edelson RL, Fink JM: The immunologic function of skin. Sci Am 252:46, 1985.

Lucky PA, Nordlund JJ: The biology of the pigmentary system and its disorders. Dermatol Clinics 3:197, 1985.

Chapter 2

Physical Examination
of the Skin

Examination of the skin should be considered in two entirely different settings: incidental examination of the skin during the course of a general physical examination and purposeful examination of the skin when cutaneous disease is known to be present. In both settings emphasis must be placed on adequacy of exposure and lighting. Many errors in dermatologic diagnosis are made because the entire skin surface is not exposed for examination. Adequate examination requires that the clothing be removed. One cannot simply unbutton a shirt or pull up a pant leg and expect to evaluate the type and extent of a skin disease satisfactorily. It is equally important that the exposed skin be well lighted. Problems with lighting often occur when the physical examination is carried out in an in-patient setting. Hospital bedside lighting is all too often designed more for reading than for general illumination. In such circumstances the patient must be moved to an examining room or other suitable area where there is more sufficient artificial or natural lighting.

INCIDENTAL EXAMINATION

During the course of a routine physical examination the skin is not ordinarily inspected in its entirety nor is it inspected all at once as a single, separate step in the examination. Generally only those portions of skin which overlie the internal organs being examined are evaluated. Thus each of these sections of skin is viewed in turn as one approaches each new organ. This approach is eminently practical though it is often far from ideal. In particular there is considerable risk that the skin will be forgotten entirely during one's enthusiasm for examination of the internal organs. I cannot count the number of times I have received a consultation request for evaluation of a long-standing skin disease only to find that the record of the initial physical examination either fails to mention the skin at all or states: "Skin ... normal." To prevent this from happening one must make a conscious, methodical evaluation. The steps in this cutaneous evaluation should include both palpation and visualization.

Palpation. In touching the skin, evaluate the texture. Feel for scaling (ichthyosis, xerosis, sun damage) and for edema (renal disease, congestive heart failure, fluid overload, hypothyroidism). Evaluate the surface moisture. Feel for sweating (fever, anxiety, hyperthyroidism) and for excess dryness (vitamin deficiency, atopic disease, disturbances in endocrine function). Evaluate the temperature. Feel for coolness (impending shock, sepsis, anxiety, hypothyroidism, deficiencies in vascular flow) and for heat (fever, hypermetabolic states, increased vascular flow).

Visualization. In looking at the skin evaluate the color. Look for paleness (anemia, shock, chronic vascular compromise), for ruddiness (Cushing's syndrome, polycythemia, carcinoid tumors), for yellowness (jaundice, carotenemia), for cyanosis (cardiopulmonary disease, methemoglobinemia), and for evidence of pigmentary change (Chapters 10 and 26). Look for excoriations which might signal the presence of pruritus as a clue for underlying systemic disease (Chapter 25).

Look at the hair for evidence of alopecia (Chapter 18) or for hirsutism (Chapter 26). Look at the fingernails for ridging, pigment banding, and splinter hemorrhages (Chapter 19).

PHYSICAL EXAMINATION OF DISEASED SKIN

In the event the patient is being evaluated because of known dermatologic disease, the skin is examined in a somewhat different fashion. Evaluation in this setting is carried out as a separate and distinct step in the physical examination. Specific abnormalities of the skin, hair, nails, and mucous membranes are noted as to distribution, palpability, color change, surface characteristics, size, margination, and configuration (Chapter 3). This extensive and elaborate evaluation of diseased skin is carried out not only to assist in making the appropriate initial diagnosis but also to document the severity and extent of the disease at a given point in time. The natural course of the disease or its response to therapy can subsequently be objectively documented.

The terminology necessary to describe the pathologic changes which may be found on physical examination is covered in the following chapter.

SELECTED READING

Lynch PJ: Examination of the skin. In Judge R, Zuidema MD, Fitzgerald FT (eds): Clinical Diagnosis. Little, Brown & Co., Boston, 1982, pp 59-76.

Chapter 3

Basic Terminology

The skin is surely the most accessible of the body's organs for examination and study. Because of this, clinicians centuries ago developed astoundingly sharp visual skills and they have left us a written heritage of precise clinical description. This emphasis on description is both good and bad: good because it has fostered skills in physical examination to the point where most skin diseases can be recognized instantly but bad because we are carrying the baggage of history in the form of confusing and archaic terminology. This terminology is often unintelligible and frustrating to those who are not dermatologists. The magnitude of the problem, however, is usually overstated. The definitions of no more than 20 words will provide the generalist with all the terminology necessary for the day-to-day practice of dermatology. This vocabulary is covered in the paragraphs which follow.

Lesion. A lesion is a general term for any single, small area of skin disease. Examples of lesions include such things as macules, patches, papules, plaques, nodules, vesicles, pustules, bullae, wheals, erosions, and ulcers.

Rash. The term rash is used to describe a more extensive process. Generally a rash is made up of many lesions; these lesions may be isolated or confluent.

Macule. A macule is a small area of color change. It has no substance and thus the borders (margination) of the macule are distinguished visually rather than through palpation. Most often macules are red, brown, yellow, or white. Macules have a diameter no greater than 1.5 to 2 cm. The surface of the macule is usually smooth but sometimes a small amount of very fine, nonpalpable scale may be present.

Patch. Macules larger than 2 cm in diameter are termed patches. Except for size, patches have all of the other attributes of macules. Patches may arise as such but are more often formed from the growth of one, or the confluence of several, centrifugally enlarging macules.

Papule. A papule is a small palpable mass less than 1.5 cm in diameter. Papules differ from macules by virtue of their substance, that is, their palpability. Most, but not all, papules are visibly elevated above the surface of the surrounding normal skin. Papules may be red, brown, yellow, white, or skin colored. Papules may be smooth surfaced or may have surface changes such as scale, crust, erosion, or ulceration. They may be flattopped, dome shaped, slope shouldered, or pointed.

Plaque. A plaque is a flattopped, palpable lesion larger than 1.5 cm in diameter. It may be considered as a papule that has enlarged in two dimensions: length and width.   The third dimension, that of height, is not greater than that of a papule.   Most, but not all, plaques are elevated above the surface of the surrounding, normal skin.   Plaques may arise as such but most are formed from the growth of one, or the confluence of several, centrifugally enlarging papules.   Plaques may have any of the color changes or surface features described for papules.

Nodule.   A nodule is a papule which has enlarged in all three dimensions: length, width, and depth.   A nodule may be considered as a spherical enlargement of a papule.   As such they are larger than 1.5 cm in diameter.   Nodules may have any of the color changes and surface features described for papules.   Nodules may be solid, edematous, or cystic.   They may be dome shaped or slope shouldered but are not flattopped.   The term "tumor" is occasionally, but inappropriately, used as a synonym for a large nodule.

Scale.   The keratinocytes of surface epithelium produce a series of proteins which are collectively known as keratin.   In nondiseased skin keratin is shed from the surface as rapidly as it is produced and thus is neither visible nor palpable.   In diseased skin the equilibrium between production and loss can be disturbed such that keratin builds up on the surface of the skin as visible and palpable scale.   The presence of scale reflects the presence of an underlying proliferative and usually thickened epithelium.

Three types of scale may be encountered.   The first is the psoriatic-type scale which is characterized by the presence of white, silver, or gray flakes.   The color occurs because of the looseness of the scale wherein an air-surface interface is present on both top and bottom of the flake.   The additional surface bends light waves a second time and creates a white opaqueness like that which occurs where the white distal edge of the fingernail freely overhangs the more proximal nail bed.   The second category is the pityriasis-type scale.   This scale has a fine, slightly white, powdery character which is inapparent until the scale is loosened from the underlying epithelium through fingernail or scalpel scraping.   The third category is lichen-type scale.   This scale is firmly adherent to the underlying epithelium and is characterized by a shiny, somewhat translucent appearance.   All scale lends a certain amount of roughness to the surface of a palpated lesion.   Thus even when scale is not readily visible, palpation sometimes offers a clue to its presence.

Crust.   Crust represents the solidification of plasma proteins which occurs when plasma water has evaporated.   Crust develops when the epithelium is disrupted to the point where plasma exudes (weeps) onto the surface of the skin and dries in place.   Crust is amorphous or granular in shape and is yellow or yellow-brown in color. However, when red blood cells accompany the extrusion of plasma, a black, hemorrhagic crust is formed.   The colloquial term for a crust is a scab.

Wheal. A wheal is a smooth surfaced, fluid filled papule in which the fluid is not macroscopically loculated. That is, a wheal is an edematous papule. Wheals arise when vascular dilation is accompanied by increased permeability. The presence of the additional interstitial fluid reduces the intensity of the redness which otherwise might have been present. As a result most wheals are pale pink in color.

Vesicle. A vesicle is also a fluid filled papule but the fluid is loculated into a visibly recognizable compartment. In short, a vesicle is a small blister. When a vesicle is punctured fluid will run out and the blister compartment will collapse. The fluid filled compartment in a vesicle may lie either at the dermal-epidermal junction or entirely within the epidermis.

Vesicles ordinarily contain clear fluid and thus are skin colored. If red blood cells are present in the fluid the vesicle will be red, blue-red, or black in color. If even a small number of white blood cells are present in the fluid the vesicle will be cloudy in color. Nearly all vesicles accumulate white blood cells as they age; thus older vesicles are usually somewhat cloudy. Vesicles with larger numbers of white blood cells are called pustules (see below).

Vesicles are fragile structures. For this reason patients with vesicular disease may lack intact vesicles and present instead with erosions. Clues which suggest that erosions were once the base of blisters include a perfectly round configuration and the presence of a collarette of devitalized roof which encircles the erosion.

Bulla. A bulla (pl. bullae) is a vesicle larger than 1 cm in diameter. Bullae that arise as single large blisters are unilocular and are round in configuration. Bullae that develop through the coalescence of several small vesicles are multilocular and are often irregular in configuration. The fluid constituency and blister colors are similar to those described for vesicles.

Pustule. A pustule is a vesicle fully packed with polymorphonuclear leukocytes. Pustules must be differentiated from cloudy vesicles. Pustules are bright white at the time of examination and historically have been so from the time they first arose. Small white papules, such as milia, which are filled with keratin may mimic the appearance of pustules. Such pseudopustules may be distinguished by the fact that they are quite firm on palpation. Moreover, such lesions, when incised, reveal solid keratin rather than liquid pus. Pustules do not, ipso facto, imply the presence of infectious process. There is often no visible difference between sterile and infected pustules.

Erosion. An erosion occurs when surface epithelium is visibly disrupted. Depending on the degree to which fluid escapes, the base of an erosion will be either red and moist or will be covered by a crust. Erosions form either by blister roof breakdown or by disruption of skin due to a traumatic event. Those erosions due to

blister roof breakdown are circular in configuration and have a
collarette of fragmented roof around the periphery of the erosion.
Those erosions formed by external trauma are linear or angular in
configuration and lack a peripheral collarette of scale. Angular
excoriations and xerotic fissures are the two most common types of
nonvesicular erosions.

Erosions are most commonly encountered in vesiculobullous
diseases (Group 1) and in eczematous diseases (Group 10).

Ulcers. Ulcers are deeper than erosions. Not only is the
epithelium disrupted but some dermal destruction has also occurred.
Ulcers have a visibly sunken appearance whereas erosions appear
rather superficial. An ulcer may have a moist red base or it may be
filled with crust and necrotic skin. When hemorrhage occurs in an
ulcer the crust -- which is thick, tough, and black -- is known as
an eschar.

Ulcers usually occur when vascular flow to the skin is
impaired. This impairment can be due to external compression
(decubitus ulcers), narrowing of the vascular lumen (vasculitis,
thrombosis, or embolism), or as a result of tissue growth
outstripping its blood supply (the ulceration of cutaneous tumors).
Ulcers are most often found in skin colored nodules (Group 3) and in
vascular reactions (Group 8).

Margination. Margination is the shape of a lesion as it is
viewed in cross section. It represents the transition from normal
to diseased skin. If that transition occurs abruptly (within the
space of about 1 mm) or if the cross section is square shouldered or
dome shaped, the lesion is said to be sharply marginated. If, on
the other hand, the transition occurs over a zone of several
millimeters or if the cross section is slope shouldered, the lesion
is said to be diffusely (or poorly) marginated. Intermediate
margination occurs when lesions have shoulders which are rolled.
Margination is particularly helpful in separating the red scaling
plaques of the papulosquamous diseases from those of the eczematous
diseases. The former tend to have sharp margination, whereas the
latter, over at least a part of their circumference, are poorly
marginated.

Configuration. Configuration is the outline of a lesion as it
is viewed from above. Lesions may have a circular, oval, linear,
angular, gyrate (polycyclic), or annular configuration. Linear and
angular configurations suggest that external factors have played an
important role in the pathogenesis of the lesions. Annular
configurations occur when clearing in the central portion of the
lesion results in a ring-like border.

Pruritus. Pruritus (please note the spelling) is the sensation
of itching. The degree of pruritus experienced by a patient depends
upon several factors. First, some diseases are inherently more
pruritic than others. Everybody with scabies and urticaria
experiences pruritus, whereas those patients with secondary syphilis

rarely if ever describe itching. Second, some individuals appear to
have a threshold for itching that is lower than that found in
others. Thus those who have inherited the atopic diathesis
experience more intense itching with any skin disease than do those
who have not. Third, lesions located in warm areas where sweat is
retained are usually more pruritic than those located elsewhere.
Thus groin, foot, and scalp lesions are more pruritic than are
similar lesions occurring elsewhere. Finally, psychologic factors
greatly influence the intensity of itching. Those who are anxious
or depressed generally experience more itching for a given skin
disease than do those who are not.

Patients experiencing pruritus may or may not respond by
scratching and rubbing. For instance, patients with lichen planus
and urticaria often complain of intense itching but they rarely
scratch to the point of excoriation. On the other hand, patients
with atopic dermatitis sometimes minimize the presence of itching
yet their skin is covered with excoriations.

Excoriation. Excoriations are scratch marks. They appear as
small linear or angular erosions which are often covered with a
hemorrhagic crust. The amount of skin disease which accompanies
excoriations is highly variable. Excoriations are confined almost
entirely to eczematous diseases (Group 10).

Lichenification. Patients who respond to pruritus with chronic,
habitual rubbing rather than with scratching develop a distinctive
thickening of the skin known as lichenification. This thickened
skin feels tough and leather-like on palpation. Visually there is
an accentuation of the normal skin markings accompanied by a mild
amount of lichen-type scale. This accentuation of the skin markings
develops because the "valleys" of the skin markings remain untouched
while the islands of skin which surround them are preferentially
rubbed. Lichenification can be viewed as analogous to the process
of callus formation which occurs on the palms and soles when they
are chronically traumatized. Lichenification is seen only in the
eczematous diseases (Group 10) and, in my view, may be considered as
a pathognomonic feature of atopic dermatitis.

When the 20 words defined above are combined with a description
of color and distribution, unknown skin lesions can generally be
assigned to one of ten specific categories through the use of a
clinical algorithm. This problem oriented diagnostic process is
discussed in Chapter 6.

Basic Therapeutics

SOAKS

Soaks are used for three purposes. First, the application of fluid to eroded or ulcerated skin restores a relatively physiologic environment to the exposed nerve endings responsible for transmitting sensations of pain and itching. Second, by softening and dissolving crusts, soaks remove solidified protein which otherwise serves as a nidus for bacterial infection. Third, removal of the crusts reduces the damaging effect of fluid entrapment, that is, it reduces maceration. The fluid used for soaking can be as elaborate as your imagination desires but for the most part tap water is quite sufficient. It has the incomparable advantages of no cost, no preparation, no staining, and no potential toxicity. Other commonly used preparations include Burow's solution (Domeboro or Bluboro packets), normal saline, and the addition of colloidal oatmeal (Aveeno) or cornstarch (Linit) to bath water.

Soaks can be carried out either by immersion or by wrapping. In a <u>wrapped soak</u>, strips of cloth (Kerlix, Kling, or cotton towels) are moistened and are wrung out to the point where they are just short of dripping wet. These wet strips are then wrapped around the

affected area and are kept continually moist by the periodic
application of additional fluid. In a hospital setting, normal
saline is conveniently used since it can be replenished through the
constant drip of an intravenous setup. Wrapped soaks, to be
effective, must be used for a minimum interval of 30 minutes.
Longer periods of application are not at all detrimental. In fact,
soaks can be left in place indefinitely if the patient can be
suitably immobilized. Such continuous soaks are a convenience for
the nursing staff since the dressings need to be changed only once
or twice a day. On the other hand, continuous soaks are somewhat
less effective for debridement since the periodic unwrapping of
intermittent soaks allows for some mechanical removal of the crust
during the changing process. Debridement is actually carried out
most effectively when the bandages are allowed to partially dry
before removal. Unfortunately, damage to normal tissue occurs all
too often during removal and for this reason "wet-to-dry" soaks are
seldom indicated.
    Immersion soaks, while offering less debridement, are easy to
carry out and may represent the only practical approach when trunk
lesions are present. A bathtub, sitz bath, or foot pan can be used
depending on the portion of the body requiring care. Immersion
soaks are carried out for 30 to 45 minutes at a time and may be
repeated several times daily. The debriding effect of an immersion
soak can be enhanced by the use of swirling water such as is
available in a whirlpool or Jacuzzi bath.
    Water temperatures are not critical with either type of soak.
Lukewarm water is usually best but cool water is more effective if
pruritus is present. Patients with chronic cutaneous ulcers will
require several weeks of soaks whereas patients with other types of
crusted or eroded lesions are best limited to only 2 or 3 days of
soaks. Soaks continued beyond this period may lead to overdrying of
the skin and worsening of the problem.

SELECTED READING

Arndt KA: Manual of Dermatologic Therapeutics: With Essentials of
    Diagnosis, 3rd edition. Little, Brown & Co., Boston, 1983.

VEHICLES AND LUBRICANTS

    Lotions. Three types of lotions are available. Shake lotions
consist of insoluble but hydrophilic powders such as zinc oxide and
talc suspended in water. Because they are suspensions rather than
solutions they must be shaken prior to use. Calamine lotion is the
only shake lotion which is widely used today. The soothing effect
of a shake lotion depends on the cooling evaporation of the aqueous
vehicle. The powder which remains "wicks" up moisture from oozing
skin surfaces and helps to dry weeping lesions. Unfortunately,
shake lotions are messy to use and repeated applications cause a

buildup of zinc oxide under which the damaging effects of maceration occur. Pharmaceutical lotions are white, liquid emulsions in which small amounts of oils are suspended in a continuous phase of water. These lotions are typified by the ubiquitous "hand lotions." Pharmaceutical lotions are mildly lubricating and can also be used for the delivery of water soluble medicinal agents to hairy areas of the body. Pharmaceutical solutions are transparent liquids containing considerable amounts of propylene glycol and alcohol. They have no lubricating value but, since they will dissolve many ingredients not soluble in water, are useful for the application of some medications to hairy areas. Pharmaceutical solutions often cause stinging or burning when they are applied to broken skin.

Creams. Creams are semisolid white emulsions too thick to pour from a bottle. For the most part they consist of oils suspended in a continuous aqueous phase. The prototypes of such products are the commercially available "vanishing" or "hand" creams. These preparations are moderately useful for lubrication and, because they lack a greasy feel, are cosmetically very acceptable. They are also widely used as a vehicle for medicinal ingredients.

Ointments. Two types of ointments are available. Hydrophilic ointments are milky white emulsions very similar in appearance to the creams described above. They contain moderate amounts of water suspended in a continuous phase of oil. The prototype of such products is rose water ointment (cold cream). These preparations are extremely useful for lubrication but, because they have a somewhat greasy feel, are considerably less cosmetically acceptable than standard creams. Widely used hydrophilic ointments include Polysorb and Aquaphor. A limited amount of water can be added to these ointments. The resultant products, such as Eucerin and Nivea, then appear almost identical to the standard creams described in the paragraph above. These ointments are also widely used as vehicles for medicinal ingredients. Hydrophobic ointments are thick, gray preparations composed entirely of oils. The prototype of such products is petrolatum (Vaseline). These preparations are extremely good lubricants but are far too greasy for most people to use. They are excellent vehicles for medicaments which are insoluble in water. Finally, because they lack propylene glycol, preservatives, stabilizers, and other chemical ingredients, they rarely cause burning or allergic sensitization on application.

SELECTED READING

McKay M: Topical dermatologic therapy. Dermatol Clinics 2:645, 1984.

SKIN LUBRICATION

Smoothness and suppleness of the skin depend largely on the presence of adequate amounts of water in the outer epidermal stratum

corneum cells. Water is furnished to the epidermis by plasma that
percolates throughout the underlying papillary dermis. This
moisture diffuses through the epidermis and is eventually lost to
the atmosphere in the form of "insensible perspiration." The amount
of moisture retained in the upper epidermis and stratum corneum is
mostly dependent on the presence of a thin lipid layer covering the
surface of the skin. These lipids, derived both from sebum and from
keratinocytes, restrict evaporative water loss.

The two major factors which adversely influence skin lubrication
are the presence of epithelial disruption (chapping and eczematous
disease) and the exposure to solvents which remove the external
lipid layer. Conversely, improvement of lubrication requires
treatment of any associated skin disease and reestablishment of the
surface lipid layer. Treatment of the eczematous diseases is
covered in Chapters 16 and 17. Reestablishment of the lipid layer
depends both on reducing the loss of naturally produced lipid and
application of additional lipid. Lipid loss can be decreased if the
number of exposures to soap and water can be reduced. Dishes can be
washed once instead of three times daily. Soap does not need to be
used for each hand washing. The wash-water temperature can be
reduced and drying of wet skin can be carried out by "patting"
rather than by rubbing with a towel. Lipid can be added to the skin
by way of the application of creams and ointments on multiple
occasions throughout the day. It is particularly useful to apply
these products while the skin is still wet and the stratum corneum
is well hydrated.

Many commercial lubricants are available. Most of these are
labeled as hand lotions or hand creams. The lotions are very
acceptable cosmetically but offer only marginal benefits except for
the preservation of adequate lubrication in nondiseased skin. Hand
creams are more appropriate than lotions for the restoration of
lipid on chapped or diseased skin. Eucerin cream is much favored by
dermatologists, but many patients find it a little hard to spread
and somewhat too greasy. Other suitable products include Keri
Creme, Moisturel, Lubriderm, and Neutrogena. Hydrophilic substances
such as urea and lactic acid are sometimes added to lubricants to
enhance their water holding capacity. Commerical preparations of
these products include Aquacare HP, Carmol, Lacticare, and
Lac-Hydrin. Unfortunately, the efficacy of these latter agents is
somewhat compromised by the fact that they may cause appreciable
stinging when applied to fissured or eroded skin.

Oils added to the bath water offer only minimal amounts of
lubrication. Perhaps the best use for these bath oils is to apply
them directly to a wet washcloth in which form they can be used as
soap substitutes. Cetaphil, used in the same manner, is another
useful soap substitute.

SELECTED READING

Wu, M-S, Yee DJ, Sullivan ME: Effect of a skin moisturizer on the
    water distribution in human stratum corneum. J Invest Dermatol
    81:446, 1983.
Imokawa G, Hattori M: A possible function of structural lipids in
    the water-holding properties of the stratum corneum. J Invest
    Dermatol 84:282, 1985.
Wehr R, Krochmal L, Bagatell F, Ragsdale W: A controlled two-center
    study of lactate 12 percent lotion and a petrolatum-based creme
    in patients with xerosis. Cutis 37:205, 1986.

TOPICAL STEROIDS

Topical steroids represent a class of corticosteroids which have
been incorporated into lotions, creams, and ointments. Their
primary pharmacologic effect is the reduction of inflammation. A
secondary antipruritic effect accrues as a result of the decreased
inflammation. Of the ten groups of diseases discussed in this book
topically applied steroids are extremely useful in one group (the
eczematous diseases), moderately useful in a second (the
papulosquamous diseases), and somewhat useful in a third (the
vesiculobullous diseases).

In using topical steroids the clinician must make four
decisions: what brand? what strength? what vehicle? and what
quantity? Brand and strength are interrelated. Table 4-1 lists a
few of the most widely sold products. They have been grouped on the
basis of my experience into rather arbitrary categories of low
potency, mid potency, and high potency products. A steroid from the
low potency group can be used for all acute and subacute eczematous
diseases. A steroid from the mid potency group can be used for
resistant eczematous diseases and for most papulosquamous diseases.
A steroid from the high potency group can be used for eczematous
diseases of the palms and soles and for resistant papulosquamous
disease. A special caveat applies to use of corticosteroids on the
face and in the groin. In these two locations only nonfluorinated,
low potency products such as hydrocortisone should be used. To do
otherwise leads all too often to the development of a rosacea-like
rash on the face and striae formation in the groin.

The choice of a vehicle for topical steroids depends on the
distribution and extent of the disease to be treated. As a general
rule creams represent the best choice. Lotions, because of their
ease of spreading, can be used in hairy areas and where large
surface areas are involved. Ointments can be used where additional
lubrication is desirable and can be substituted for creams when
patients indicate that stinging on application has been a problem.
In addition, for a given strength of steroids, ointments are
slightly more efficacious than creams. This advantage is based on
the fact that the partition coefficients for ointments allow for

TABLE 4-1
TOPICAL STEROIDS

HIGH POTENCY

   Clobetasol proprionate 0.05% (Temovate cream/oint)

   Betamethasone Diproprionate 0.05% (Diprolene oint)

   Halcinonide 0.1% (Halog cream/oint/soln)

   Fluocinonide 0.05% (Lidex cream/oint/soln; Topsyn gel)

MID POTENCY

   Triamcinolone 0.1% (Kenalog, Aristocort cream/oint)

   Fluocinolone 0.025% (Synalar, Fluonid cream/oint)

   Flurandrenolide 0.5% (Cordran cream/oint/soln)

   Betamethasone Valerate 0.1% (Valisone cream/oint/soln)

   Betamethasone Diproprionate 0.05% (Diprosone cream/oint/soln)

   Desonide 0.05% (Tridesilon cream/oint)

   Desoximetasone 0.25% (Topicort cream)

   Amcinonide 0.1% (Cyclocort cream)

   Clocortolone 0.1% (Cloderm cream)

LOW POTENCY

   Desonide 0.05% (Desonide cream)

   Hydrocortisone Valerate 0.2% (Westcort cream)

   Hydrocortisone 0.5 to 1.0% (Hytone, Cort-Dome)

   (Note: 0.5% is available without prescription)

---

better transfer of the active ingredient from the vehicle into the
lipid layer of the skin.

Most topical steroids come in a small and a large size.
Generally the small size is about 15 grams and the large size is
about 60 grams. For limited disease, such as that which occurs on
the hands and feet, the small size will be sufficient. For larger
areas, or where it is anticipated that treatment will be carried out
for weeks at a time, the large size will offer better economy.

Patients have generally been instructed to apply topical
steroids three or four times daily. It is, however, becoming
increasingly apparent that equally good results can be obtained with
as few as one or two applications per day. One of these
applications ought to occur directly after bathing since at this
time penetration is slightly better and spreading occurs more
easily. Topical steroids, like all topical medications, should be
spread as thinly as possible.

Penetration and thus the clinical efficacy of topically applied
steroids can be enhanced by the addition of occlusive techniques.
Such occlusion can be obtained through the use of plastic or latex
gloves for disease of the hands, Baggies for disease of the feet,
wrapped plastic film for disease of the arms or legs, and a vinyl
sweat suit for disease of the trunk. Unfortunately, occlusion,
while enhancing efficacy, leads to problems such as atrophy,
miliaria, and folliculitis. In general, consultation should be
obtained before the generalist introduces the use of occlusive
techniques.

Long term use of topical steroids raises a question about the
potential risk of systemic absorption and consequent development of
systemic effects. This does not seem to be a problem when low
potency steroids such as hydrocortisone are used even over large
body surface areas. Mid and high potency steroids cause no trouble
when used over small areas but some detrimental effect on the
pituitary-adrenal axis can be demonstrated when whole body
application is carried out. But even in these circumstances concern
is rarely warranted at the practical level unless occlusive
techniques are being used. As might be expected, extra care should
be taken when children are treated since their large surface
area-to-volume ratio magnifies the effect of whatever amount is
absorbed.

SELECTED READING

Guin JD: Complications of topical hydrocortisone. J Am Acad
    Dermatol 4:417, 1981.
Cook LJ, Freinkel RK, Zugerman C, Levin DL, Radtke R: Iatrogenic
    hyperadrenocorticism during topical steroid therapy: Assessment
    of systemic effects by metabolic criteria. J Am Acad Dermatol
    6:1054, 1982.
Robertson DB, Maibach HI: Topical corticosteroids. Int J Dermatol
    21:59, 1982.

Weston WL: Topical corticosteroids in dermatologic disorders.
 Hosp Prac 19:159, 1984.
Parish LC, Witkowski JA, Muir JG: Topical corticosteroids. Int J
 Dermatol 24:435, 1985.

INTRALESIONAL STEROIDS

   Intralesionally injected steroids can be used for the treatment
of some diseases which are resistant to the effect of topically
applied steroids. This approach is particularly useful for acne
cysts, hypertrophic scars, alopecia areata, discoid lupus
erythematosus, lichen simplex chronicus, and, to a limited degree,
in psoriasis and lichen planus. Dermatologists generally prefer the
use of triamcinolone acetonide (Kenalog) because of its very long
depot effect. This preparation is available in a stock strength of
10 mg per cc. The stock solution must be diluted down to an
appropriate working strength of 3 to 5 mg per cc. Normal saline is
the usual diluent though lidocaine can also be used. A tuberculin
syringe with a 26- to 30-gauge needle is used for the injection.
Approximately 0.1 cc of the working solution is injected at each
injection site. Injection sites should be spaced at 1 cm
intervals. A total of no more than 10 mg is injected during any one
office visit to prevent any possibility of systemic effect.
   The injection is performed by inserting the needle parallel to
the skin in a manner similar to that used for conventional skin
tests. If the plunger is very easily compressed or if no tissue
distention appears during injection, the needle point is too deep.
This results in little or no therapeutic effect. On the other hand,
if too much pressure is required or if blanching and dimpling of the
skin occurs, the needle point may be too superficial. In such
instances atrophy to the point of ulceration can develop. Air
pressure guns similar to those used for mass vaccinations can be
used in lieu of a syringe and needle. This air pressure technique
is somewhat less painful but depth of the injected steroid is not as
easy to control and there is greater risk of postinjection
infection. With either technique, postinjection atrophy often
occurs. This atrophy is reversible but resolution requires 12
months or more.

SELECTED READING

Gottlieb NL, Riskin WG: Complications of local corticosteroid
 injections. J Am Acad Dermatol 243:1547, 1980.
Callen JP: Intralesional steroids. J Am Acad Dermatol 4:149, 1981.
Broughton R: Corticosteroid injections into the hands and feet.
 Cutis 33:575, 1984.

TOPICAL ANTIPRURITICS

Several approaches are available for the topical treatment of pruritus. Topically applied steroids are particularly useful for the treatment of pruritus associated with eczematous disease. Their effectiveness presumably occurs as a by-product of their anti-inflammatory action. For this reason no benefit is recognized until 24 to 48 hours after the applications have first begun. Topical steroids have little or no effect on pruritus associated with noninflammatory diseases.

Topically applied anesthetics act more quickly but their effect is less than dramatic and it is of rather short duration. Some of the more commonly used anesthetics include benzocaine (Americaine), dibucaine (Nupercainal), dimethisoquin (Quotane), lidocaine (Xylocaine), and pramoxine (Pramasone). Allergic contact sensitization can occur with all but the latter two. Topically applied antihistamines, probably because of their anesthetic effect, are also widely used. Benadryl mixed with calamine lotion (Caladryl) is the prototypic preparation. It too has a reasonably high risk of allergic sensitization.

Finally there is a miscellaneous group of antipruritic products containing menthol, phenol, and camphor. Any one or a combination of these agents may be added in 0.25 to 0.5% amounts to standard lotions and creams. The mechanism by which these agents work is unknown, although in the case of phenol it is probably due to a necrotizing effect on nerve endings. Care should be taken with the application of these agents since toxicity has been reported when large amounts have been absorbed through the skin.

Other approaches to the treatment of pruritus include the use of systemically administered antihistamines and corticosteroids. These agents are discussed later in this chapter. The general subject of pruritus is discussed in Chapter 25.

TOPICAL TARS

Prior to the advent of corticosteroids, coal tar preparations were the major medications used in the treatment of skin disease. Today their use is confined to the treatment of psoriasis, seborrheic dermatitis of the scalp, and some instances of chronic eczematous disease. Ointments containing coal tar in a concentration of 1 to 5% or a shale tar, anthralin (Lasan, Anthra-Derm), in a concentration of 0.1 to 0.5% can be used in the treatment of psoriasis. Problems with staining and odor generally limit the usefulness of these two products. However, several commercial products containing derivatives of coal tar, such as Alphosyl, Estar, and Balnetar, are more cosmetically acceptable and can be used at home. Tar shampoos such as Zetar, T-Gel, and Sebutone can be used for the treatment of both psoriasis and

seborrheic dermatitis of the scalp. Tar products also have some
limited usefulness in the treatment of chronic eczematous disease.
They do have the advantage of low cost and do avoid the problem of
absorption seen with steroids but they are cosmetically less
acceptable than topical steroids and are probably less effective as
well.

SELECTED READING
Olansky S: Whole coal tar shampoo. A therapeutic hair repair
    system. Cutis 25:99, 1980.
Ashton RE, Andre P, Lowe NJ, Whitefield M: Anthralin: Historical
    and current perspectives. J Am Acad Dermatol 9:173, 1983.

TOPICAL ANTIBACTERIALS

    There is considerable controversy regarding the use of topically
applied antibacterials in the treatment of skin disease. Most
physicians no longer use them in the treatment of impetigo, but
there is perhaps a place for them in the treatment of infected cuts,
hang nails, and folliculitis. A few clinicians use them,
particularly in combination with topical steroids, on eczematous
skin disease where the rate of bacterial colonization (if not true
infection) is rather high. The efficacy of this approach is
unproven but they are at the very least unlikely to do any harm.
Typical products include bacitracin, mycitracin, neomycin,
gentamycin, and combination products such as Neosporin and
Polysporin. Combinations of steroids and antibacterials include
products such as Neo-Synalar and Cordran N. Most of these
antibacterials, when used on broken skin for long periods of time,
have a moderately high rate of allergic sensitization. For this
reason many dermatologists prefer to use the nonsensitizing
erythromycin and chloramphenicol ointments if long term treatment is
contemplated.

SELECTED READING
Wilkinson RD, Collins JP, Raymond GP, et al: Therapy of infected
    dermatitis: Comparative response to two corticosteroid
    antimicrobial creams. J Am Acad Dermatol 2:207, 1980.

TOPICAL ANTIFUNGAL AGENTS

    Historically the topical antifungal agents were divided into two
groups: those effective against dermatophytes (exemplified by
tolnaftate) and those effective against yeasts (exemplified by
nystatin). However, the development of ciclopirox (Loprox),
haloprogin (Halotex), clotrimazole (Lotrimin, Mycelex), miconazole
(Micatin, Monistat), and econazole (Spectazole), which are equally
effective against both yeasts and dermatophytes, has simplified this

area of therapy. They are, although somewhat more expensive, now
the treatment of choice for both infections. Several of these
preparations are over-the-counter products. Nystatin (Mycostatin)
suspension or clotrimazole (Mycelex) troches represent the treatment
of choice for oral candidiasis. The combination steroid-antifungal
agent Lotrisone is useful in the treatment of candidal paronychia
and some other forms of resistant candidiasis. Tinea capitis and
onychomycosis require the use of orally administered griseofulvin or
ketoconazole but other forms of superficial fungal infection can
usually be treated topically with a 3-week course of twice daily
applications.

SELECTED READING

Wortzel MH: A double-blind study comparing the superiority of a
   combination antifungal (clotrimazole)/steroidal (Betamethasone
   diproprionate) product. Cutis 30:258, 1982.
Smith EB: Topical antifungal agents. Dermatol Clinics 2:109, 1984.

SUNSCREENS

Sunburn and photoinduced carcinogenesis occur as the result of
irradiation in the UVB (280 to 320 nanometer) range of ultraviolet
light. Blockage of these wavelengths can be obtained through the
use of sunscreens containing benzophenones, padimate-O,
para-aminobenzoic acid (PABA), and esters of PABA. Efficacy of
these products is determined by measuring their sun protective
factor (SPF). This factor is calculated as the ratio of minutes of
sunlight necessary to produce minimal redness in sunscreen protected
skin versus unprotected skin. Thus if redness develops in 15
minutes when no sunscreen is used but appears only after 150 minutes
following sunscreen use, that sunscreen is said to have an SPF of
10. Sunscreens with an SPF less than 10 offer only partial
protection; those with an SPF above 10 are almost totally
protective. Some tanning occurs with all of these products due to
their relative inability to block UVA (320 to 400 nanometer) type
ultraviolet light.

An additional measure of sunscreen effectivensss is the degree
to which it protects after heavy sweating or swimming. This
property is called substantivity. Currently there is no standard
means of measuring substantivity but it is known that for all
sunscreens substantivity is improved when they are applied 1 hour or
more prior to the onset of sweating or swimming. The combination of
excellent protection and substantivity can be enhanced when
sunscreens with an SPF of 15 or better are applied every day on a
once daily basis.

The sunscreens discussed above are designed for the UVB spectrum
and offer little protection for the longer wavelengths of the UVA
spectrum. These longer wavelengths are responsible for some skin

diseases such as porphyria cutanea tarda, solar urticaria, polymorphous light eruption, and some medication reactions. UVA irradiation, through the process known as photoaugmentation, may even plan a role in skin aging and carcinogenesis. Partial protection in the UVA spectrum can be obtained with the products discussed above but complete UVA protection requires the use of opaque materials such as zinc oxide or titanium dioxide (A-fil, RVPaque).

SELECTED READING

Kligman LH, Akin FJ, Kligmam AM: Sunscreens promote repair of ultraviolet radiation-induced dermal damage. J Invest Dermatol 81:98, 1983.

Diffey BL, Farr PM: An evaluation of sunscreens in patients with broad action-spectrum photosensitivity. Br J Dermatol 112:83, 1985.

Pathak MA, Fitzpatrick TB, Greiter FJ, Kraus EW: Principles of photoprotection in sunburn and suntanning, and topical and systemic photoprotection in health and diseases. J Dermatol Surg Oncol 11:6, 1985.

Stern RS, Weinstein MC, Baker SG: Risk reduction for nonmelanoma skin cancer with childhood sunscreen use. Arch Dermatol 122:537, 1986.

Pathak MA: Sunscreens: Topical and systemic approaches for the prevention of acute and chronic sun-induced skin reactions. Dermatol Clinics 4:321, 1986.

SYSTEMIC ANTIBACTERIALS

More than 90% of all cutaneous bacterial infections are caused by the gram positive organisms Staphylococcus aureus and group A streptococci. Orally administered phenoxymethyl penicillin (Pen VK) 1.0 gram per day is the treatment of choice for streptococcal infection. Orally administered oxacillin (Prostaphilin) or dicloxacillin (Dynapen, Veracillin), or nafcillin (Unipen) 1.0 gram per day is preferred for the treatment of staphylococcal infections. Orally administered erythromycin (EES, Erythrocin, E-Mycin) 1.0 gram per day is quite effective against both staphylococcal and streptococcal infections. Erythromycin is usually the treatment of choice when the identity of the infecting organism is not known and is always the treatment of choice when patients are allergic to penicillin products. Second line antibiotics for skin infections include tetracycline derivatives such as minocycline (Minocin, Vectrin) and doxycyclin (Vibramycin) and cephalosporins such as cephalexin (Keflex) and cephradine (Anspor, Velosef). All of these second line medications share the considerable disadvantage of very high cost.

Most cutaneous infections such as impetigo, furunculosis,
folliculitis, and cellulitis can be treated empirically without
incurring the cost of cultures. Cultures should be obtained,
however, in situations of recurrent infection, resistant infection,
infection occurring in a hospital setting, and infection occurring
in immunocompromised individuals. Antibiotics are used rather
differently in the treatment of acne. This subject is discussed in
Chapter 8.

SELECTED READING

Wilson WR, Cockerill FR III: Tetracyclines, chloramphenicol,
   erythromycin, and clindamycin. Mayo Clin Proc 58:92, 1983.
Wright AJ, Wilkowske CJ: The penicillins. Mayo Clin Proc 58:21,
   1983.
Thompson RL, Wright AJ: Symposium on antimicrobial agents – Part
   II. Cephalosporin antibiotics. Mayo Clin Proc 58:79, 1983.
Elewski BE, Lamb BAJ, Sams WM Jr, Gammon WR: In vivo suppression
   of neutrophil chemotaxis by systemically and topically
   administered tetracycline. J Am Acad Dermatol 8:807, 1983.
Washington JA II, Wilson WR: Erythromycin: A microbial and
   clinical perspective after 30 years of clinical use (second of
   two parts)*. Mayo Clin Proc 60:271, 1985.
Feingold DS, Wagner RF Jr: Antibacterial therapy. J Am Acad
   Dermatol 14:535, 1986.

SYSTEMIC ANTIFUNGAL AGENTS

Griseofulvin is an orally administered antibiotic which provides
effective treatment for most dermatophyte fungal infections.
Absorption of griseofulvin from the gastrointestinal tract is less
than ideal, but it can be enhanced when particle size is decreased
during the manufacturing process. Two forms of griseofulvin are in
current use. The first is called "microsized" and is the form of
griseofulvin used when a prescription for the generic product is
written. Dosage with this form of griseofulvin is generally 1.0
gram per day divided into a morning and evening dose taken with
meals. The second utilizes an even smaller particle size which has
been suspended in polyethylene glycol (Gris PEG, Fulvicin P/g).
Suggested dosage with these products is 500 to 750 mg per day.
Griseofulvin is delivered to the stratum corneum by way of
transepidermal water loss and through the deposition of sweat
containing griseofulvin on the surface of the skin. Concentration
of the drug in the stratum corneum is thus higher than can be
obtained in the plasma.
     Systemically administered griseofulvin can be used in all cases
of tinea capitis and onychomycosis; topical antifungal therapy is
not effective for these two conditions. Griseofulvin is also useful
in instances of tinea corporis which are too extensive for topical

therapy. Griseofulvin is not effective in the treatment of cutaneous yeast infections such as candidiasis or pityriasis (tinea) versicolor nor is it effective in the treatment of systemic fungal infections.

Griseofulvin has an unjustifiably bad reputation for the frequency and severity with which side effects occur. Gastrointestinal upset and headaches develop in about 10% of patients, but they are usually not severe enough to warrant discontinuation of the medication. Urticaria occurs in 1 or 2% of patients; this does require discontinuation of use. Photosensitivity eruptions, proteinuria, and leukopenia occur with great rarity. Most clinicians do not obtain urine and blood tests for patients taking griseofulvin for less than 3 months. Griseofulvin is contraindicated in patients with all types of porphyria and it should be used with extreme care in patients taking warfarin-like anticoagulants.

Ketoconazole represents a great advance in the treatment of fungal and yeast infections. Advantages include greater efficacy in resistant dermatophyte infections, effectiveness against yeast as well as dermatophyte infections, and once daily dosage. Unfortunately, these are nearly balanced by its very high cost, potential for significant hepatoxicity, and antiandrogenic properties when taken in high doses. As a result it probably represents the systemic treatment of choice only for griseofulvin resistant infections, short term therapy for pityriasis (tinea) versicolor, some systemic fungal diseases, and unusual cases of onychomycosis.

Ketoconazole obtains its antifungal effect by interfering with the integrity of the fungal cell walls. It is generally given for cutaneous infections in a single morning dose of 200 mg. Rarely, twice that dose will be required. Long term administration, such as would be required for routine nail infections, is discouraged because of some remaining concern over toxicity.

Flucytosine (Ancobon) is available for the treatment of serious yeast infections due to candidiasis and cryptococcus. It is chemically related to fluorouracil and thus has potential hematologic toxicity. Moreover, resistance of organisms to this medication occurs frequently. As a result of these considerations there is probably little reason for its use in dermatologic disease.

Amphotericin B and miconazole administered intravenously are primarily indicated in the treatment of systemic fungal disease and are not discussed here.

SELECTED READING

Jones SE: Ketoconazole. Arch Dermatol 118:217, 1982.
Roberts DT: The current status of systemic antifungal agents. Br J Dermatol 106:597, 1982.

Hay RJ, Midgeley G: Short course ketoconazole therapy in pityriasis
    versicolor. Clin Exp Dermatol 9:571, 1984.
Pont A, Graybill JR, Craven PC, et al: High-dose ketoconazole
    therapy and adrenal and testicular function in humans. Arch
    Intern Med 144:2150, 1984.
Hay RJ, Clayton YM, Griffiths WAD, Dowd PM: A comparative double
    blind study of ketoconazole and griseofulvin in
    dermatophytosis. Br J Dermatol 112:691, 1985.

SYSTEMIC ANTIVIRAL AGENTS

Topical antiviral agents have been available for some time, but
except for their use in ophthalmic herpes simplex infection, they
have not been useful in viral skin infections. Intravenously
administered vidarabine and acyclovir are of great importance in the
treatment of systemic herpes infections, but here, too, they are
rarely appropriate for ordinary cutaneous infections. In contrast,
the recent availability of acyclovir for oral administration
represents a real breakthrough in antiviral therapy.

Acyclovir given orally in a dose of 200 mg five times a day is
now the treatment of choice for initial episodes of herpes
genitalis. It can also be used in similar dose for the treatment of
recurrent episodes and is perhaps of even greater usefulness when
taken prophylactically (at a dose of 200 mg three times a day) for
the prevention of recurrent disease. Its use in this setting is
discussed in greater detail in Chapter 7.

The role for oral acyclovir in herpes labialis is less certain.
It probably is effective but since most patients do not experience
great disability the high cost of therapy is ordinarily not
warranted. Likewise, its use in herpes zoster is controversial.
The varicella-zoster virus is more resistant than is the herpes
simplex virus and as a result rather large doses are required to
demonstrate a clinical effect. With this in mind, acyclovir is
likely not warranted in ordinary herpes zoster infections. Herpes
simplex and herpes zoster infections in those who are significantly
immunocompromised generally require hospitalization for intravenous
acyclovir administration.

Acyclovir itself is not an active antiviral agent. When
administered it is converted to the active, phosphorylated form of
the drug by the action of virally coded thymidine kinase. The
active form interferes with DNA polymerase and in so doing prevents
viral replication. Host cells are relatively unaffected because
they lack a thymidine kinase which can phosphorylate the parent
acyclovir compound. Moreover, human cellular DNA polymerase is more
resistant to drug effect than is viral DNA polymerase.

Concern exists regarding the potential for the development of
viral resistance to acyclovir. Fortunately, so far this has not
proven to be a practical, clinical problem.

SELECTED READING

Hermans PE, Cockerill FR III: Symposium on Antimicrobial Agents -
Part IV. Antiviral agents. Mayo Clin Proc 58:217, 1983.
Chadwick EG, Shulman ST: Advances in antiviral therapy:
Acyclovir. Pediatr Dermatol 2:64, 1984.
Dolin R: Antiviral chemotherapy and chemoprophylaxis. Science
227:1296, 1985.

SYSTEMIC STEROIDS

Systemically administered corticosteroids are useful in those
situations where the severity or extensiveness of a cutaneous
disease precludes topical application. They may be given orally or
intramuscularly.

Prednisone is the oral corticosteroid most often used. It is
cheap, relatively short acting, and available in a variety of
convenient sizes. For most dermatologic diseases, prednisone is
used in the form a a "burst." In this form of therapy 40 to 60 mg
of prednisone is given in a single early morning dose each day for 7
to 10 days. At that point therapy is discontinued without
tapering. Bursts such as this are especially useful in the
treatment of eczematous disease where complete (although often
transient) response can be expected. Toxicity is rarely a problem
when prednisone is used in this manner. In fact, with the exception
of occasionally encountered psychologic changes, serious side
effects are practically unheard of. With some caution, bursts of
prednisone can even be used in most patients with mild hypertension,
treated diabetes, and healed ulcerative disease of the
gastrointestinal tract.

Some clinicians believe that a beneficial effect equivalent to
that of an oral burst of prednisone can be obtained through the
intramuscular injection of 40 to 80 mg of the depot-type steroid
triamcinolone acetonide (Kenalog). Those who utilize this form of
therapy claim that, because of the small number of milligrams used,
side effects are infrequent and problems with patient compliance are
completely avoided. However, many patients do develop cutaneous
purpura and women may experience changes in menstrual flow.
Moreover, pituitary-adrenal suppression does last for 2 to 3 weeks.
These difficulties have prevented the development of widespread
enthusiasm for this approach.

Long term administration of steroids is almost never indicated
except in the treatment of pemphigoid, pemphigus, exfoliative
erythrodermatitis, and the more serious forms of vasculitis and
lupus erythematosus. Unfortunately, within months of daily
administration, one or more problems such as the development of
hypertension, glucose intolerance, potassium wasting, sodium
retention, edema formation, osteoporosis, cataract formation,
pituitary-adrenal suppression, and infection secondary to immune

suppression can be expected. The likelihood of these side effects
is somewhat reduced if the entire daily dose of prednisone is
administered in the early morning. Even less risk occurs if the
disease in question can be controlled with alternate day
administration of a short acting steroid such as prednisone.

SELECTED READING

Storrs FJ: Intramuscular corticosteroids: A second point of view.
J Am Acad Dermatol 5:600, 1981.

Gallant C, Kenny P: Oral glucocorticoids and their complications.
J Am Acad Dermatol 14:161, 1986.

ANTIHISTAMINES

Antihistamines are primarily used in the treatment of urticaria
and for the amelioration of pruritus due to various causes. Two
major categories of antihistamines are available: H1 and H2
blockers.

The approximately 30 H1 antagonists are subdivided into several
chemical groups but there is relatively little clinical difference
among them. Familiarity with three or four different antihistamines
should be sufficient for the treatment of most problems.
Diphenhydramine (Benadryl) in a dosage of 150 to 200 mg per day is
the most widely used antihistamine. It is quite potent but its use
is accompanied by considerable sedation. It is now available
generically as an over-the-counter product. Chlorpheniramine
(Chlor-Trimeton, Teldrin) 12 to 16 mg per day is equally potent and
has the advantages of low cost. It, too, is available without a
prescription. Cyproheptadine (Periactin) 12 to 16 mg per day has an
antiserotonin effect as well as an antihistamine effect. Some
clinicians believe this gives it a somewhat broader anti-inflammatory effect. Hydroxyzine (Atarax, Vistaril) 100 to 200 mg per day
protects better against histamine-induced wheal formation than any
other antihistamine. Hydroxyzine also has a significant
tranquilizing effect. It is the antihistamine most widely preferred
by dermatologists, but it is, unfortunately, quite expensive.
Terfenadine (Seldane) administered in a dose of 60 mg twice a day is
the least sedating H1 blocker available. High cost prevents its
more widespread use.

The dosages given above for these antihistamines can be viewed
as approximations. The key to their successful use is to advance
the dose gradually until clinical improvement occurs or until
sedation or anticholinergic side effects (dry mouth, blurred vision,
and impaired micturition) become troublesome. Some sedation occurs
with administration of all antihistamines but this can be minimized
by having patients take most of their daily dose at suppertime and
bedtime. Generally sedation becomes less noticeable after the first
week of therapy. Patients should be warned about lengthened

reaction times while driving or operating machinery. Alcohol increases these problems and should be avoided during antihistamine therapy.

The two H2 antagonists available in this country are cimetidine (Tagamet) and ranitidine (Zantac). They are marketed for the treatment of gastrointestinal ulcerative disease of the upper gastrointestinal tract. In spite of this they are in widespread use for many other conditions. Blood vessels of the skin do have H2 receptors but treatment of urticaria with H2 blockers alone is usually ineffective. Some studies have, however, shown a synergistic effect when these agents are used along with standard H1 antagonists. There is little to choose between the two medications. Ranitidine, the more expensive of the two, appears to cause fewer side effects.

SELECTED READING
Fisher AA: The antihistamines. J Am Acad Dermatol 3:303, 1980.
Freston JW: Cimetidine. I. Developments, pharmacology, and
    efficacy. Ann Intern Med 97:573, 1982.
Zeldis JB, Friedman LS, Isselbacher KJ: Ranitidine: A new
    H2-receptor antagonist. N Engl J Med 309:1368, 1983.
Flowers FP, Araujo OE, Nieves CH: Antihistamines. Int J Dermatol
    25:224, 1986.

PSYCHOTROPIC AGENTS

Considerable controversy exists regarding the degree to which psychologic factors can adversely affect the skin. But even those who doubt the etiologic effect of psychic disability recognize that the presence of skin disease often results in the development of anxiety or depression. Whether cause or effect, these psychologic factors can, most of the time, be handled by a simple, common sense approach: warmth, a willingness to listen, and support. When more than this is needed the clinician must be ready either to treat the patient with psychotropic medication or to offer appropriate referral.

The benzodiazepines such as chlordiazepoxide (Librium), diazepam (Valium), and flurazepam (Dalmane) are useful adjuncts in the treatment of associated anxiety. They are particularly helpful in the control of pruritus and will often work where antihistamines alone have failed. As in the case with antihistamines, the usefulness of the benzodiazepines is often limited by the side effect of drowsiness. This can be partially circumvented by the administration of chlordiazepoxide (10 to 25 mg) or diazepam (5 to 10 mg) at suppertime and, if necessary, again at bedtime. Flurazepam is designed primarily as a sedative. Thus it is used, in a dose of 15 to 30 mg, only at bedtime. These medications are particularly helpful in the control of nighttime scratching which is

so characterically present in patients with atopic dermatitis. They
are also worth trying in chronic urticaria which is unresponsive to
conventional antihistamine therapy. Habituation, of course, is a
problem of considerable importance. This risk can be lessened by
avoiding their use in people with past drug dependency problems, by
limiting the number of pills prescribed, and by sharp restriction on
refills. Enthusiasm exists in some quarters regarding the use of
the newer, shorter acting benzodiazepines such as alprazolam (Xanax)
and triazolam (Halcion), but consensus has not yet developed
regarding their advantages over the older, well established, and
generically available products.

Phenothiazines such as chlorpromazine (Thorazine) and
trifluoperazine (Stelazine) are at least as effective as the
benzodiazepines. They are used less often because of a greater
frequency of side effects and because of a widespread (but, I think,
mistaken) belief that they are too potent to be used by
nonpsychiatrists. The phenothiazines have a chemical structure
which is very close to that of some of the antihistamines. It is
possible that the efficacy of both groups of drugs depends on their
mixed antihistaminic and tranquilizing effect.

Depression is a problem which is overlooked to an even greater
degree than is anxiety. I believe that it is present in at least 10
to 20% of patients with serious dermatologic disease. Mild
depression often improves as the skin disease clears and, of course,
requires no specific therapy. Depression of greater severity
deserves greater attention. Patients should be offered the
opportunity for psychotherapy or medical treatment or both.
Endogenous depression is thought to be more amenable to treatment
with medication than are other forms of depression but many
clinicians believe that a therapeutic trial is worthwhile regardless
of diagnosis. The tricyclics amitriptyline (Elavil) or doxepin
(Sinequan, Adapin) given in a single daily dose at bedtime are most
often used. The usual starting dose with either is 25 to 50 mg but
this can gradually be increased to 150 mg as necessary. The
tricyclics are extraordinarily effective antihistamines and appear
to be particularly effective in the treatment of resistant chronic
urticaria. Imipramine (Tofranil) is also effective and may be
somewhat less sedating. Both physician and patient need to remember
that the maximum effect of these medications is not apparent until
they have been taken for 2 to 3 weeks. Side effects of drowsiness
and confusion are fairly common, but other more serious
cardiovascular and central nervous system side effects are only
rarely seen.

SELECTED READING
Greenblatt DJ, Shader RI, Abernethy DR: Current status of
    benzodiazepines (first of two parts). N Engl J Med 309:354,
    1983.

Richelson E: Antimuscarinic and other receptor-blocking properties
of antidepressants. Mayo Clin Proc 58:40, 1983.
Richardson JW III, Richelson E: Antidepressants: A clinical update
for medical practitioners. Mayo Clin Proc 59:330, 1984.
Black JL, Richelson E, Richardson JW III: Antipsychotic agents: A
clinical update. Mayo Clin Proc 60:777, 1985.
Gupta MA, Gupta AK, Haberman HF: Psychotropic drugs in dermatology.
A review and guidelines for use. J Am Acad Dermatol 14:633,
1986.

PSORALENS AND PUVA THERAPY

The psoralens are a group of photosensitizing furocoumarins.
They are found in a variety of plants and as such are occasionally
responsible for accidental photocontact ("phytophoto") dermatitis.
Their photosensitizing potential was first used medically some 30
years ago when they were given to stimulate sunlight-induced melanin
formation in patients with vitiligo. Their efficacy in this disease
is due to the fact that they allow "resting" melanocytes located
deep in the hair follicles to become responsive to the small amount
of long wavelength ultraviolet light (the UVA wavelengths) which
reaches the deep dermis. Patients with vitiligo are usually given
methoxsalen (Oxsoralen) in a dose of 20 to 40 mg 2 hours prior to a
measured exposure of natural or synthetic ultraviolet light.
Topical applications of methoxsalen solution 0.1 to 1.0% can be
used for patients with very small areas of vitiligo. Cutaneous
burns occur with disturbing frequency when sunlight is used as the
source of photoenergy; this problem is minimized when the recently
developed fluorescent light bulb which produces only high intensity
UVA wavelengths is used. This combination of psoralens and UVA
light (PUVA therapy) is now the standard approach to psoralen usage.
PUVA therapy is extremely effective in the treatment of
psoriasis and in the early stages of mycosis fungoides. It has some
usefulness in alopecia areata, atopic dermatitis, pityriasis
lichenoides, lichen planus, and some types of pruritus. Acute side
effects have been limited to the induction of pruritus, "sunburn,"
and occasionally blistering. These can be almost entirely avoided
by careful metering of the ultraviolet light dose. The potential
for long term toxicity is somewhat greater. Skin cancers, which are
known to be related to chronic sunlight exposure, probably occur
with increased frequency in patients given PUVA therapy but this
problem will take many years to assess. Laboratory animals can
develop eye damage in certain circumstances but the importance of
this problem in tumors has not yet been determined. Because of this
potential toxicity, suitable eye protection must, of course, be used
during therapy.

SELECTED READING

Farber EM, Abel EA, Cox AJ: Long-term risks of psoralen and UV-A
    therapy for psoriasis. Arch Dermatol 119:426, 1983.
Roelandts R: Mutagenicity and carcinogenicity of methoxsalen plus
    UV-A. Arch Dermatol 120:662, 1984.
Stern RS, Parrish JA, Fitzpatrick TB: Ocular findings in patients
    treated with PUVA. J Invest Dermatol 85:269, 1985.
Abel EA, Reid H, Wood C, Hu C-H: PUVA-induced melanocytic atypia:
    Is it confined to PUVA lentigines? J Am Acad Dermatol 13:761,
    1985.

DAPSONE

The sulfone Dapsone is a sulfonamide with both antibiotic and
anti-inflammatory properties. This product has been used in the
treatment of leprosy for 40 years and for the past 25 years it has
also been used as an extraordinarily effective anti-inflammatory
agent in the treatment of dermatitis herpetiformis. It is at the
present also receiving widespread experimental use for a variety of
other inflammatory diseases such as vasculitis, pyoderma
gangrenosum, and relapsing polychondritis. The mechanism through
which its anti-inflammatory effect occurs is unknown but one
hypothesis suggests that it is mediated through lysosomal
stabilization. The usual dose of Dapsone when it is used for
dermatitis herpetiformis and other inflammatory diseases is 100 to
200 mg per day. Once the maximum clinical benefit is obtained the
dose is reduced to maintenance levels of 50 mg or less per day.
Dapsone, like other sulfa derivatives, is accompanied by a
relatively large number of side effects. Some erythrocyte hemolysis
and macrocytosis occurs in all patients who take the medication and,
in those who are G6PD deficient, hemolysis may be severe.
Methemoglobinemia also occurs in all patients but at the dosage of
Dapsone usually used it is not clinically significant. Peripheral
neuritis is seen in a small number of patients and is especially
likely with higher dosages. Hepatotoxicity and granulocytopenia
have been reported as occurring in a few patients.

SELECTED READING

Bernstein JE, Lorincz AL: Sulfonamides and sulfones in dermatologic
    therapy. Int J Dermatol 20:81, 1981.

CYTOTOXIC AGENTS IN DERMATOLOGIC DISEASE

A variety of cytotoxic agents are used for the treatment of
autoimmune diseases such as pemphigus, pemphigoid, dermatomyositis,
and lupus erythematosus. The most commonly administered medications
include azathioprine (Imuran), cyclophosphamide (Cytoxan), and
methotrexate. For the most part these medications are used only for

patients nonresponsive to steroids or in instances where steroid
side effects require a lowering of the steroid dose. An exception
to this occurs in the treatment of psoriasis where methotrexate can
be considered as a first line drug for widespread, debilitating
disease.

Methotrexate when used in psoriasis is usually given as a once
weekly oral dose of 25 mg. Most patients will show a very good
response by the end of the first month of therapy. In these
individuals the dose is gradually reduced to a maintenance level
which generally averages about 15 mg per week. Patients with less
reponsive disease sometimes require fractionation of the dosage.
The most common acute side effects occurring with methotrexate
include nausea, aphthous like ulcers of the mouth, abnormal liver
function studies, and transient bone marrow depression. All of
these appear to be dose related and can be managed by appropriate
reduction in the amount administered at the time of the next
treatment. Hepatotoxicity is a major long term side effect.
Recognition of this problem appears to require periodic liver biopsy
since, despite the presence of major structural changes, liver
function abnormalities as measured by conventional tests may not be
present. Liver biopsy in patients who have taken methotrexate for
several years regularly reveals some degree of inflammation and
fatty infiltration. About 10% of patients who have taken
methotrexate for 10 years will also develop mild to moderate
fibrosis. So far there has been no problem with drug induced
carcinogenesis or opportunistic infection.

Discussion regarding the use of azathioprine and cyclophosphamide falls outside the scope of this book.

SELECTED READING
Roenigk HH Jr, Auerbach R, Maibach HI, Weinstein GD: Methotrexate
    guidelines - revised. J Am Acad Dermatol 6:145, 1982.
Jolivet J, Cowan KH, Curt GA, Clendeninn NJ, Chabner BA: The
    pharmacology and clinical use of methotrexate. N Engl J Med
    309:1094, 1983.
McDonald CJ: Cytotoxic agents for use in dermatology. I. J Am Acad
    Dermatol 12:753, 1985.

TOPICAL CYTOTOXIC THERAPY

Topically applied cytotoxic agents can be effective in the
treatment of some premalignant and malignant skin diseases. Actinic
keratoses on the face and scalp respond rather well to topically
applied fluorouracil (Efudex and Fluoroplex). Applications of
fluorouracil in a 1 to 5% concentration are carried out on a twice
daily basis. After several days of application, areas of dysplastic
skin become painfully inflamed. In spite of this, daily
applications are continued until a total of 3 weeks of therapy has

been accomplished. In the weeks following cessation of therapy the inflammation gradually resolves and the keratoses disappear. Occasionally during this period basal or squamous cell carcinomas, which were previously hidden by numerous keratoses, become apparent. The results obtained are cosmetically excellent but they are not permanent; retreatment may be necessary in 2 to 3 years.

Topically applied nitrogen mustard is used in the treatment of mycosis fungoides. A 10-mg ampule of nitrogen mustard (Mustargen) is mixed with 50 to 100 cc of tap water and this diluted working solution is applied to the entire surface of the skin (the face and scalp excluded) three times a week. Applications are continued until the lesions resolve at which time the frequency of application can be reduced to once weekly. This maintenance program must be continued indefinitely or the disease will reappear. Allergic sensitization to nitrogen mustard occurs with some frequency. The mechanism by which nitrogen mustard treatment is effective is unknown but it is more likely due to the modulation of immunologic factors than it is to a direct cytotoxic effect.

SELECTED READING

Goette DF: Topical chemotherapy with 5-fluorouracil. J Am Acad Dermatol 4:633, 1981.
Jansen GT: Local use of fluorouracil. Dermatol Clinics 2:245, 1984.
Bennett R, Epstein E, Goette D, et al: Current management using 5-fluorouracil: 1985. Cutis 36:218, 1985.

RETINOIDS

Vitamin A deficiency results in the development of hyperkeratosis and scaling skin lesions. Not surprisingly, this observation led many clinicians to treat various types of keratinizing disorders with vitamin A. Some beneficial effects were noted but vitamin A toxicity often supervened before adequate therapy had been accomplished. This led to a search for safer variants of the vitamin A molecule. The first clinically successful retinoid was transretinoic acid (Retin-A) which, when topically applied to the face in acne patients, results in extrusion ("dekeratinization") of the follicular plugs responsible for the initiation of acne lesions. Considerable unwanted inflammation occurs concomitantly with this keratolytic effect; but, in spite of this drawback, topically applied transretinoic acid remains a first line medication in the treatment of acne. More recently two new retinoids, 13-cis-retinoic acid (Accutane) and the aromatic retinoid etretinate, have become available for oral use. The former has shown remarkably good results in the treatment of acne and both produce considerable improvement in some of the papulosquamous diseases such as psoriasis, lichen planus, pityriasis rubra pilaris,

Darier's disease, and ichthyosis. A somewhat less good effect seems to occur during the treatment of certain cutaneous malignancies.

The dosage of 13-cis-retinoic acid used in acne patients is 0.5 to 1.5 mg per kg. For practical purposes a decision is usually made to use either 40 mg or 80 mg per day. The lower dose is associated with fewer side effects and thus has better patient compliance. Unfortunately, the interval until return of sebaceous gland function and the reappearance of acne is shorter (6 to 18 months) than it is when the larger dose is used. A consensus regarding the dosage of etretinate to be used in the papulosquamous diseases has not as yet been reached. It most likely will fall in the range of 0.5 to 1.0 mg per kg.

Many toxic effects are associated with the oral use of retinoids. Patients taking 13-cis-retinoic acid for acne regularly develop severe xerosis and chelitis. Less often myalgia, arthralgia, conjunctivitis, epistaxis, and hair loss are experienced. Triglyceride levels increase in these patients and must be monitored. Cholesterol levels may also rise and some disturbance in liver function studies may be noted. Long term administration is accompanied by idiopathic calcification of the spine in an unknown percentage of patients. Of greatest importance is the fact that the retinoids are among the most potent teratogens ever used in medicine. Retinoids may not be given until it is certain that a patient is not already pregnant and pregnancy must then be prevented until 2 months after 13-cis-retinoic acid is discontinued and, because of long term fat storage, until 2 years after etretinate is discontinued.

SELECTED READING

Thomas JR III, Doyle JA: The therapeutic uses of topical vitamin A acid. J Am Acad Dermatol 4:505, 1981.

Dicken CH, Connolly SM: Systemic retinoids in dermatology. Mayo Clin Proc 57:51, 1982.

Wolska H, Jablonska S, Bounameaux Y: Etretinate in severe psoriasis. Results of double-blind study and maintenance therapy in pustular psoriasis. J Am Acad Dermatol 9:883, 1983.

Bollag W: Vitamin A and retinoids: From nutrition to pharmacotherapy in dermatology and oncology. Lancet, April 16:860, 1983.

Jones DH, King K, Miller AJ, Cunliffe WJ: A dose-response study of 13-cis-retinoic acid in acne vulgaris. Br J Dermatol 108:333, 1983.

Dicken CH: Retinoids: A review. J Am Acad Dermatol 11:541, 1984.

Lammer EJ, Chen DT, Hoar RM, et al: Retinoic acid embryopathy. N Engl J Med 313:837, 1985.

Pochi PE: Isotretinoin for acne. N Engl J Med 313:1013, 1985.

Vahlquist A: Clinical use of vitamin A and its derivatives --
    physiological and pharmacological aspects. Clin Exp Dermatol
    10:133, 1985.
Vahlquist C, Michaelsson G, Vahlquist A, Vessby B: A sequential
    comparison of etretinate (Tigason) and isotretinoin (Roaccutane)
    with special regard to their efforts on serum lipoproteins. Br
    J Dermatol 112:69, 1985.

CYCLOSPORINE

    Cyclosporine is a remarkable new immunotherapeutic agent. It is
currently approved only for the treatment of graft versus host
reactions in organ transplantation but is likely to prove helpful in
other settings as well. The advantages of this medication include
the fact that it is not related to the corticosteroids and thus
allows avoidance of the many toxicity problems associated with long
term steroid administration. Moreover there is little bone marrow
toxicity such as is seen with cyclophosphamide and azathioprine.
Unfortunately, there is considerable risk of hypersensitivity
reactions and the development of renal toxicity but the latter can
apparently be minimized through careful monitoring of serum levels.
    The pharmacologic action of cyclosporine occurs through its
effect on T helper lymphocytes where, by inhibiting production of
growth type factors, it dampens the response of suppressor T cells
and decreases B cell activity.
    Cyclosporine is currently being used experimentally in
dermatology for the treatment of cutaneous T cell lymphoma,
immunobullous disease, and other autoimmune conditions.

SELECTED READING
Cohen DJ, Loertscher R, Rubin MF, et al: Cyclosporine: A new
    immunosuppressive agent for organ transplantation. Ann Intern
    Med 101:667, 1984.
Page EH, Wexler DM, Guenther LC: Cyclosporin A. J Am Acad Dermatol
    14:785, 1986.

Chapter 5

Basic Diagnostic and Therapeutic Techniques

POTASSIUM HYDROXIDE (KOH) PREPARATIONS

Fungal hyphae can be found in affected tissues taken from superficial fungal diseases such as candidiasis, pityriasis (tinea) versicolor, and dermatophyte infections of the skin, hair, and nails. The potassium hydroxide (KOH) preparations which identify these hyphae are both sensitive and specific. Scale, pustules, blister roofs, and clippings taken from hair and nails may be examined with this technique. Most often KOH examination will be carried out during the evaluation of scaling disorders. In such instances scrapings are obtained after the affected skin has been moistened with an alcohol sponge or with tap water. Then, before the lesion dries, the sharp edge of a No. 15 scalpel blade, held perpendicular to the skin, is scraped across the surface. The moistened scale which sticks to the edge of the blade is then transferred to a microscope slide. One drop of a 10 to 20% solution of potassium hydroxide (KOH) is then placed over the material on the slide. A coverslip is added. If the scale is fine and has been spread thinly on the slide, the preparation can be examined immediately. If the scale is thick, or if fragments of hair or nails are to be examined, gentle heating of the slide may be necessary in order to get a layer of cells thin enough to examine.

In examining the slide the condenser is racked to its lowest position and the intensity of the light source is reduced. These two maneuvers increase the contrast between the fungal hyphae and the underlying epithelial cells. The medium power objective is used for scanning the field and the high power objective is used to confirm the presence of suspected hyphae.

In pityriasis (tinea) versicolor, fungal hyphae are short, stubby, and vaguely "Y" shaped (Fig. 5-1). Small round spores are numerous and are collected in clusters around the hyphae. The terms "grapes on a branch" and "spaghetti and meatballs" are often used to describe these hyphae and spores.

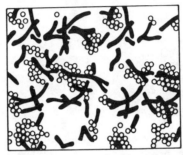

Figure 5-1.   The hyphae and spores of pityriasis (tinea) versicolor. The hyphae are short, stubby, and branched. Small spores are clustered around the hyphae. Background skin cells are not shown in this figure.

In dermatophyte and candida infections the hyphae are thinner and longer (Fig. 5-2). Few if any spores are present. Most observers cannot easily separate the pseudohyphae of candida infections from the true hyphae of dermatophyte infections and a decision as to which of the two infections is present usually depends on the clinical presentation or subsequent culture.

Artifacts are commonly found and may be confused with hyphae. Cotton threads are thicker and lack parallel sides and branching. Hairs have parallel sides but they too lack branching. The edges of epithelial cells sometimes overlap and appear to form a continuous, branching line. In such a situation compression of the coverslip against the slide will cause the cells to change position, thus breaking up the appearance of a single line.

The unequivocal presence of hyphae on a KOH preparation identifies the disease in question as being of fungal origin. Therapy can be initiated on the basis of this finding without waiting for the report of a fungal culture.

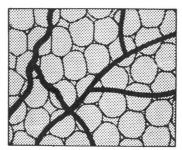

Figure 5-2. The hyphae of a dermatophyte fungal infection. The hyphae are long, thin, and branching. A background of circular epithelial cells is shown.

SELECTED READING

Rippon JW: Medical Mycology, 2nd edition. W.B. Saunders Co., Philadelphia, 1982.

Head E: Laboratory diagnosis of the superficial fungal infections. Dermatol Clinics 2:93, 1984.

FUNGAL CULTURES

There is some controversy as to whether or not fungal cultures are always necessary in situations where fungi have been identified on KOH preparations. Certainly they should be obtained in cases of deep fungal infection, onychomycosis, or tinea capitis (where KOH preparations are difficult to interpret) and when therapy requires systemically administered medications. On the other hand, cultures may not be necessary for tinea corporis, tinea cruris, and tinea pedis since KOH preparations are easy to carry out and topical therapy is usually effective.

In instances where fungal culture is desired, scraped scale, clipped nails, or plucked hairs can be collected in any clean container (such as a urine collection cup) for transportation to the microbiology laboratory where technicians implant them in Sabouraud's or other suitable medium.

The yeasts, Candida sp., grow quickly and can be identified in as few as 72 hours. The dermatophytic fungi require 1 to 3 weeks of growth before positive identification can be obtained. The yeast Pityrosporum sp. responsible for pityriasis (tinea) versicolor cannot be grown in ordinary microbiologic laboratories.

SELECTED READING

Rippon JW: Medical Mycology, 2nd edition. W.B. Saunders Co., Philadelphia, 1982.

Head E: Laboratory diagnosis of the superficial fungal infections.
    Dermatol Clinics 2:93, 1984.

BACTERIAL CULTURES

Bacterial cultures are not often necessary for the diagnosis and treatment of the common bacterial skin infections. In fact, they are sometimes more confusing than helpful. The problem arises because cultures taken from moist, eczematous skin lesions very often recover "pathogenic" bacteria which are merely colonizing diseased skin. Antibacterial therapy based on such cultures has little or no effect on the ultimate outcome of the disease, suggesting that these organisms are unimportant from a standpoint of pathogenesis. Cultures should be obtained, however, whenever hospital-acquired organisms are suspected, whenever patients are immunosuppressed, and whenever initial therapy leads to treatment failure.

A particular note of caution should be made regarding the performance of blood cultures in patients with exfoliative erythrodermatitis. Needle punctures through diseased skin, no matter how carefully the skin is prepared, are quite likely to be contaminated. Thus, positive cultures in such patients should be interpreted with extreme care.

Cultures are obtained with swabs provided in the packets which accompany commercially prepared transport media. Crusts should be lifted so that purulent material beneath the crust is sampled. Pustules can be opened sterilely and the drop of fluid which exudes can be touched with the swab. Care should be taken to avoid contamination with the surrounding skin. Needle aspiration can be carried out when larger vesicular or bullous lesions are present.

Plaques of suspected cellulitis cannot be easily cultured. Some clinicians recommend the injection and subsequent aspiration of sterile saline but because of low yields I have never found this approach helpful.

SELECTED READING

Noble WC: Microbiology of Human Skin, 2nd edition. Lloyd-Luke
    Medical Books Ltd., London, 1981.

TZANCK PREPARATIONS (CUTANEOUS CYTOLOGY)

Cytologic examination can be of considerable help in rapid identification of the bullous lesions of pemphigus and vesicular lesions due to herpesvirus infections. Such examinations, called Tzanck smears, depend on the recovery and identification of abnormal cells removed from the blister. To obtain such cells the roof of the blister is cut and lifted away. The fluid contained in the blister is allowed to run off and the base of the blister is gently scraped with the sharp edge of a No. 15 scalpel blade. The cells adherent to the blade are then transferred to a glass slide and are allowed to air dry. These cells are then stained with Giemsa or Wright's stain and the slide is examined under the microscope. The presence of rounded-up, acantholytic cells suggests the presence of pemphigus, whereas the presence of multinucleated giant cells identifies the process as that of herpesvirus infection: herpes simplex, herpes zoster, or varicella. Unfortunately, all three of these viral infections result in an identical microscopic appearance and thus cannot be individually identified on the basis of the Tzanck smear.

SELECTED READING

Solomon AR: The Tzanck smear. Viable and valuable in the diagnosis of herpes simplex, zoster, and varicella. Int J Dermatol 25:169, 1986.

VIRAL CULTURES

The availability of cultures for the herpesviruses has increased appreciably in recent years. It is now practical and appropriate to obtain cultures from vesicular and erosive lesions of the mouth and genitalia. Such cultures are particularly indicated when sexually transmitted disease is suspected and when patients are immunosuppressed as a result of disease or therapy. Cultures are obtained through the application of a swab to the erosion or base of the vesicle. These swabs must then immediately be placed in special carrying medium before conveyance to the microbiology laboratory. Culture results are rapidly available for suspected cases of herpesvirus infection since these viruses can be grown in 24 to 72 hours. Even more rapid results can sometimes be obtained when smears made from swabs are examined with fluorescent labeled antibodies.

SELECTED READING

Weller TH: Varicella and herpes zoster. N Engl J Med 309:1362, 1983.
Straus SE (moderator): Herpes simplex virus infection: Biology, treatment, and prevention. Ann Intern Med 103:404, 1985.

FLUORESCENT LIGHT (WOOD'S LAMP) EXAMINATION

A Wood's lamp is a low output UVA ("black light") lamp which has been filtered such that most of the radiation is approximately 360-nm wavelength. Wood's lamp examination is carried out in a darkened room.
Patients with tinea capitis due to Microsporum sp. will demonstrate sharply marginated, bright blue-green patches of

fluorescence when the lesions on their scalp are exposed to light from a Wood's lamp. Unfortunately, the proportion of tinea capitis cases due to Microsporum audouinii and M. canis has gradually decreased to the point where only about 10% of patients with tinea capitis will show this characteristic fluorescent pattern.

Hypopigmented, white lesions are considerably more prominent under the light from a Wood's lamp than they are under most other lighting conditions. Thus better identification of pityriasis (tinea) versicolor, vitiligo, and the ash leaf spots of tuberous sclerosis can be obtained when patients with these diseases are examined with a Wood's lamp.

Porphyrin compounds reveal a characteristic coral red fluorescence when illuminated by light from a Wood's lamp. If the porphyrin concentration is high enough, freshly voided urine from a patient with porphyria cutanea tarda will show this distinctive fluorescent pattern. Wood's lamp examination is considerably less valuable in the diagnosis of other diseases of porphyrin metabolism.

Finally, patients with erythrasma, a trivial and uncommon bacterial infection of intertriginous skin, will show red fluorescence of the skin when examined with a Wood's lamp.

SELECTED READING

Jillson OF: Wood's light: An incredibly important diagnostic
    tool. Cutis 28:620, 1981.

PATCH TESTING

Patch testing is helpful in identifying allergic contact dermatitis among those patients with otherwise nondistinctive eczematous eruptions. However, as is so true for many diagnostic tests, patch testing, because of Bayes's theorem, is more useful in confirming a suspected clinical diagnosis than it is when used as a screening technique.

Patch testing can be carried out with a suspected contactant itself ("use test") or with the chemical constituents of the contactant. The former is usually more practical since it does not require the purchase and periodic updating of a patch test kit. Use tests are suitable for most nonindustrial contactants such as clothing, cosmetics, and medications where the item in question has been designed for direct application to the skin. Use tests are considered inappropriate when evaluating industrial and laboratory chemicals because of the possible development of an unexpectedly severe reaction. In carrying out a use test the suspected contactant is taped in place so that it is held tightly against the skin for 48 hours. At the end of 48 hours (or earlier if the patient experiences severe itching) the bandages or tapes are removed and the site of application is examined. Positive reactions will be red, raised, and pruritic. Flat, red reactions are interpreted as indeterminant and are not ordinarily considered clinically important. Negative reactions, of course, show no visible change at all. Care should be used so that reactions to the tape are not misinterpreted as reactions to the contactant.

Patch test kits are available for more sophisticated types of testing. These kits contain appropriately diluted concentrations of the most commonly encountered contact antigens. They are generally used either to screen for possible contactants in eczematous disease of unknown etiology or for identification of a single, specific antigen in patients with positive use tests. The complexity of this type of testing together with the need to continually replace outdated material makes the use of patch test kits impractical for most generalists.

A positive patch test does not automatically confirm a diagnosis of contact dermatitis any more than a positive tuberculin skin test proves that a patient's pulmonary disease is due to tuberculosis. Coincidental positive reactions can occur in both instances. Proof that a patient has allergic contact dermatitis requires both the presence of a positive patch test and improvement of the patient's condition when the suspected contactant is removed from the patient's environment.

SELECTED READING

Adams RM: Patch testing -- A recapitulation. J Am Acad Dermatol 5:629, 1981.
Dahl MV: Pitfalls of patch testing. In Callen JP, et al (eds): Dermatology, vol 2. G.K. Hall Medical Publishers, Boston, 1984, p 255.

LIGHT TESTING FOR PHOTOSENSITIVITY

A number of skin diseases are either caused by or are aggravated by exposure to ultraviolet light. Generally such reactions are apparent to the patient and clinician alike since the distribution conforms to a sunlight exposure pattern. Specifically such reactions most often develop on the face (excluding the areas shaded by the nose and chin) and arms. In the broadest sense, photosensitivity diseases can be caused by either UVA or UVB light. These diseases can often be separated clinically by the fact that reactions owing to UVA occur with light passing through window glass whereas those owing to UVB do not. More advanced testing is possible using light sources with appropriate filters. A special variant of such testing involves the use of photopatches through which photo induced contact dermatitis can be recognized. A generalist need only be aware that light testing for photosensitivity reactions is available on appropriate referral.

SELECTED READING

Epstein JH: Photoxicity and photoallergy in man. J Am Acad
    Dermatol 8:141, 1983.
Emmett EA: Evaluation of the photosensitive patient. Dermatol
    Clinics 4:195, 1986.

SEROLOGIC TESTS FOR SYPHILIS

Two classes of serologic tests for syphilis (STS) are
available: those which use a nonspecific antigen and those which
use a specific, treponemal antigen. The two nonspecific tests in
most widespread use are the rapid protein reagin (RPR) test and the
Venereal Disease Research Laboratory (VDRL) test. Both are easy to
perform and are inexpensive. The sensitivity of these two tests for
the presence of infectious syphilis is excellent. The specificity
is also good though occasional false-positive reactions are
encountered.

The most widely available test using a specific treponemal
antigen is the fluorescent treponemal antigen (FTA-Abs) test. This
test is technically more difficult to perform but because of its
excellent specificity it is regularly used as a final arbiter in
diagnosis of syphilis. It is not usually quantitated. The more
recently developed microhemagglutination assays for antibodies to
Treponema pallidum can be quantitated but these tests are not yet
widely available.

The VDRL, RPR, and FTA-Abs tests generally become positive 7 to
14 days after a syphilis chancre has appeared. Thereafter,
essentially all patients with primary and secondary syphilis will
have positive tests. Patients with signs and symptoms suggestive of
infectious syphilis and a positive STS are assumed to have the
disease and treatment can be carried out on this basis. Once
infectious syphilis has been treated, quantitative STS are
periodically obtained. The titer gradually drops and by the end of
2 years, assuming no reinfection, all the tests will become negative.

A positive RPR or VDRL is sometimes found in the absence of
clinical evidence for syphilis. In such instances the FTA-Abs test
should be performed. If the FTA-Abs test is negative the patient
most likely has a false-positive serologic reaction. These
false-positive reactions most commonly occur in the presence of
collagen vascular disease but they may also be found in patients
with malaria, leprosy, and various parasitic or viral diseases. If
no explanation for a false-positive reaction can be found, the STS
should be repeated a month or so later. If the test has reverted to
negative nothing further need be done. If it is still positive the
entire work-up for diseases known to be associated with positive
reactions should be repeated.

On the other hand if the FTA-Abs test is positive the patient
almost certainly has or has had syphilis. A very few instances of

false-positive FTA-Abs tests have been reported in the presence of lupus erythematosus, dysproteinemias, and malignancy, but for practical purposes the presence of two positive FTA-Abs tests is tantamount to a diagnosis of syphilis. The first step in evaluation of a patient with a positive FTA-Abs test is to inquire about serologic tests which may have been done in the past such as before marriage or during military service. If previous tests were positive, if the patient was adequately treated, and if the VDRL titer remains constant and low, one can assume that the patient, although clinically cured, is sero-fast. Such patients require no additional therapy but periodic quantitative STS ought to be carried out since a rising titer may be the only clue to reinfection. If a past history of serologic tests is not available or if previous tests were negative a presumptive diagnosis of syphilis is made and the patient is checked for stigmata of congenital or tertiary syphilis. If none are present, a diagnosis of sero-fast latent syphilis can be made. In all these instances one must be sure that appropriate therapy has been administered and that the patient is followed with periodic quantitative tests as described above.

SELECTED READING
Hart G: Syphilis tests in diagnostic and therapeutic decision making. Ann Intern Med 104:368, 1986.

IMMUNOFLUORESCENT TECHNIQUES

Immunofluorescent techniques are extremely useful in the diagnosis of several dermatologic diseases. Such tests are relatively expensive but they are of immense importance and ought to be obtained whenever possible. All university medical centers and most private dermatopathology laboratories have the facilities to carry out these tests. Transport solutions, such as Michel's solution, are easily available so that specimens of skin to be tested for direct immunofluorescence can be mailed if necessary. Two types of immunofluorescent testing are available: the direct technique and the indirect technique.

Direct immunofluorescent testing is carried out on skin specimens. With this technique one attempts to identify immunoglobulin or complement, or both, which have been deposited within the skin as part of the disease process. A regular skin biopsy is performed but instead of the specimen being placed in Formalin it is either immediately frozen in liquid nitrogen or is placed in transport solution. In the laboratory, fluorescein labeled antibodies to IgG, IgM, IgA, complement components, and fibrin are layered over the tissue. If any of these substances are present the antibodies will adhere to the tissue and will be visible on fluorescent microscopy. Positive direct immunofluorescent tests are expected in six diseases described in this book: dermatitis herpetiformis, pemphigoid, pemphigus, lupus erythematosus, lichen planus, and some forms of vasculitis.

In dermatitis herpetiformis, perilesional skin will contain globules of IgA located in the superficial papillary dermis. In a few cases the deposits of IgA are found instead in a linear pattern at the dermal-epidermal junction. Complement (C3) occasionally is present in the same site as the globular or linear deposits of IgA.

In pemphigoid, IgG and C3 are found at the dermal-epidermal junction of lesional and perilesional skin In pemphigus, IgG and occasionally C3 are found within the epidermis neatly outlining the cytoplasmic membrane of the epidermal cells.

In the skin lesions of both discoid and systemic lupus erythematosus C3 and IgG are present at the dermal-epidermal junction in a pattern somewhat similar to that seen with pemphigoid. In about 70% of patients with systemic lupus erythematosus these same deposits may be found on sun exposed but nonlesional skin.

In lichen planus, globular deposits of fibrin and IgM are often found in the papillary dermis. In the neutrophilic types of vasculitis IgG, C3, and fibrin are generally found in and around the affected vessels.

Indirect immunofluorescent studies identify specific antibodies circulating within the patient's plasma. These antibodies are directed against individual antigens found within the patient's skin. When direct studies are performed, the patient's serum is layered over an appropriate substrate such as slices of epithelium (for the bullous diseases), certain tumor cells (for the antinuclear factors of lupus erythematosus), or specific organisms (such as T. pallidum for syphilis). If the patient's serum contains antibodies they will adhere to the antigen present in the substrate. To visualize these attached antibodies a second layer of fluorescein tagged antibodies to human immunoglobulin is applied. Under fluorescent microscopy any tagged antibody adherent to human immunoglobulin will then be visible.

Almost all patients with pemphigus will have circulating antibodies directed toward antigens on the outer surface of epithelial cell membranes. Approximately 70% of patients with pemphigoid will have circulating antibody directed against antigens present within the basement membrane zone of the dermal-epidermal junction. Most patients with primary syphilis and all patients with secondary syphilis will have circulating antibodies which will bind to T. pallidum fixed on microscopic slides (the FTA-Abs test). More than 90% of patients with systemic lupus erythematosus will have antibodies which bind to one or more antigens present within cell nuclei.

A rough estimation of the amount of antibody present in the patient's serum can be determined by making serial dilutions of the serum before layering it over the substrate. The number reported

(the titer) is the weakest dilution at which fluorescence can still
be identified. Thus the higher the titer, the greater the amount of
antibody present. To a limited degree, changes in these titers
correlate with changes in the activity of the disease and can, with
caution, be used to determine the degree of response to therapy.

SELECTED READING

Ongley RC: Immunofluorescent microscopy in dermatology:
   Diagnostic applications. Int J Dermatol 21:233, 1982.
Beutner EH, Chorzelski JP, Jablonska S: Immunofluorescence tests.
   Clinical significance of sera and skin in bullous diseases. Int
   J Dermatol 24:405, 1985.

CUTANEOUS ANESTHESIA

Anesthesia is required for excisional and electrosurgical
procedures on the skin. If anesthesia is needed only momentarily
(such as for a simple incision and drainage) Freon or ethyl chloride
sprays can be used. For all longer procedures, injected anesthesia
should be used. Almost all dermatologists currently use lidocaine
(Xylocaine) because of its almost instantaneous effect and because
it rarely causes allergic reactions. It can be used alone, but it
is also prepackaged with epinephrine for use when better hemostasis
or longer duration of action is desired. Lidocaine with epinephrine
probably should not be used for anesthesia of the fingers or toes
because of the possible development of digital ischemia.

Lidocaine in a 0.5 to 0.1% concentration is injected
intradermally using a tuberculin syringe and a 26- to 30-gauge
needle. Usually 0.5 to 1.0 cc will be all that is necessary to
obtain an anesthetized field 2 cm in diameter. A burning discomfort
is noticeable during injection; this can be minimized by injecting
at a slow rate. When injecting the anesthesia, care should be taken
that the tissue is not overly distended as this tends to interfere
with good suture closure.

Allergic reactions to lidocaine are extraordinarily rare but
occasionally patients will indicate that for one reason or another
they cannot receive lidocaine. In most instances careful checking
will reveal that their problem occurred with procaine (Novocain)
rather than with lidocaine. Cross reactions between these two
products are not a problem. However, if there is doubt about the
nature of a previous reaction, an alternate anesthetic must be
chosen. Injectable diphenhydramine (Benadryl) or even normal saline
can be used but neither one approaches the effectiveness of
lidocaine. Toxic side effects can occur when very large amounts of
lidocaine are used but this is not often a consideration for minor
surgery of the skin.

SELECTED READING
Arndt KA: Manual of Dermatologic Therapeutics, 3rd edition.
Little, Brown & Co., Boston, 1983, pp 201-202.

HEMOSTASIS

Control of bleeding is not often a problem during minor skin
surgery. Most bleeding is due to capillary or venous oozing and can
be handled by pressure, chemical cauterants, or the insertion of
Gelfoam.
Application of pressure is the simplest approach to the control
of oozing. Constant pressure for 5 minutes will almost always
achieve hemostasis. Alternatively, a protein coagulant, such as
ferric chloride or ferric subsulfate (Monsel's solution), can be
applied. To do this, a cotton tipped applicator is first moistened
with the solution and then is firmly applied to a clear, dry field
with a twisting motion. This allows the cauterant solution to
directly contact and coagulate the tip of the blood vessel.
Application of Monsel's solution to a bloody field without pressure
simply leads to the development of a black hemoglobin coagulum which
is totally ineffective for hemostasis. Application of Monsel's
solution to nonanesthetized skin results in transient stinging.
Some clinicians prefer the use of 20% aluminum chloride solution
to Monsel's solution because the latter occasionally leaves a small
visible deposition of iron pigment. I have never encountered this
complication. Silver nitrate sticks are also sometimes used for
hemostasis but they are considerably less effective than either
aluminum chloride or Monsel's solution.
Bleeding from a punch biopsy site may require special
consideration. In most cases the placement of a single suture to
close the defect will result in hemostasis. But, in the event
closure is not desired, a small pledget of Gelfoam can be stuffed
into a defect with a forceps. The pledget should be wedged tightly
so that it cannot fall out easily. The inserted Gelfoam acts as a
matrix on which a solid clot is formed. Later, the Gelfoam is
spontaneously absorbed; there is no need for subsequent removal.
Gelfoam works better than Monsel's solution within the defect left
by a punch biopsy simply because it is difficult to apply the latter
to the cut ends of blood vessels in such a small, narrow space.
Rarely a small arteriole or "spurter" will be transsected.
Bleeding of this type will require ligation or electrocoagulation of
the vessel.

SELECTED READING
Arndt, KA: Manual of Dermatologic Therapeutics, 3rd edition.
Little, Brown & Co., Boston, 1983, p 206.

SKIN BIOPSY

Skin biopsy is often required to confirm a clinical diagnosis. It is a simple, relatively inexpensive procedure. The general rule regarding its use should be: "If any doubt exists, biopsy!" Biopsies can be performed in several ways: shave excision, punch excision, or elliptical excision. All three techniques require the use of cutaneous anesthesia.

Shave biopsy is carried out by making a horizontal slice through the skin such that the No. 15 scalpel blade just passes below the expected depth of the lesion (Fig. 5-3). This technique is particularly useful for those elevated lesions in which the pathology is confined to the superficial portion of the skin. In some instances a shave biopsy can be curative as well as diagnostic. Because the skin is not deeply cut, problems with bleeding rarely occur. Likewise, there is little or no postoperative scarring. Unfortunately, if the depth of the pathology is misjudged the lesions may be transsected at a level too superficial for identification. Hemostasis is easily obtained with chemical cauterants.

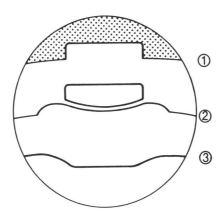

Figure 5-3. Shave biopsy. 1, a line drawing of a superficial lesion such as a seborrheic keratosis. 2, the same lesion with the base "puffed up" with injected lidocaine. The line of transsection made by the scalpel blade lying parallel with the surface of the skin is also shown. 3, the slightly dish shaped defect left after the edema caused by the lidocaine injection has subsided.

A punch biopsy (Fig. 5-4) can be carried out almost as quickly and easily as a shave biopsy. This technique is best used for lesions in which the histologic changes are expected to extend to the mid or lower portions of the dermis. It is not necessary to include any adjacent normal skin when carrying out a punch biopsy. The punch used for such biopsies can be envisioned as a very small cookie cutter. This instrument is placed perpendicular to the skin and with downward pressure, the punch is turned with a rotary motion such that a cylinder of skin is cut. Stabilization of the skin in the area to be cut assures a smoothly cut and better formed specimen. The skin should be cut completely through to the depth of the subcutaneous layer. The depth of the cut can be judged by removing the punch and observing the central piece of tissue. One is certain that the skin has been cut entirely through when the central piece of tissue has shrunken away from the sides and appears "loose" in the hole. At that point the cylinder of skin is gently lifted with a forceps on the tip of a needle and the underlying connection to subcutaneous fat is cut with a sharply pointed small scissors. The defect left by the removal of the skin cylinder can either be left open or can be closed with a single 5-0 suture. If the defect is left open, a small block of dental Gelfoam or caustic such as Monsel's solution should be inserted to ensure hemostasis. In most instances a 3- or 4-mm punch will give both an adequate piece of tissue and a suitably small scar.

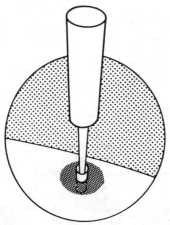

Figure 5-4. Punch biopsy. The skin punch is held perpendicular to the surface of the lesion. A small core is cut from the lesion when the punch is rotated with downward pressure.

If it is necessary to remove a piece of tissue 5 mm or more in diameter an elliptical excision ought to be performed (Fig. 5-5). Such excisions are also useful when the pathology to be evaluated

extends to the levels of the subcutaneous fat since the cylinder cut
by a punch often is too tapered to include an adequate sample of
panniculus. Prior to carrying out an elliptical excision markings
should be placed on the surface of the skin such that the long axis
of the identified ellipse lies in a wrinkle line. The length of the
ellipse should be 2.5 to 3 times the required width. Once the skin
is suitably marked and anesthetized the cut is made with a No. 15
scalpel blade. The blade should be held perpendicular to the
surface of the skin throughout the cut so that the edges of the cut
are not beveled. The cut should be completely through the dermis;
some subcutaneous fat should be visible at the bottom of the piece
of skin when it is removed. Hemostasis is rarely a problem.
Pressure alone is usually sufficient but bleeding vessels may be
tied off or coagulated if necessary. If the ellipse is large the
edges of the cut should be undermined to reduce suture tension.
Most elliptical excisions can be closed with a single layer of 5-0
monofilament nylon but in some instances a subcutaneous layer of
absorbable suture material such as Vicryl will be required. Skin
surface sutures should be removed within 5 days on the face but in
other areas it may be necessary to leave the sutures in for 7 to 14
days in order to obtain adequate wound strength.

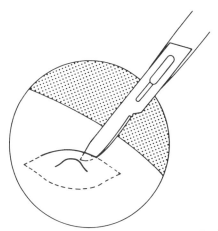

Figure 5-5. Elliptical excision. This technique should be used
when the tissue to be removed is larger than 4 mm in diameter or
when the pathology of a lesion is expected to lie at a point deeper
than the mid dermis.

    Tissue removed by any one of the three biopsy techniques
described above should be placed immediately in a 10% Formalin

solution for transport to the pathology laboratory. A urine
collection cup (it need not be sterile) is a cheap and easily
available container for this purpose.

SELECTED READING
Peters MS, Winkelmann RK: The biopsy.   Dermatol Clinics 2:209, 1984.

ELECTROSURGERY

There are many instances when electrosurgery (with or without
curettage) can take the place of excisional removal of lesions.
Electrosurgery can be performed more quickly than excision because
there is little bleeding and suture closure is not carried out.
However, because the wound heals by secondary intention, healing
time is long (2 to 3 weeks) and the resultant scar is larger than it
would be following excision. Moreover, since the tissue being
treated is destroyed there is no tissue specimen which can be
histologically examined for adequacy of the resection margins.

The machinery used for electrosurgery can be either a monopolar
device, such as the Hyfrecator, which requires no grounding plate or
a bipolar device such as the Bovie, which requires that the patient
be grounded. In both instances the destructive effect is obtained
by way of a rapidly oscillating electrical field which disrupts
cells both thermally and mechanically.

In carrying out monopolar electrosurgery one may either let a
spark jump from the tip of the needle to the tissue to be destroyed
(electrofulguration) or one may touch the tip of the needle directly
to the tissue (electrodesiccation) (Fig. 5-6). The former results
in a pattern of wide, flat destruction and is appropriate for
superficial lesions whereas the latter gives a more spherical
pattern of destruction and is useful for deeper lesions. Curettage
to remove destroyed tissue is usually carried out in conjunction
with either technique (Fig. 5-7). The use of a curet prior to
electrosurgery gives a better sense of the type and margins of the
pathologic process whereas use of a curet after electrosurgery
results in fewer problems with hemostasis. The dermal curet, unlike
an ear curet, has a cutting edge, but this edge is not nearly as
sharp as that found on a scalpel blade. This semisharp edge allows
for easy removal of soft cancerous tissue but it will not easily cut
through normal collagen. The experienced operator develops a
feeling for the difference in substance between tumor and normal
collagen. This allows one to determine tumor margins with a high
degree of accuracy. Curettage can also be carried out without
accompanying electrosurgery. This process results in somewhat less
scar formation but since the destruction is less the rate of
recurrence for lesions so treated is higher. For this reason
curettage without electrosurgery is usually reserved for benign
lesions such as seborrheic keratoses and warts.

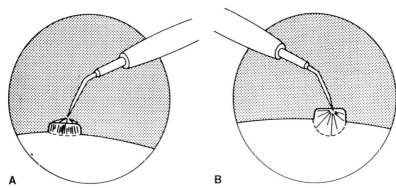

A   B

<u>Figure 5-6</u>. <u>A</u>, electrofulguration. The tip of the needle does not
touch the surface of the lesion. Sparks flow in a wide, flat
pattern causing a superficial destruction pattern. <u>B</u>,
electrodesiccation. The tip of the Hyfrecator needle touches the
surface of the lesion. Little or no visible sparking occurs and the
destruction pattern is more spherical than that obtained with
electrofulguration.

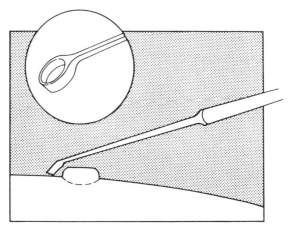

<u>Figure 5-7</u>. A dermal curet is used for the scraping removal of
benign and malignant skin lesions. The circular cutting edge is
semisharp: sharp enough to cut through soft pathologic tissue but
not sharp enough to cut through normal connective tissue.

Considerable care should be exercised when using electrosurgery on patients with pacemakers as the radio field which is created has the potential for disrupting pacemaker function. At the practical level this never occurs when short, intermittent bursts of electrical current are used.

SELECTED READING

Edens BL, Bartlow GA, Haghighi P, et al: Effectiveness of curettage and electrodesiccation in the removal of basal cell carcinoma. J Am Acad Dermatol 9:383, 1983.

Sebben JE: Electrosurgery and cardiac pacemakers. J Am Acad Dermatol 9:457, 1983.

Jackson R, Laughlin S: Electrosurgery. Dermatol Clinics 2:233, 1984.

CHEMICAL CAUTERANTS

Chemical cauterants such as phenol and trichloracetic acid are very useful for the destruction of benign, superficial lesions. The advantages of chemical cauterants are twofold: first, no injected anesthesia is required; and, second, bleeding does not occur during therapy. In using either preparation the solution is applied with the wooden end of a cotton tipped applicator or with a miniature cotton swab such as the urethral Calgiswab. The applicator should be brushed against the neck of the bottle to be sure that there is no loose drop which could accidentally fall from the tip. The lesion is then barely moistened with the solution; none of the solution is allowed to touch the surrounding normal skin. Generally there is no discomfort for the first 60 to 90 seconds after application. The operator can thus treat several lesions before the patient is aware of the process. This is a property which is clearly advantageous when small children with multiple lesions must be treated. Pain after application reaches a maximum in about 5 to 15 minutes and thereafter subsides fairly quickly. Most patients find the overall degree of discomfort quite tolerable. Within several days of treatment necrotic tissue forms at the site of application. This dead tissue sloughs spontaneously and complete healing takes place in approximately 10 days. The cosmetic appearance at the treated area is generally excellent but occasionally a small amount of scarring is visible. The destruction caused by spillage of even a drop or two of these fluids is very great and one cannot overemphasize the care which must be taken during their use. These solutions are best used on nonscaling, benign lesions such as condyloma acuminata, molluscum contagiosum, skin tags, and some warts. Seborrheic keratoses can be treated if they are not too keratotic. Most warts must be trimmed to reduce the amount of overlying keratin before chemical cauterants are used. Cauterants

are not used for malignant lesions because the destruction is
insufficiently deep to assure cure.

SELECTED READING

Arndt KA: Manual of Dermatologic Therapeutics, 3rd edition.
Little, Brown & Co., Boston, 1983, p 304.

CRYOTHERAPY

The use of freezing temperature to cause cell death and tissue
destruction (cryotherapy) has the same two advantages possessed by
cauterants: prior anesthesia by injection is not required and
bleeding during therapy does not occur. Cryotherapy has the
additional advantage of potentially deeper destruction so that the
technique can also be used for malignant lesions. On the other
hand, cryotherapy shares with electrosurgery and cauterants the
disadvantages of prolonged healing times and lack of tissue for
histologic examination. Cryotherapy is easily used for benign
lesions; but, for the treatment of malignant lesions, needles
containing thermocouples must be placed under the lesion in order to
offer certainty that the totality of the lesion has been adequately
frozen.

Cryotherapy can be carried out in three ways. Most commonly a
cotton tipped applicator is used to transfer liquid nitrogen (at a
temperature of approximately -200°C) from a Thermos-type bottle to
the lesion. Since the liquid nitrogen evaporates quickly, the
cotton tipped applicator must be redipped and reapplied multiple
times to get an adequate freeze. The lesions blanches as it is
frozen and this blanching must be maintained for at least 30
seconds. The depth of the freeze is regulated by the degree of
pressure applied to the cotton tipped applicator as much as by the
length of time the lesion is frozen. To minimize the risk of
scarring the applicator is usually applied without pressure; the tip
of the applicator is simply rested on the lesion.

A second approach employs a liquid nitrogen spray. A metal
spray tip is affixed to a Thermos-type bottle containing liquid
nitrogen. Expansion of the liquid nitrogen forms sufficient
pressure to expel the nitrogen in a narrow fine spray. This spray
is applied to the lesion for a total of 15 to 30 seconds. Sprayed
liquid nitrogen can be applied quickly to multiple lesions but it
requires some skill to confine the freeze precisely to the treated
lesion.

Finally, liquid nitrogen can be circulated through a metal probe
such that the tip of the probe approaches the temperature of the
nitrogen itself. The machinery for this application is quite
expensive but this approach offers the highest possible degree of
control over the size and depth of the tissue to be treated.

Discomfort is only moderately great during the freeze but becomes somewhat greater as the tissue thaws. For this reason it is not usually suitable for use in young children. A blister, often hemorrhagic in appearance, usually develops at the treated site the day after treatment. If the depth of the freeze was sufficient the lesion will be found in the roof of the blister. At this point the blister roof and contained lesion can be trimmed away or, for greater comfort to the patient and for preservation of sterility, the blister can be left intact until the roof sloughs spontaneously 7 to 14 days later. Postinflammatory hypopigmentation, sometimes of a permanent nature, sometimes occurs at the treated site; but frank scarring is rarely encountered.

SELECTED READING

Shepherd J, Dawber RPR: The historical and scientific basis of cryosurgery. Clin Exp Dermatol 7:321, 1982.
Kuflik EG, Lubritz RR, Torre D: Cryosurgery. Dermatol Clinics 2:319, 1984.

MOHS SURGERY

Mohs surgery represents a unique approach for microscopically controlled removal of malignant lesions. Under suitable local anesthesia thin horizontal slices of tumor are excised in a staged, saucerized fashion. Each slice is mapped through edge marking and is examined under frozen section by the surgeon as soon as it is removed. In this way remaining malignant tissue is immediately identified and further sections can be removed from appropriate locations at the excision margins. This approach to tumor removal conserves the greatest possible amount of normal tissue and offers the patient the best possible likelihood of complete removal. Mohs surgery is most often used for tumors recurrent after more conventional therapy and for primary removal at certain troublesome locations such as the canthi of the eyelids and nasal folds. The defect left after Mohs surgery can be closed primarily (using flaps and grafts if necessary) or can be left to heal by way of secondary intention. Cure rates approaching 100% are possible as a result of this unique approach to surgical excision.

SELECTED READING

Amonette RA: Microscopic control of skin cancer. Mohs' technique: Chemosurgery and fresh tissue surgery. Dermatol Clinics 2:219, 1984.

LASER SURGERY

The word "laser" is an acronym for light amplification by stimulated emission of radiation. The wavelengths of

electromagnetic energy used in this modality occur in the infrared
and visible portions of the spectrum. Several different types of
lasers are currently available, each having its own set of
advantages and disadvantages. However, all laser therapy is
characterized by preciseness of margination, good control over depth
of destruction, and freedom from problems of hemostasis. Argon
lasers, which emit light that is preferentially absorbed by
pigmented lesions, appear to be particularly useful for vascular
lesions. Carbon dioxide lasers, on the other hand, destroy whatever
is encountered within the focused beam and are therefore useful in
treating a wide array of benign and malignant lesions. More precise
guidelines for use of laser surgery will develop gradually as the
number of machines in use increases and the cost per treatment
decreases.

SELECTED READING

Goldman L: Current developments in laser dermatologic surgery.
    Dermatol Clinics 2:293, 1984.

Chapter 6

The Problem Oriented Algorithm

One of the most intimidating aspects of clinical medicine is the awesome amount of material to be learned. Medical students and house officers are exposed to massive amounts of new information during each specialty rotation. While each student recognizes that total understanding is impossible one invariably asks oneself "what of this material must I know?" and "how best can I learn it?" All too often answers for these questions are not offered. Instead an unorganized morass of information containing both relevant and irrelevant material is presented in an almost random fashion. In some instances students are simply told to read a textbook which is far too large to be completed during a single rotation. In other instances, a series of lectures is given by a succession of relatively uninterested individuals who have prepared little and teach poorly. In still other instances the instruction is purely patient oriented and depends entirely on whatever mix of patients enter the office, clinic, or hospital. In circumstances such as these learning is more clearly related to the quality of students than to the "excellence" of the teaching.

Remedies for the problems listed above depend on answers to several specific questions. First, which of the multitude of diseases presented will be most important to your practice of medicine? Second, which aspects of the diseases judged to be important are so critical as to be committed to memory and which can be safely left to be subsequently retrieved from reference sources? Third, how can one organize the material to be learned such that an unrecognized disease can be easily and assuredly identified? My thoughts regarding the answers to these questions are contained in the paragraphs below.

Limiting the Number of Diseases. It has been estimated that there are approximately 2000 separately named diseases in dermatology. Clearly not all of these are equally important to the medical student or to the house officer preparing for a career in a field other than dermatology. One approach to the identification of the most important diseases would involve considering the frequency with which they are encountered. This is not terribly hard to do since the frequency with which diseases occur falls into a geometric progression. Thus a very small number of diagnoses cover a very large number of patient visits. I estimate that for dermatologic problems, 10 diseases account for 50% of the patients seen, 25 diseases for 75% of the patients seen, and 50 diseases for more than 90% of the patients seen. However, frequency alone is insufficient to determine importance. Potential seriousness, high likelihood of

contagion, and amenability to therapy represent additional
characteristics which must be considered. With these considerations
in mind I have compiled a list of the 50 most common conditions and
have added to these an additional 25 serious, contagious, or curable
uncommon diseases for a total of about 75 diseases (Table 6-1) which
I believe will be important in general medical practice.

    The Most Important Aspects of Specific Diseases. A remarkable
amount of information regarding the history, epidemiology, genetics,
etiology, pathogenesis, clinical hallmarks, laboratory features,
prognosis, and therapy is known for every disease in medicine.
Clearly not all of this information can be learned for every disease
and, in fact, it is not practical to learn all of this even for
those diseases determined to be most important as outlined in the
paragraph above. I believe that it is most sensible to put the
major emphasis on those aspects of a disease which allow for its
recognition. After all, once recognized it is relatively easy to
use the readily available reference sources to obtain accurate,
up-to-date information regarding the other aspects of a patient's
disease. In emphasizing recognition let us concentrate on what
might be called "diagnostic hallmarks." For diseases of internal
organs these diagnostic hallmarks will incorporate features of
patient history, physical examination, and laboratory medicine. In
the case of dermatologic disease we are more fortunate. This is so
because the organ involved, the skin, is so readily available for
clinical examination. Indeed, I believe that the majority of skin
diseases can be correctly diagnosed solely on the basis of
inspection and palpation. Thus, in dermatology, if one thoroughly
learns the morphologic hallmarks of the 75 diseases found in Table
6-1 it should be possible to correctly diagnose the patient's
problem about 95% of the time. After that, all other necessary
information about the disease can be quickly looked up in a standard
reference source. Not only does this reduce the amount of material
to be learned, it also focuses one's attention on precisely those
aspects of a disease that will never change -- the clinical
features. For this reason, once these features are learned you will
have a store of knowledge which will remain useful over your
clinical lifetime.

    Organization of One's Knowledge. Of course, four or five
diagnostic features for each of 75 diseases still add up to more
information than can easily be carried, unorganized, in memory.
What is needed is a road map that guides you to smaller, more
manageable segments of this information. Such a road map is called
an algorithm.

    Traditionally diseases have been classified on the basis of
etiology or pathogenesis. Thus most textbooks include chapters on
infectious diseases, metabolic disease, inherited diseases,
malignancies, etc. This approach is intellectually attractive but
is useless in terms of helping a clinician diagnose an unrecognized

TABLE 6-1
DERMATOLOGIC DISEASES

I. Vesiculobullous Diseases
    A. Vesicular disease
       1. Herpes simplex
       2. Varicella-zoster
       3. Vesicular tinea pedis
       4. Dyshidrosis
       5. Dermatitis herpetiformis

    B. Bullous disease
       1. Pemphigus vulgaris
       2. Pemphigoid
       3. Erythema multiforme bullosum
          (Stevens-Johnson syndrome)
       4. Poison-ivy-type contact dermatitis
       5. Bullous impetigo

II. Pustular Diseases
    A. True (soft) pustules
       1. Acne vulgaris
       2. Rosacea (acne rosacea)
       3. Bacterial folliculitis
       4. Fungal folliculitis
       5. Candidiasis

    B. Pseudopustules
       (See white papules, Group IV)

III. Skin Colored Papules and Nodules
    A. Keratotic (rough surfaced lesions)
       1. Warts: verruca vulgaris, paronychial,
          and plantar warts
       2. Actinic keratoses
       3. Corns and calluses

    B. Nonkeratotic (smooth lesions)
       1. Warts: genital warts, flat warts
       2. Basal cell carcinoma
       3. Squamous cell carcinoma
       4. Epidermoid ("sebaceous") cysts
       5. Lipomas
       6. Molluscum contagiosum

TABLE 6-1 (cont'd)
_____

IV. White Lesions
     A. White patches and plaques
         1. Pityriasis alba
         2. Pityriasis (tinea) versicolor
         3. Vitiligo

     B. White papules
         1. Milia
         2. Keratosis pilaris
         3. Molluscum contagiosum

. V. Brown-Black Lesions
     A. Brown-black macules, papules, and nodules
         1. Freckles
         2. Lentigines
         3. Nevi: junctional, compound, and intradermal
         4. Dysplastic nevi
         5. Melanoma
         6. Seborrheic keratoses
         7. Dermatofibromas

     B. Brown patches and plaques
         1. Cafe-au-lait patches
         2. Giant congenital nevi

     C. Generalized hyperpigmentation

VI. Yellow Lesions
     A. Smooth yellow lesions
         1. Xanthelasma
         2. Necrobiosis lipoidica diabeticorum

     B. Rough yellow lesions
         1. Actinic keratoses
         2. Any crusted lesion (see vesiculobullous and
         eczematous diseases)

VII. Red Papules and Nodules
     A. Red papules
         1. Insect bites
         2. Cherry angiomas
         3. Pyogenic granulomas
         4. Granuloma annulare
_____

TABLE 6-1 (cont'd)

    B. Red nodules
        1. Furuncles
        2. Inflamed epidermoid cysts
        3. Cellulitis (erysipelas)
        4. Hidradenitis suppurativa

VIII.   Vascular Reactions
    A. Transient erythemas
        1. Urticaria and angioedema

    B. Persistent erythemas
        1. Erythema multiforme
        2. Erythema nodosum

    C. Purpuric erythemas
        1. Leukocytoclastic vasculitis

IX.   Papulosquamous Diseases
    A. Prominent plaque formation
        1. Psoriasis
        2. Tinea: corporis, capitis, pedis, and cruris
        3. Lupus erythematosus: discoid type
        4. Parapsoriasis and mycosis fungoides

    B. Nonconfluent papules
        1. Pityriasis rosea
        2. Lichen planus
        3. Secondary syphilis

X.   Eczematous Diseases
    A. Excoriations prominent
        1. Atopic dermatitis (neurodermatitis, lichen
            simplex chronicus, infantile eczema)
        2. Dyshidrotic eczema
        3. Stasis dermatitis
        4. Scabies (scabetic eczema)

    B. Little or no excoriation
        1. Seborrheic dermatitis
        2. Irritant contact dermatitis
        3. Allergic contact dermatitis
        4. Xerotic eczema

    C. Eczematous reaction patterns

---

condition. In effect, such books are useful only once you have a
diagnosis! The classification used in this book is instead a
problem oriented one. Diseases which share prominent clinical
features (i.e., look alike) are grouped together regardless of
whether or not they share a common etiology, pathogenesis, etc. The
ten groups chosen for this book are listed in Table 6-1 and are also
used as the chapter titles for the next ten chapters. In this
format, for example, those viral diseases, such as herpes simplex,
which present with vesicles will be found in a different category
than those, such as warts, that present as skin colored papules.
Moreover, since some diseases have a variable clinical presentation
or have more than a single prominent clinical feature, it will
sometimes be necessary to list a disease in two or more categories.
For example, scabies, which sometimes is vesicular and sometimes
eczematous, is listed both with the vesiculobullous diseases and
with the eczematous diseases.

The algorithm itself is the road map which guides the clinician
to the correct group and, within the group, allows for the
identification of the two or three most likely diagnoses: in effect
creating a list of differential diagnoses. This algorithm
(depicted in Table 6-2) consists of a series of questions, the
answers to which require accurate description of the morphologic
features of the disease in question. Unfortunately, the possession
of a map does not guarantee that one will not occasionally lose the
way. However, precise use of terminology, constant practice, and a
modicum of common sense help to assure accurate use of the
algorithm. Guidance in these areas is contained in the remaining
paragraphs in this chapter.

USE OF THE DIAGNOSTIC ALGORITHM

QUESTION 1a: ARE THE LESIONS SOLID OR FLUID FILLED?

Are blisters present? The recognition of large blisters is
relatively easy; small vesicles are often not so apparent. If in
doubt about the vesicular nature of a lesion, the roof should be
opened with a scalpel blade or needle tip. The lesion is said to be
vesicular if the fluid runs out and the compartment collapses. On
the other hand, edematous papules (wheals) when pierced exude a drop
of fluid but remain unchanged in size and shape. The presence of
even a few blisters (regardless of the appearance of the rest of the
eruption) is sufficient to identify the process as a member of the
vesiculobullous group.

Blistering diseases are sometimes misclassified when patients
present with vesicles or bullae whose roofs have been destroyed. In
such instances only erosions will be found. The roundness of the
erosions and the presence of roof fragments in a collarette around
each erosion should alert the examiner to the original blistering

TABLE 6-2
ALGORITHM FOR UNKNOWN SKIN DISEASE

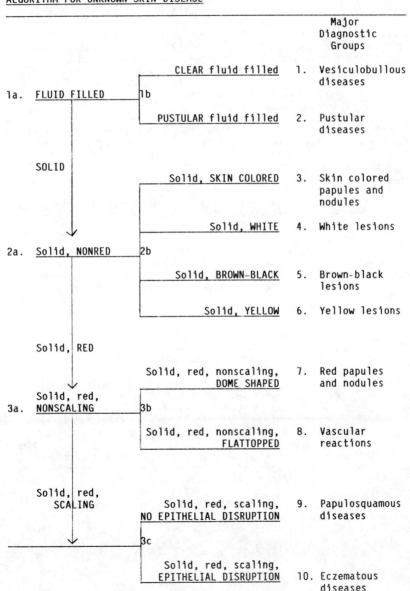

nature of the process. Patient history regarding the blistered
appearance of the lesions at the onset of the disease would, of
course, also be helpful.

The amount of inflammation at the base of blistering lesions
varies appreciably. Some blistering diseases arise from normal
appearing skin whereas in others the amount of inflammation greatly
overshadows the presence of a few small vesicles. Regardless of the
ratio between inflammation and vesiculation, these latter diseases
are still classified with the diseases of the vesiculobullous group.

If the lesions are fluid filled, Question 1b should be answered;
if the lesions are solid, proceed directly to Question 2a.

QUESTION 1b: IS THE BLISTER FLUID CLEAR OR PUSTULAR?

Diseases which belong to Group 1, the vesiculobullous diseases,
usually have blisters that are filled with clear fluid. There are,
however, two variants which are classified within this group:
blisters filled with slightly cloudy fluid and blisters filled with
blood tinged fluid. Cloudy blisters occur as the result of
neutrophil accumulation during the process of blister aging; such
lesions contain too few neutrophils to be considered pustular.
Hemorrhagic blisters occur when vascular disruption is a part of the
underlying disease process. Hemorrhagic fluid is most often found
in herpes zoster, pemphigoid, and some cases of neutrophilic
vasculitis. The blistering diseases are further subdivided on the
basis of size into those that are primarily vesicular and those that
are primarily bullous. The individual diseases are listed in Table
6-1 and are discussed in Chapter 7.

The lesions of Group 2, the pustular diseases, contain bright
white or yellow-white fluid. Moreover, in contrast to the late
occurring cloudiness of vesiculobullous diseases, the pustular
diseases must have had this white appearance from the time of their
inception. The pustular lesions are further divided according to
the consistency of the contents into those which contain fluid pus
(true pustules) and those which contain semisolid material
(pseudopustules). The latter overlap appreciably with the solid
white lesions of Group 4 and some are listed in both categories.
The pustular diseases are listed in Table 6-1 and are discussed in
Chapter 8.

QUESTION 2a: ARE THE LESIONS RED OR SOME OTHER COLOR?

In arriving at this point one has excluded all of the blistering
diseases; the remainder of the algorithm is devoted to solid
lesions. The question at this branch primarily revolves around
color: are the lesions red or are they nonred? This is usually
quite apparent. Difficulty occurs only when the lesions are covered
with appreciable scale. Scaling lesions are classified on the basis

of the color of the underlying lesion, not on the color of the
scale.   If the entire lesion seems to be made up of scale (as
happens with calluses, actinic keratoses, and some warts) the
underlying lesion is assumed to be skin colored.
If the lesions are nonred, Question 2b should be answered; if
the lesions are red, proceed directly to Question 3a.

QUESTION 2b: WHICH COLOR, OTHER THAN RED, ARE THE LESIONS?

Skin Colored Lesions. These lesions are placed in Group 3. The
determination as to whether or not lesions are skin colored depends
on the degree to which the color of the lesion matches the hue of
the surrounding normal skin. The absolute color of the lesion is
less important. Thus in a dark skinned patient a brown lesion is
considered skin colored if it is neither darker nor lighter than the
patient's normal skin. Likewise in a very fair skinned person a
skin colored lesion may be nearly white. Skin colored lesions are
further divided into those which are rough surfaced and those which
are smooth surfaced. These diseases are listed in Table 6-1 and are
discussed in Chapter 9.
White Lesions. These lesions are placed in Group 4. White
lesions are easy to recognize in all but the fairest skinned
patients. In such individuals, examination in a darkened room with
a Wood's light is helpful as it increases the contrast between the
white lesions and normally pigmented skin. The white lesions are
further divided into those which are papular and those which are
composed of patches or plaques. These diseases are listed in Table
6-1 and are discussed in Chapter 10.
Brown-Black Lesions. These lesions are placed in Group 5. To
be placed in this group lesions must be darker in pigmentation than
the surrounding skin. The absolute color of the condition in this
group varies appreciably. They may be as light as the tan color of
freckles or as dark as the black color of some seborrheic
keratoses. The diseases in this group are further divided on the
basis of size and elevation. The brown-black lesions are listed in
Table 6-1 and are discussed in Chapter 11.
Yellow Lesions. These lesions are placed in Group 6. Yellow
lesions are easy to recognize except sometimes in dark skinned
patients when the normal brown pigment partially obscures the yellow
color with a beige hue. Yellow lesions are further divided into
those that are smooth surfaced and those that are rough surfaced.
Since the roughness in the latter subgroup is generally due to
crusting there is considerable overlap with crusted lesions from the
vesiculobullous and eczematous diseases. The yellow lesions are
listed in Table 6-1 and are discussed in Chapter 12.

QUESTION 3a: ARE THE RED LESIONS SCALING OR SMOOTH?

All of the remaining diseases (Groups 7 through 10) are
basically red and separated on the basis of whether or not scale is
present. This determination is not always easy as several pitfalls
exist. First, it must be recognized that three categories of scale
exist: psoriasis-type, pityriasis-type, and lichen-type.
     Psoriasis-type scale is the easiest to recognize. It consists
of macroscopic flakes (or discs) of scale that are white, gray, or
silver in color. This opaque whiteness occurs because of the
looseness of the scale which in turn results in the bending of light
waves by both the top and bottom air-surface interfaces. This is
the same phenomenon which accounts for the whiteness of the distal
tip of the fingernail where it extends freely beyond the point of
attachment of the nail bed. Pityriasis-type scale is made up of
extremely fine flakes. Generally it is not visible unless it is
stirred up by scraping with the fingernail or scalpel blade. When
this is done, the scale takes on a light-white powdery appearance.
Lichen-type scale is flat and compacted against the underlying
epithelium. This results in a shiny, almost translucent
appearance. The reflective aspect of this flat scale sometimes
gives a glistening sheen which, unless palpated, can be mistaken for
moistness of the surface.
     Second, scale which ought to have been present may be obscured
by actions carried out by the patient. Washing, followed by
vigorous drying, just prior to examination can do this as can the
application of hand cream or other lubricants. Finally, if the
lesions in question have been partially treated the scaling may have
resolved as part of the early resolution of the lesion.
     Thus, before deciding whether or not scale is present one must
ask the patient about the prior presence of scale, inspect the
lesion for flakes or shininess, and palpate the lesions for
roughness or powdery surface.
     If the lesions are determined to be nonscaling, Question 3b
should be answered; if scale is present, Question 3c should be
answered.

QUESTION 3b: ARE THE NONSCALING, RED LESIONS DOME SHAPED OR FLAT-
     TOPPED?

Separation of the two groups of nonscaling red lesions can
sometimes be difficult. While it is true the erythematous papules
and nodules (Group 7) are usually dome shaped and the vascular
reactions (Group 8) are usually flattopped, secondary
characteristics may have to be considered. Some of these rules of
thumb include the following. First, solitary lesions are nearly
always assigned to the erythematous papules and nodules. Second,
nonblanchable (purpuric) lesions are always assigned to the vascular

reactions. Third, coalescence of lesions favors assignment to the
vascular reactions. One apparent exception to this last rule is the
frequency with which the papules of granuloma annulare (a Group 7
disease) take on a confluent, annular configuration. However, in
this situation the confluence is generally not complete; the
confluent papules often retain sufficient individual identity to be
identified as such.
    The diseases of Groups 7 and 8 are listed in Table 6-1; the
erythematous papules and nodules are discussed in Chapter 13 and the
vascular reactions are discussed in Chapter 14.

QUESTION 3c: IS EPITHELIAL DISRUPTION PRESENT OR ABSENT?

    In my experience clinicians have more problems separating the
papulosquamous diseases (no epithelial disruption) from the
eczematous diseases (epithelial disruption present) than they do
with any other part of the algorithm. Most of the problem seems to
revolve about the difficulty in recognizing the more subtle signs of
epithelial disruption (Table 6-3). The linear or angular erosions
of excoriation are readily recognized as representing epithelial
disruption but the presence of weeping or the occurrence of crusts
is often overlooked. Even more often missed are the fine red lines
which represent minute fissures and the presence of a yellow hue in
accumulated scale. The former occurs in xerotic eczema and some
forms of irritant contact dermatitis when drying of the epithelium
leads to shrinkage and separation of islands of epithelial cells.
The latter occurs in many types of subacute eczematous disease when
weeping through microscopically disrupted epithelium is just
sufficient to color the scale but is not enough to leave a moist
surface or form crusts.
    Two other rules of thumb help in differentiating papulosquamous
from eczematous diseases. First, papulosquamous diseases are
sharply marginated around the entire circumference of each lesion
whereas eczematous diseases are either poorly marginated entirely or
have a sharp margination around only a portion of each lesion.
Second, lichenification (see Chapter 3 for definition), if present,
is a pathognomonic feature of eczematous lesions.
    The final area of confusion in separating the papulosquamous
from the eczematous diseases revolves around uncertainty of
assignment when what appears to be a papulosquamous disease has
become secondarily eczematized. This problem is covered in greater
detail under secondarily eczematized lesions in Chapter 16, but in a
situation such a this, it is best to assign the condition to the
eczematous diseases, treat the itch-scratch cycle, and then reassign
the disease on a subsequent visit when the eczematous features have
cleared.
    The papulosquamous diseases are assigned to Group 9. They are
listed in Table 6-1 and are discussed in Chapter 15. The eczematous

TABLE 6-3
SIGNS OF EPITHELIAL DISRUPTION IN ECZEMATOUS DISEASES

---

1. Erosions (especially excoriations)
2. Wetness of the surface (weeping)
3. Crust formation
4. Thin red fissures
5. Yellow scale

---

diseases are assigned to group 10. They are listed in Table 6-1 and are discussed in Chapter 16.

CONCLUSIONS

Answers to the questions discussed above will, in the vast majority of instances, allow for the placement of an unknown disease into one of the ten major disease groups (Table 6-1). Each of the next ten chapters discusses one of the major groups together with the diseases which belong within it. Moreover, the discussion of each disease is preceded by a list of three or four diagnostic hallmarks which, when taken in aggregate, define the disease. These diagnostic hallmarks can be easily scanned such that, when faced with an unrecognized dermatologic problem within one of the ten groups, a few diseases can be quickly identified as being among the most likely diagnoses. One's list of differential diagnoses is built in this fashion; a single, specific diagnosis usually becomes apparent after reading the full description of the several suspected diseases.

Years of using this system have convinced me that a problem oriented approach is readily learned and is remarkably accurate. Failure to arrive at the correct diagnosis means either that the patient's disease is too uncommon or unimportant to be included on the preselected list of 75 diseases or that a wrong turn was made when the questions of the algorithm were answered. This latter error is best rectified by going back over the questions searching for a branching point where, because of confusing clinical data, a somewhat arbitrary choice of branches had been made. With this review the alternate branch can be taken and a new group of diagnoses will be made available for consideration.

Finally, it must be recognized that algorithms of all types are simply guidelines. It is the arbitrariness of algorithms that allows for the desired simplification of complex and confusing problems. For this reason they are extremely valuable for neophytes. As one gathers experience and confidence they become less useful. In fact, slavish adherence to such algorithms can lead to a "cookbook" approach which is at best inaccurate and at worst anti-intellectual. One can only hope that clinicians using this book will think of the diagnostic algorithm as analogous to training wheels on one's first bicycle. They are to be discarded just as soon as sufficient confidence and expertise are achieved lest they otherwise interfere with the development of further skills.

SELECTED READING

Burton JL: The logic of dermatological diagnosis. Clin Exp Dermatol 6:1, 1981.

Branch WT Jr, Collins M, Wintroub BU: Dermatologic practice: Implications for a primary care residency curriculum. J Med Educ 58:138, 1983.

Margolis CZ: Uses of clinical algorithms. JAMA 249:627, 1983.

Barrows HS: Problem-based, self-directed learning. JAMA 250:3077, 1983.

Johnson ML, Johnson KG, Engel A: Prevalence, morbidity, and cost of dermatologic diseases. J Am Acad Dermatol 11:930, 1984.

Lynch PJ, Edminster SC: Dermatology for the nondermatologist: A problem oriented approach. Ann Emerg Med 13:603, 1984.

Wolf FM, Gryppen LD, Billi JE: Differential diagnosis and the competing hypothesis heuristic. JAMA 253:2858, 1985.

Chapter 7

Group 1: The Vesiculobullous Diseases

GROUP IDENTIFICATION

Recognition of the vesiculobullous diseases is usually not difficult. Specifically, those cutaneous lesions which on examination contain any number of intact, clear, fluid filled blisters should be assigned to this group. Problems can arise if, in a blistering process, all the roofs have been broken. In this situation the presence of perfectly round erosions with a thin collarette of scale (representing the peripheral remnants of the roof) should provide a clue to the vesiculobullous nature of the process.

Pustular lesions should, of course, be assigned to the pustular group but sometimes it is difficult to differentiate an aging vesicle containing cloudy fluid from a true pustule. Generally, however, true pustules are pure white or yellow-white rather than gray or cloudy. Moreover, pustules will have been white right from the time of their inception. Hemorrhagic blisters can be encountered in both the vesiculobullous group and the vascular reaction group. The presence of nearby nonvesicular petechiae favors assignment to the vascular reaction group.

HERPES SIMPLEX

DIAGNOSTIC HALLMARKS

1. Distribution: perioral, genital, and perigenital skin
2. Tight clustering of small vesicles
3. Recurrent episodes in the same location

CLINICAL PRESENTATION

Cutaneous infection with <u>Herpesvirus</u> <u>hominis</u> results in the appearance of small vesicles of uniform size and shape. Two clinical patterns are commonly seen: herpes labialis and herpes genitalis.

Herpes labialis consists of a clustered group of three to eight very small vesicles at the vermillion border of the lips. Occasionally the grouped vesicles are found in other locations on the face. The individual vesicles are 1 to 3 mm in diameter and are so closely set that sometimes the appearance is that of a single, irreguarly shaped multiloculated bulla. The vesicles usually appear to arise from normal skin but occasionally a narrow ring of erythema surrounds the base. The vesicles of herpes simplex are quite fragile and patients often present with one or more erosions rather than with intact vesicles. The erosion is usually 1.0 to 1.5 cm in diameter. The configuration of the erosion is distinctive since it reflects the multiple vesicles which led to its formation and is thus irregular rather than round in outline. The eroded surface may be covered by a loosely adherent yellow crust. Clinical separation of such a crusted lesion from that of impetigo may be difficult and depends on the history of a preceding multivesicular stage.

The lesions of herpes labialis are relatively asymptomatic but patients often describe a pre-eruptive sensation of mild burning or tingling which precedes the appearance of the vesicles by several hours. Regional lymphadenopathy, which is usually somewhat tender, is sometimes present.

The lesions of herpes genitalis are entirely analogous to those of herpes labialis. Multiple small vesicles suddenly appear on genital or perigenital skin. They differ from herpes labialis in that more vesicles may be present and the tightness of clustering may be less. This is particularly true in women in whom, especially in initial attacks, 20 or more vesicles may be scattered in a random, bilateral distribution over the entire vulva. These severely painful initial episodes may be accompanied by lymphadenopathy, malaise, meningismus, urethritis, cystitis, and cervicitis. Recurrent lesions in both men and women are less troublesome but still remain more painful than the recurrent lesions of herpes labialis.

Because of trauma from movement and the rubbing of clothing, intact vesicles are not often seen. Here too, the irregular shape of the resultant erosion is a clue to the fact that the lesion was originally composed of clustered, confluent vesicles.

The diagnosis of herpes simplex is usually made on a clinical basis. A suspected diagnosis can be confirmed, if desired, by means of a Tzanck smear, viral culture, or biopsy (see Chapter 5).

Uncommon Clinical Presentations. In some children, initial exposure to herpesvirus results in widespread oral and genital lesions with fever and malaise. This syndrome of primary herpes infection is fortunately rather rare.

Herpes simplex infection occurring in patients with atopic disease or Darier's disease sometimes develops into a disseminated cutaneous infection known as eczema herpeticum or Kaposi's varicelliform eruption.

Older patients with depressed immune response and patients treated with cancer chemotherapeutic drugs may have difficulty clearing their herpes simplex lesions. In such instances seemingly trivial infections develop into chronic, burrowing ulcers.

Finally, recurrent, clustered herpes simplex infection sometimes occurs on other than perioral or genital skin. These infections appear as bright red inflammatory plaques 3 to 6 cm in diameter. Vesiculation is often rather inapparent; the lesions appear eczematous or urticarial instead. Such lesions are particularly common on the sacrum and buttocks. Rarely, recurrent herpes simplex occurs entirely as an intraoral process with no lip involvement. These lesions must be differentiated from recurrent aphthous ulcers (see Chapter 20).

COURSE AND PROGNOSIS

Individual episodes of recurrent herpes labialis last 5 to 10 days. During the first few days viral particles are present and contagion is possible. By the third or fourth day the vesicles have usually broken and crusting develops. Healing occurs without scarring. Repeated episodes, occurring as a result of viral reactivation rather than reinfection, follow sunburn, coryza, fever, and psychologic stress. These recurrent episodes tend to involve the same skin location each time and may continue intermittently for many years.

Individual episodes of herpes genitalis last 7 to 18 days; this longer duration occurs as a result of the extra heat, maceration, and trauma which are present in the groin. Viral particles are present during the first 5 to 7 days and contagion is likely during this time. Healing eventually occurs without scarring. Approximately 50% of the patients will have one or more recurrences. Generally these develop at the same site as the original lesion. Recurrent episodes are related to trauma during intercourse, vaginitis, menses, and psychologic stress. These recurrences are less severe than the original infection and, by the end of 3 years, approximately half of the affected individuals will cease having recurrent episodes.

For purposes of counseling one generally assumes that there is no risk of contagion during the asymptomatic intervals between attacks. Actually, some asymptomatic viral shedding, especially in women, does occur, but it is not known to what degree these patients are contagious. Proof of a patient's status as a "shedder" or "nonshedder" would require multiple viral cultures done during asymptomatic intervals.

PATHOGENESIS

Herpes simplex infections are due to the enveloped DNA virus Herpesvirus hominis types I and II. These two organisms are identical in appearance under electron microscopy but differ somewhat biochemically and antigenically. Both are transferred as a result of close human-to-human contact. Type I infections tend to occur in childhood and are extremely common. Antibody studies suggest that, by the time of adult life, a very large proportion of the population has been infected. Type II infections tend to occur in early adult life. They are considerably less common, affecting 10 to 20% of sexually active adults. Antibody studies suggest that the likelihood of infection is directly related to the number of sexual partners. Approximately 80% of the cases of herpes labialis will be due to type I infection and about 20% to type II infection. These proportions are reversed for herpes genitalis. It is extremely important to realize that the initial infection with either type of virus may be entirely asymptomatic and that the pool of those infected is considerably larger than the number of people who experience visible lesions.

Following initial infection (which may be either symptomatic or asymptomatic) the virus resides in a latent, nonreplicating phase in one or more of the dorsal root ganglia. Reactivation of the infection results in the movement of viral particles along the sensory nerves such that within a matter of hours they arrive at the terminal branches within the skin. At that point viral particles infect the nuclei of epithelial cells where they reproduce and infect adjoining cells. After several days of replication the cell mediated immune response of the host halts the process and slow resolution of the disease ensues. Humoral immune response does not seem to control cutaneous infection since recurrent episodes can take place in the face of high antibody titers. Antibody response, however, does seem to play a role in restricting the viral infection to the skin. Those without antibody response are at considerable risk of developing herpes encephalitis or other systemic infection.

Immune responsiveness to type I infection confers only a modest degree of protection against subsequent type II infection.

From an epidemiologic standpoint it should be recognized that there are several mechanisms through which a person might develop his or her first clinically recognizable infections. Such infection might occur as a result of 1) exposure to a clinically infected person 3 to 5 days earlier, 2) exposure to an asymptomatic viral shedder 3 to 5 days earlier, or 3) reactivation of a latent infection which had originally occurred asymptomatically months or even years earlier. As a result of these latter two mechanisms, contact tracing in individuals with herpes genitalis often is unproductive.

THERAPY

The development of the antiviral antibiotic acyclovir several years ago has greatly improved the therapeutic possibilities for patients with herpes simplex infections. Initial attacks of herpes genitalis (and herpes labialis if they are sufficiently symptomatic) can be treated with the oral administration of acyclovir in a dosage of 200 mg taken five times per day. This treatment rapidly reduces the severity of symptoms and reduces the number of days of viral replication appreciably. Similar improvement occurs when recurrent episodes are treated, especially if therapy can be initiated during the prodromal stage.

Patients who experience multiple episodes of recurrent herpes genitalis can also be treated prophylactically. In this situation 200 mg of acyclovir is taken three times a day. Such treatment reduces the recurrence rate essentially to zero and probably (though not certainly) stops asymptomatic shedding. However, uncertainty about the safety of long term administration and concerns about the possible development of viral resistance have led to the recommendation that such prophylactic therapy be interrupted at the end of 6 months of continuous administration. There is unfortunately no long term effect on the recurrence rate once the medication has been stopped and for this reason new episodes generally ensue a short time after discontinuation. Most of these patients are then started on one or more additional 6-month periods of acyclovir usage.

For some patients acyclovir therapy may not be desirable or practical. Patients with mild initial episodes, patients with infrequent recurrences, and patients in monogamous relationships may find that concerns about safety, viral resistance, and high cost outweigh potential benefits. For these patients local, symptomatic treatment with soaks followed by a thin layer of a bland cream or ointment may be all that is necessary.

The recurrence rate for herpes labialis is most effectively reduced through the frequent application of sunscreen to the lips and by the avoidance of local mechanical trauma. It is harder to reduce the recurrence rate of herpes genitalis. Reduction in genital trauma through the use of condoms in the male and treatment of even trivial vaginitis in the female is helpful as is the use of added lubrication during intercourse. However, perhaps of greatest effectiveness is the reduction in stress that seems to account for such a large percentage of recurrent episodes.

An important component of therapy for patients with genital herpes is the provision of advice to reduce the likelihood of transfer to a sexual partner. Certainly intercourse ought to be avoided during symptomatic episodes. It is probably safe for infected men to have intercourse when no lesions are present since asymptomatic shedding in men seems to occur very infrequently. This is probably not true for women because intermittent shedding from the cervix seems to occur in a larger percentage of affected individuals. Women, therefore, should use a diaphragm and should encourage their consorts to use a condom. The degree of protection offered by these mechanical barriers is not known with certainty, but empirical observations suggest that it is quite good.

SELECTED READING

Conant MA, Spicer DW, Smith CD: Herpes simplex virus transmission: Condom studies. Sex Transm Dis 11:94, 1984.

Straus SE, Rooney JF, Sever JL, et al: Herpes simplex virus infection: Biology, treatment, and prevention. Ann Int Med 103:404, 1985.

Marlowe SI: Medical management of genital herpes. Arch Dermatol 121:467, 1985.

Corey L, Spear PG: Infections with herpes simplex viruses (second of two parts). N Engl J Med 314:749, 1986.

Guinan ME: Oral acyclovir for treatment of suppression of genital herpes simplex virus infection. J Am Acad Dermatol 255:1747, 1986.

VARICELLA-ZOSTER INFECTIONS

DIAGNOSTIC HALLMARKS

Varicella (Chickenpox)
1. Distribution: trunk with centrifugal spread
2. Randomly located, nonclustered vesicles on a red base
3. History of contagion

Herpes Zoster
1. Distribution: unilateral; trunk in children, face and trunk in adults
2. Multiple "plaques" of clustered vesicles along a single dermatome
3. Pain precedes the eruption in adults
4. Occasional hemorrhage into vesicles

CLINICAL PRESENTATION

Initial infection with the varicella-zoster virus results in a widespread vesicular eruption known as varicella or chickenpox. Reactivation (or possibly reinfection) of the same virus results in a more localized infection known as herpes zoster or "shingles."

Varicella. Clinical evidence of infection begins with a prodrome of fever and malaise 10 to 14 days after exposure to the virus. Shortly thereafter vesicles begin to develop on the central portions of the trunk and face. These vesicles are 3 to 5 mm in diameter and they are surrounded by a thin ring of erythema. The vesicles are randomly distributed and clustering does not occur. As individual vesicles resolve, new ones appear in a centrifugal pattern such that vesicles develop on the arms and legs 2 to 3 days after the trunk lesions have first appeared. A few vesicles may be found in the mouth but mucosal involvement is not prominent. Vesicles are also almost always present in the scalp. Pruritus is often severe in children but this is less prominent in adults. As the individual vesicles age, the fluid within them becomes cloudy and the roof begins to sag, causing an umbilicated appearance. By the end of the first week the early vesicles have become crusted; eventually all of the lesions heal with little or no scarring.

Diagnosis is based on the epidemiology and clinical appearance of the disease. Confirmation of a clinical diagnosis may be obtained through Tzanck smears or by viral culture (see Chapter 5).

Herpes Zoster. Viral reactivation (or possibly reinfection) in an individual previously exposed to the varicella-zoster virus results in the development of herpes zoster. In this disease small vesicles, 3 to 5 mm in diameter, occur in clustered patterns. Each cluster consists of 5 to 20 vesicles which are found in a linear distribution along a single dermatome. The eruption occurs unilaterally with little or no crossover at the midline.

Any dermatome can be involved but in children and young adults the thoracic dermatomes are most commonly infected. In older adults the first branch of the trigeminal nerve is frequently involved. Individual vesicles have a narrow ring of erythema around them. Where the clustering of vesicles is tight this erythema becomes confluent and the vesicles appear to arise from an underlying erythematous base.

The fluid within the vesicles is initially clear although a small amount of hemorrhage may be noted in some of the blisters. Vesicular fluid becomes somewhat cloudy as the vesicles age. Because of blister roof fragility the vesicles often rupture, resulting in clusters of irregularly shaped erosions. In adults, pain generally precedes the appearance of the vesicles and may continue after they have resolved as postherpetic neuralgia. In childhood zoster, pain is not usually a significant factor. New crops of vesicles continue to occur along the dermatome for several days but by the end of the first week new vesicles have stopped forming and resolution of the earliest vesicles has begun.

Atypical Clinical Manifestations. Disseminated herpes zoster sometimes occurs in individuals who have depressed cell mediated immune responsiveness. In these patients lesions begin along a dermatome but by the third or fourth day vesicles begin to appear outside of the original dermatome. The scattered lesions occurring outside of the dermatome are identical in appearance with those seen in chickenpox. Disseminated zoster is particularly likely to occur in individuals with advanced Hodgkin's disease; it is associated with a very grave prognosis.

Patients with facial zoster sometimes develop an accompanying eye infection. This seems particularly likely to occur if the tip of the nose (representing nasociliary nerve infection) is involved.

Patients with varicella or disseminated zoster occasionally develop systemic infection most usually in the form of pneumonia or encephalitis. Motor nerve infection with accompanying paralysis is also occasionally seen. Herpes simplex infection can sometimes cause a dermatomal vesicular eruption identical in appearance to that of zoster.

The diagnosis of varicella and herpes zoster can almost always be made on the basis of history and physical examination. Laboratory confirmation, if such is required, can be obtained by way of Tzanck smears and viral cultures (see Chapter 5).

COURSE AND PROGNOSIS

Varicella (chickenpox) infections resolve spontaneously within 7 to 14 days. Contagion is unlikely after the first week. Healing generally takes place without scarring but a few small pits may be left at the site of secondarily infected vesicles. Following resolution of varicella, viral particles remain indefinitely in a latent form within the sensory ganglia. Subsequent reactivation of the virus results in the appearance of herpes zoster. Reinfection from an external source is believed by some to also cause the appearance of zoster but it is undoubtedly an uncommon explanation for such infection.

The lesions of herpes zoster in children resolve spontaneously in 10 to 14 days but may remain active for 14 to 21 days in adults.

Scarring following the resolution of zoster is rarely seen in children but is occasionally found in adults. Neuralgia neither precedes nor follows zoster in children. Pain before, during, and after infection in older adults can, however, be extraordinarily severe.

Most patients will experience only a single episode of zoster but approximately 5% of patients will develop one or more recurrences.

PATHOGENESIS

The varicella-zoster virus, <u>Herpesvirus varicellae</u>, is a DNA virus of the herpesvirus group. Initial exposure to this virus occurs via droplet spread and results in a viremia with subsequent skin and mucous membrane infection. Viral replication takes place in the nuclei of epithelial cells and continues until the process is halted by development of immunologic response. The antibody formation which occurs seems to be important in preventing internal, systemic dissemination of the disease but apparently plays little or no role in the development of the skin lesions. Interferon and other T cell mediated responses, on the other hand, are responsible for controlling the severity and spread of the infection within the skin. When the lesions of varicella heal, viral particles remain in the sensory ganglia where they stay indefinitely in an inactive, latent phase. The virus may be reactivated under a variety of circumstances, at which point skin lesions, in the form of zoster, appear. The trigger which sets off reactivation is not known although depression of cell mediated immune responsiveness and the occurrence of trauma to the ganglia or nerve root may play some role. Nerve destruction is greater in zoster than it is in herpes simplex and this is presumably the reason for the clinical problem of pre- and postherpetic neuralgia.

THERAPY

Marked limitations exist in our ability to treat varicella zoster infections. Zoster immune globulin offers some protection against the development of initial infection but it is probably not useful in the treatment of established infection. Vidarabine and interferon administered systemically are somewhat effective in the treatment of active disease but their use is restricted to those immunosuppressed patients who would otherwise develop very severe infection. Acyclovir is beneficial when given intravenously but is less effective when administered orally, presumably because sufficient serum levels cannot be obtained via this route. Systemically administered steroids given early in the course of herpes zoster decrease the incidence of postherpetic neuralgia but seem to have no other beneficial effect on the active infection. On a day-to-day basis most treatment for varicella and zoster is on a symptomatic basis. The itching of chickenpox can be treated with either topical antipruritic agents or with the administration of antihistamines (see Chapter 4). Soaks and systemically administered analgesics may be necessary to alleviate the discomfort of herpes zoster occurring in older adults. Postherpetic neuralgia is extraordinarily difficult to treat. Intracutaneously injected triamcinolone, oral administration of tricyclic antidepressants, transcutaneous electrical stimulation of nerves, and surgical sectioning of affected nerves are possible approaches for those unrelieved by analgesics.

SELECTED READING

Weller TH: Varicella and herpes zoster. Changing concepts of the
    natural history, control, and importance of a not-so-benign
    virus (first of two parts). N Engl J Med 309:1362, 1983.
Liesegang TJ: The varicella-zoster virus: Systemic and ocular
    features. J Am Acad Dermatol 11:165, 1984.
Gershon AA, Steinberg SP, Gelb L: Clinical reinfection with
    varicella-zoster virus. J Infect Dis 149:137, 1984.
Balfour HH Jr: Acyclovir therapy for the herpes zoster:
    Advantages and adverse effects. J Am Acad Dermatol 255:387,
    1986.

VESICULAR TINEA PEDIS

DIAGNOSTIC HALLMARKS

1. Distribution: plantar aspect of the foot
2. Associated fungal infection of the toenails and fourth web space
3. Positive KOH from vesicle roof

CLINICAL PRESENTATION

Fungal infections can occur anywhere on the body, but blister formation as a component of fungal infection occurs only on the plantar surfaces of the feet. The vesicles of tinea pedis are usually confined to the instep but they are accompanied by red scaling lesions on the remainder of the plantar surface and by lateral web space cracking and fissuring. Onychomycosis is also often present. The vesicles of tinea pedis are 5 to 10 mm in diameter and they are usually clustered tightly, sometimes to the point where they form a large, multilocular bulla. Relatively little inflammatory change is found around the base of the blisters. The fluid contained in the vesicles is usually somewhat cloudy. Severe vesicular fungal infections of the feet are sometimes accompanied by a sterile vesicular or eczematous eruption on the hands. This process of autosensitization (see Chapter 16) is known as the dermatophytid, or "id," reaction.

A clinical diagnosis of vesicular tinea pedis should be supported by objective evidence of fungal infection. This is most easily carried out by way of a KOH preparation (see Chapter 5). A small pointed scissors is used to trim away a vesicle roof. The roof is then placed on a microscope slide and is covered with several drops of 10 to 20% potassium hydroxide solution. The preparation is set aside for approximately 20 to 30 minutes in order for the roof to dissolve sufficiently for fungi to be visualized. Alternately, the roof can be sent for fungal culture but this results in a delay of 2 weeks before confirmation is available.

COURSE AND PROGNOSIS

Tinea pedis rarely occurs in children but it is a rather common problem in teenagers and adults. Men are affected several times more frequently than are women. The infection, once present, is chronic with intermittent periods of exacerbation and remission. Trauma to the feet accompanied by heat and sweating will activate a previously quiescent infection. Individual episodes of vesicular tinea pedis, unless treated, can progress to chronic foot eczema (see Chapter 17).

PATHOGENESIS

Vesicular tinea pedis is almost always caused by the dermatophyte fungal organism, Trichophyton rubrum. A surprisingly large proportion of the human population carries T. rubrum on its feet and this in turn leads to high contamination levels on floors. Most contagion appears to occur because of bare foot contact with such contaminated floors but to a limited degree person-to-person contagion is probably also possible. Simple contact with the fungal organisms is not sufficient to cause infection. Broken skin and a warm moist environment must also be present. With this in mind it is no wonder that the sweaty, traumatized feet of physically active individuals are so often infected. Atopics and other individuals with defective cell mediated immune responsiveness are particularly subject to infection. Once present, the organisms live indefinitely in the thick dead layers of the stratum corneum. For the most part this is a symbiotic relationship with little evidence of host response until the equilibrium is disturbed. At that point fungal proliferation develops and an inflammatory response is triggered.

THERAPY

Topical antifungal agents do not work particularly well in the treatment of vesicular tinea pedis. Griseofulvin or possibly ketoconazole (see Chapter 4) should be given for a period of about 3 weeks. This usually results in resolution of visible disease but total eradication of organisms is generally not possible no matter how long the antifungal agent is taken. Long term topical antifungal therapy should be substituted once the patient is asymptomatic in order to minimize fungal proliferation. Environmental factors also ought to be optimized. The feet should be kept as cool and dry as possible. Leather soled shoes and cotton blend socks are helpful. Tennis type shoes, because of their nonporous rubber soles, should be avoided except for use during a specific athletic event.

DYSHIDROSIS

DIAGNOSTIC HALLMARKS

1. Distribution: tips and sides of the digits; palms and soles
2. Clustering of minute, noninflammatory vesicles
3. History of recurrent episodes

CLINICAL PRESENTATION

Dyshidrosis consists of minute, noninflammtory vesicles located along the lateral sides and tips of the digits. Individual vesicles are rarely more than a single millimeter in size but as the disease increases in severity tight clustering can lead to coalescence and the formation of multiloculated bullae. In children, the toes, and in adults, the fingers, are most often affected. In either instance palmar or plantar skin may become involved as the disease progresses. The dorsal surfaces of the hands and feet are never involved initially, but subsequent eczematous spread to these locations is possible when the disease evolves into a chronic condition (see Chapter 16).

Because of their location and size, the vesicles of dyshidrosis have a morphology quite different from those found in the other vesicular diseases. First, the vesicles are deeply situated and thus early on are not elevated above the surface of the surrounding skin. Second, the thick stratum corneum which constitutes the vesicle roof lends an opaque, rather than translucent, color to the vesicle. Third, the size of individual vesicles is only about 1 mm. Finally, the thick roof and deep location give the vesicles a certain toughness; they do not break open easily.

The range of symptoms in dyshidrosis varies greatly. Some individuals are asymptomatic; others describe pruritus or pain or both. If pruritus leads to scratching, the dyshidrosis (a noninflammatory disease) is converted into its inflammatory counterpart, dyshidrotic eczema (see Chapter 16). Patients with mild dyshidrosis will have only occasional intermittent attacks and

the skin returns to normal between episodes. When attacks occur
frequently the vesicular phase will be accompanied by the constant
presence of xerosis, desquamation, cracking, and fissuring. This
dry, chapped appearance, which is essentially that of irritant
contact dermatitis, is prolonged and worsened by exposure to
solvents such as soap and water.

The diagnosis of dyshidrosis is based on clinical findings.
Biopsy is not ordinarily helpful and there are no confirmatory
laboratory tests.

COURSE AND PROGNOSIS

Dyshidrosis sometimes begins in childhood but most often the
initial appearance is found in early adult life. Thereafter
intermittent episodes can be expected. The interval between
episodes is highly variable. As mentioned above some individuals
are free of disease for months at a time whereas others have almost
continuous involvement. The severity and frequency of episodes
gradually decrease in late adult life and the disease is rarely seen
after age 60.

PATHOGENESIS

The word dyshidrosis is derived from "dys" meaning improper and
"hidrosis" meaning sweating. The word was coined because it was
originally thought that dyshidrosis represented sweat retention
(miliaria) in obstructed sweat ducts. However, even though sweat
ducts are occasionally found entering the vesicles on histologic
examination, it is now believed that vesicle formation is only
coincidentally related to sweating. An attractive hypothesis
suggests that dyshidrosis is simply a variant of atopic dermatitis
which occurs only on the hands and feet but proof for this
supposition is lacking.

Stress and anxiety appear to play an important role in the
precipitation of individual episodes but it is not clear whether
they alone are sufficient to cause the disease. In my experience
the presence of dyshidrosis correlates very well with the
internalization of stress and anger. Furthermore I believe the
disease is particularly likely to be found in individuals with
obsessive-compulsive traits. Such individuals often have difficulty
relaxing even during relatively nonstressful intervals. Perhaps it
is not surprising that I have found, using informal surveys, that
the prevalence of dyshidrosis in medical students is about four
times that of the "normal" population! Hyperhidrosis of the palms
and soles often accompanies the presence of dyshidrosis but this may
be related to the fact that such sweating is ordinarily under
psychologic, rather than thermal, control.

THERAPY

Dyshidrosis is a difficult condition to treat. Topical steroids, possibly because of poor penetration, are of limited usefulness. Enhanced effectiveness can be demonstrated if patients wear plastic or Latex gloves over the topically applied steroids (see occlusive therapy, Chapter 4). Unfortunately, sweating and irritation under these gloves often negate the beneficial effect of better steroid absorption. Patients with moderate to severe involvement are probably best treated with a "burst" of systemic steroids (see Chapter 4). This approach is momentarily very effective, but, as might be expected, it does not delay the recurrence or reduce the severity of subsequent episodes.

In my experience, treatment of patients with frequent, severe episodes requires attention to related psychologic factors. In some instances a simple explanation of the relationship between stress and the disease is sufficient. For others tranquilizers, professional counseling, or behavior modification techniques may be necessary.

The chapping, cracking, and fissuring which often accompany and sometimes persist after the vesicular phase will require the liberal application of lubricants six to eight times per day. These can be applied directly over topical steroids when both components require concomitant treatment. When the feet are involved additional modification of the environment is required. Leather soled shoes should be substituted for rubber soled "tennis" type shoes and cotton blend socks should replace those made totally of synthetic fibers. Moreover, shoes and socks should be removed as frequently as possible to allow for sweat evaporation and the application of lubricants.

SELECTED READING
(See references under dyshidrotic eczema in Chapter 16.)

DERMATITIS HERPETIFORMIS

DIAGNOSTIC HALLMARKS

1. Distribution: elbows, knees, sacrum, and scapular areas
2. Herpetic-like clustering of vesicles
3. Immunofluorescent studies: granular deposits of IgA in the papillary dermis
4. Rapid response to dapsone therapy

CLINICAL PRESENTATION

As its name implies, dermatitis herpetiformis, a very uncommon condition, is characterized by the presence of clustered, small

vesicles. The individual vesicles are usually 2 to 6 mm in
diameter, but occasionally larger blisters are present. The
clusters, each containing 5 to 20 vesicles, are most often found on
the buttocks, sacrum, scapulae, and extensor surfaces of the arms
and legs. They occur bilaterally and exhibit considerable
symmetry. There is usually a brisk inflammatory response around the
vesicles such that they appear to be arising from an erythematous
plaque. Pruritus is generally intense and it is accompanied by
vigorous scratching. For this reason, most patients have few intact
vesicles and present instead with multiple, clustered, excoriated
papules. When excoriations are more prominent than vesicles the
disease takes on an eczematous appearance (see Chapter 16). New
lesions appear in crops even while old lesions are healing.
Excoriated lesions generally heal with a hypopigmented center and a
surrounding collar of hyperpigmentation.
    Asymptomatic small bowel disease regularly occurs in association
with dermatitis herpetiformis. Bowel biopsy reveals changes similar
to, but milder than, those found in gluten enteropathy. Autoimmune
disease of several types, including glomerulonephritis and thyroid
disease, have also been noted in patients with dermatitis
herpetiformis.
    A suspected clinical diagnosis must be confirmed by biopsy. The
presence of a subepidermal vesicle with plentiful perivesicular
neutrophils on routine histology is suggestive; the finding of
granular IgA deposits in the papillary dermis of perilesional skin
on direct immunofluorescent examination is pathognomonic.

COURSE AND PROGNOSIS

    Dermatitis herpetiformis occurs most commonly in young and
middle aged adults. It is a chronic disease which lasts
indefinitely. The pruritus is extremely debilitating if the disease
is left untreated but otherwise there is little morbidity. The
gluten enteropathy remains asymptomatic in most patients. A very
few patients have developed intestinal lymphomas late in the course
of the disease.

PATHOGENESIS

    Genetic factors are presumably important since approximately 80%
of patients have the HLA markers of B8 and DW3. Familial cases are,
however, uncommon, suggesting that one or more precipitating factors
are also necessary. The regular presence of IgA and the frequent
presence of complement components in the papillary dermis suggest
that immune factors play a role but the antigen responsible for this
deposition has not been positively identified. It is likely that
the antigen is related to gluten perhaps with cross reactivity
between gluten and small connective tissue microfibrils. At the

clinical level gluten sensitivity certainly seems to play some
important role since in most cases a gluten free diet leads to
improvement in both the skin and small bowel. Immune complexes and
various other antibodies are often found in the circulation of
patients with dermatitis herpetiformis but their meaning is
presently unknown.

THERAPY

Nearly all patients with dermatitis herpetiformis respond
immediately and completely to treatment with sulfapyridine or
dapsone. The former is used in a dosage of 2.0 grams per day and
the latter, which is generally the medication of first choice, is
used in a dosage of 100 to 200 mg per day. With either drug the
dosage is tapered to maintenance levels once response has occurred.
Remissions once obtained can usually be continued indefinitely as
resistance to medication does not seem to occur. Strict adherence
to a gluten free diet will in many cases allow the dose of dapsone
to be lowered and in some cases it can be discontinued altogether.
Unfortunately, patient compliance with such diets is usually rather
poor.

SELECTED READING
Leonard J, Haffenden G, Tucker W, et al: Gluten challenge in
    dermatitis herpetiformis. N Engl J Med 308:816, 1983.
Ljunghall K, Scheynius A, Jonsson J, et al: Gluten-free diet in
    patients with dermatitis herpetiformis. Arch Dermatol 119:970,
    1983.
Buckley DB, English J, Molloy W, Doyle CT, Whelton MH: Dermatitis
    herpetiformis: A review of 119 cases. Clin Exp Dermatol 8:477,
    1983.
Huff JC: The immunopathogenesis of dermatitis herpetiformis. J
    Invest Dermatol 84:237, 1985.
Cunningham MJ, Zone JJ: Thyroid abnormalities in dermatitis
    herpetiformis. Prevalence of clinical thyroid disease and
    thyroid autoantibodies. Ann Intern Med 102:194, 1985.

MISCELLANEOUS VESICULAR DISEASES

Scabies is inherently a vesicular disease. However, the degree
of pruritus is extremely severe and most patients scratch to the
point where nearly all of the burrows have been obliterated. This
vigorous scratching thus results in an eczematous appearance. For
this reason scabies is covered primarily in the section of
eczematous disease (Chapter 16).

Hand, foot, and mouth disease is an infection in infants and
children due to certain serotypes of Coxsackie A and B virus. It is
characterized by the presence of a dozen or so small vesicles on the

fingers, toes, palms, soles, and mucous membranes of the mouth. These vesicles are distinctive in their somewhat elongated, grayish appearance. Spontaneous resolution occurs in several days without sequellae.

Transient acantholytic dermatosis (Grover's disease) is a disease of unknown etiology characterized by the presence of small erythematous vesicopapules. These lesions are found scattered in a random fashion over the chest and back of middle aged and older adults. Biopsy reveals a characteristic acantholytic pattern.

In pityriasis lichenoides of the acute type (Mucha-Habermann disease) some of the small erythematous papules may be capped with a small vesicle. These papules are randomly spread over the trunk and extremities. Hypopigmentation and small pitted scars are sometimes found at the site of healed lesions.

Insect bites, particularly those due to fleas, sometimes have a vesicle located at the summit of the inflammatory papule. The distribution (usually on the legs) and epidemiology generally suggest the correct diagnosis.

Small hemorrhagic vesicles are often seen in patients with neutrophilic vasculitis of the small vessel type (see Chapter 14). The lesions of gonoccocemia are sometimes more vesicular than pustular (see Chapter 8). The papules of molluscum contagiosum are never vesicular, but their glistening, translucent appearance sometimes fools the unwary and accounts for the lay term "water warts."

SELECTED READING

Hu CH, Michel B, Farber EM: Transient acantholytic dermatosis (Grover's disease). Arch Dermatol 121:1439, 1985.

PEMPHIGUS VULGARIS

DIAGNOSTIC HALLMARKS

1. Distribution: oral mucous membranes and upper trunk
2. Multiple shallow erosions which heal very slowly
3. Biopsy: acantholytic intraepidermal bulla
4. Immunofluorescent studies: IgG deposited in the intracellular space around epidermal cells

CLINICAL PRESENTATION

The bullae of pemphigus vulgaris arise from normal appearing skin; there is essentially no surrounding inflammation. The blisters are also extraordinarily fragile. For that reason intact bullae are found only during the first day or two of their existence. Thereafter the blister roof is broken leaving a bright red or crusted shallow erosion which requires weeks or months to heal. The initial lesions are usually found on the upper trunk and back; but, since new lesions develop faster than old ones heal, there is gradual extension elsewhere with special predilection for the face, groin, and axillae. The prominence of these crusted erosions often suggests eczematous disease and obscures the fact that the patient has, in fact, a bullous condition.

Oral mucous membrane lesions are practically always present and they frequently precede appearance of the cutaneous lesions by weeks to months. These oral lesions begin as blisters, but they, too, quickly break down to form shallow erosions. The oral erosions of pemphigus are particularly likely to occur in the posterior mouth. The accompanying discomfort interferes with eating and the resultant malnutrition contributes to the extreme debilitation which develops in untreated patients.

A suspected clinical diagnosis must be confirmed by biopsy. Light microscopy reveals a characteristic suprabasilar intraepidermal vesicle with loss of epidermal cell cohesion (acantholysis). Direct immunofluorescent studies carried out on perilesional skin demonstrate a pathognomonic pattern of IgG deposition in a network-like pattern surrounding the epidermal cells. Complement components are sometimes present. More than 90% of patients will also have specific circulating autoantibodies. These antibodies can be demonstrated on indirect immunofluorescent study (see Chapter 5) in which case they are noted to fix to antigens which lie on the cytoplasmic membrane of epithelial cells. The titer of these antibodies corresponds partially to the severity of the disease. Thus reduction in the antibody titer can be used as an adjunct to monitor the response of the disease to therapy.

Atypical Presentations. Pemphigus foliaceus is an uncommon form of pemphigus in which the intraepidermal clefting occurs high in the epidermis rather than just above the basal layer. Patients with pemphigus foliaceus develop erosions which are more superficial than those found in pemphigus vulgaris. Oral involvement is less often present and patients do not become as debilitated. Some patients with pemphigus foliaceus have a considerable degree of facial erythema and may, in addition, have a variety of lupus-like autoantibodies. The combination of these findings is known as the Senear-Usher syndrome. A form of pemphigus found in Brazil (fogo selvagem) has epidemiologic features which suggest an infectious etiology.

COURSE AND PROGNOSIS

Pemphigus begins most commonly in mid to late adult life. It is a chronic, severely debilitating disease which, left untreated, inevitably leads to death. With vigorous, early treatment the mortality rate is approximately 10%. Other autoimmune diseases are found with unexpected frequency in patients with pemphigus and a rather small, but probably significant, number of patients have thymomas and a variety of other internal malignancies.

PATHOGENESIS

Pemphigus is considered to be an autoimmune disease. Specific IgG antibodies and sometimes complement component are deposited at the precise site of epidermal cell damage; these same antibodies are regularly found in the circulation. Moreover, the antibodies, when isolated and injected into a suitable substrate, cause an epidermal lesion identical with that found in the original disease. The acantholysis caused by these antibodies appears to develop as a result of the release of proteolytic enzymes. This process does not appear to require, though it may be optimized by, the activation of complement. The antigen(s) responsible for this autoimmune reaction have not been completely identified but they appear to be located on the exterior surface of the cytoplasmic membrane of certain epithelial cells. Further evidence of an autoimmune etiology includes the frequent association of pemphigus with other autoimmune diseases and the occasional presence of a thymoma. Genetic factors as reflected by the presence of certain HLA antigens and a high incidence in certain Jewish populations are probably also important. Perhaps most interesting of all is the observation that some medications, most notably penicillamine, can induce in certain individuals a disease indistinguishable from idiopathic pemphigus.

THERAPY

The landmark studies of Lever 30 years ago proved that pemphigus need not inevitably lead to death. He showed that very high doses of orally administered steroids (120 to 240 mg of prednisone per day) would almost always bring the disease under control. Unfortunately, the long term, high dose administration of steroids which is required causes its own morbidity and mortality. In fact, the mortality associated with pemphigus today is mostly due to drug toxicity rather than to the disease itself. There are several ways in which this potential toxicity can be minimized. In some patients it is possible to administer their steroids on an alternate day schedule and for others the steroid dose can be greatly reduced through the addition of steroid sparing immunosuppressive agents such as methotrexate, azathioprine, or cyclophosphamide. Finally, for patients with relatively mild disease it is sometimes possible to obtain remission through long term administration of gold salts. This latter approach is particularly attractive because drug induced immunosuppression does not seem to occur.

SELECTED READING

Ahmed AR: Pemphigus vulgaris: Clinical features. Dermatol Clinics
    1:171, 1983.
Avalos E, Patel H, Anhalt GJ, Diaz LA: Autoimmune injury of
    squamous epithelium by pemphigus autoantibodies. Br J Dermatol
    111:359, 1984.
Lever WF, Schaumburg-Lever G: Treatment of pemphigus vulgaris.
    Results obtained in 84 patients between 1961 and 1982. Arch
    Dermatol 120:44, 1984.
Bystryn J-C: Adjuvant therapy of pemphigus. Arch Dermatol 120:941,
    1984.
Singer KH, Hashimoto K, Jensen PJ, et al: Pathogenesis of
    autoimmunity in pemphigus. Ann Rev Immunol 3:87, 1985.

PEMPHIGOID

DIAGNOSTIC HALLMARKS

1. Distribution: often starts on the extremities but usually
    becomes generalized
2. Tense, tough blisters usually arising from normal skin
3. Individual lesions heal spontaneously while new blisters
    continue to appear
4. Immunofluorescent studies: IgG and C3 in a linear pattern
    at the dermal-epidermal junction

CLINICAL PRESENTATION

Patients with pemphigoid characteristically develop the disease
after the age of 60. Crops of large bullae, 2 to 5 cm in diameter,
appear first on the extremities but within a short period of time
begin to develop on the trunk as well. Occasionally blisters are
also seen on the scalp, palms, soles, and oral mucous membranes.

In most instances the bullae arise from normal appearing skin
but a few may develop on an erythematous background. When lesions
of this latter type predominate, distinction from bullous erythema
multiforme or even dermatitis herpetiformis may be difficult. The
blisters, unlike those of pemphigus, are histologically located in a
subepidermal location. For this reason the roofs are not easily
broken and the bullae often stay intact for many days. Thus, as a
general rule, intact blisters outnumber erosions whereas the reverse
is true in pemphigus.

The bullae are usually filled with clear fluid but occasionally
some are tinged with blood. Old lesions heal as rapidly as new
lesions appear. For this reason accompanying debilitation is not as
prominent as it is in patients with pemphigus. Some patients are
completely asymptomatic but itching often is present and
occasionally it is very severe.

A clinical diagnosis must be confirmed by biopsy. Light microscopy reveals a subepidermal blister with a perilesional inflammatory infiltrate containing a large number of eosinophils. At the electron microscopic level the split appears to occur within the lamina lucida portion of the basement membrane zone. Biopsies of perilesional skin for direct immunofluorescence reveal a band of immunoglobulin and complement at the dermal-epidermal junction. The immunoglobulin deposited is usually IgG, but in a small percentage of cases, other immunoglobulins are found instead. C3 is the most common of the complement components found. Approximately 70% of patients will also have circulating autoantibodies directed at the basement membrane zone. These can be demonstrated with indirect immunofluorescent studies (see Chapter 5).

Pemphigoid Variants. IgA pemphigoid (linear IgA bullous disease of adults) presents with blisters which are smaller in size than those of classical pemphigoid. Some authorities prefer to consider this disease a variant of dermatitis herpetiformis but other than its responsiveness to dapsone therapy the two diseases have little in common. Cicatricial pemphigoid is a rare disease in which erosive disease of mucosal surfaces (particularly the eyes and the mouth) is followed by scarring. Cutaneous bullae are not prominent but when they occur they too may heal with scarring.

Localized pemphigoid is similar to conventional pemphigoid except that the lesions remain restricted to a single segment of the body. This variant most commonly occurs on the lower legs of older women.

COURSE AND PROGNOSIS

Pemphigoid is a chronic disease which persists indefinitely. New lesions develop as rapidly as old lesions heal such that 10 to 20% of the skin surface is continually involved. Debilitation due to the disease itself is not great but it is additive to that due to advanced age and other intercurrent disease. Death due to superimposed infection or to toxicity associated with steroid therapy occurs in 5 to 10% of patients.

PATHOGENESIS

Pemphigoid is an autoimmune disease directed toward a protein antigen which is located within the basement membrane zone at the dermal-epidermal junction. Immunoglobulin and complement components are almost always found at this location and 70% of patients also have circulating antibodies which fix to the dermal-epidermal junction of certain epithelial tissues. Complement activation appears to be necessary in order for blisters to be formed. Model systems for the experimental creation of blisters have recently been described.

Genetic factors seem to be less important than for the other immunobullous diseases. There are no racial or national groups which seem particularly predisposed to the disease and HLA typing has failed to reveal patterns which consistently differ from those of the normal population.

A small number of patients with pemphigoid appear to have an associated systemic malignancy. However, these patients are of advanced age and when matched against similarly aged control groups the incidence of tumors does not seem to be statistically increased.

THERAPY

Systemically administered corticosteroids are usually the treatment of choice for patients with pemphigoid. Initially prednisone is administered in a single morning dose of 60 to 80 mg. Thereafter, depending on the rapidity of response, the dosage is gradually tapered to a maintenance level of approximately 20 to 40 mg per day. At this point an attempt should be made to switch to alternate day therapy. If this cannot be accomplished, a steroid sparing immunosuppressive agent such as azothioprine or cyclophosphamide is usually added. Some patients do show a response to dapsone therapy but the degree of improvement (except in the IgA variant) is usually not great. Occasionally dapsone can be used with steroids in an attempt to reduce the dose of the latter. There are a few patients who have only occasional lesions. In such individuals it is sometimes appropriate to use no internal therapy at all and thus avoid the considerable risk of side effects which accompanies the treatment program outlined above.

SELECTED READING

Sams WM Jr, Gammon WR: Mechanism of lesion production in pemphigus and pemphigoid. J Am Acad Dermatol 6:431, 1982.
Stanley JR: Bullous pemphigoid. Dermatol Clinics 1:205, 1983.
Anhalt GJ, Patel H, Diaz LA: Mechanisms of immunologic injury: Pemphigus and bullous pemphigoid. Arch Dermatol 119:711, 1983.
Naito K, Morioka S, Ikeda S, Ogawa H: Experimental bullous pemphigoid in guinea pigs: The role of pemphigoid antibodies, complement, and migrating cells. J Invest Dermatol 82:227, 1984.
Liu H-NH, Su WPD, Rogers RS III: Clinical variants of pemphigoid. Int J Dermatol 25:17, 1986.
Ahmed AR, Hombal SM: Cicatricial pemphigoid. Int J Dermatol 25:90, 1986.

ERYTHEMA MULTIFORME BULLOSUM

DIAGNOSTIC HALLMARKS

1. Distribution: trunk, palms, soles, mouth

2. Tense blisters arising from the center of an erythematous
    base
3. Presence of some target-type lesions

CLINICAL PRESENTATION

Most patients with erythema multiforme do not develop bullous
lesions (see Chapter 14). When blisters do occur they are present
from the onset of the illness and are a marker for a rather severe
course. Bullae can occur anywhere on the body but are particularly
likely to be found on the hands and feet. Unlike those that occur
in pemphigus and pemphigoid, the bullae of erythema multiforme
always arise on an erythematous base. Generally the blisters form
from the center ("bull's-eye") of a ringed or target-type lesion,
but occasionally the bullae arise more eccentrically from a
nonringed, erythematous plaque. Individual lesions range in size
from 1.5 to 3 cm in diameter.   The amount of itching present is
highly variable, ranging from none at all to an intensity which
interferes with sleep.

Mucosal surfaces of the mouth, eyes, and genitalia are usually
involved with widespread, painful erosions. These mucosal lesions
may result in photophobia, urinary retention, and decreased intake
of food and water.

The diagnosis of bullous erythema multiforme is made on a
clinical basis. Biopsy may be helpful but it is rarely
pathognomonic. There are no characteristic immunofluorescent
findings.

Erythema Multiforme Bullosum Variants. Patients with erythema
multiforme who develop bullous cutaneous lesions and erosive mucosal
lesions in association with fever, malaise, and toxicity are said to
have the Stevens-Johnson syndrome. An even more severe variant, in
which the bullous trunk lesions become confluent to form huge,
irregularly shaped, burn-like erosions, is known as toxic epidermal
necrolysis. In both of these conditions patients become extremely
sick and there is a mortality rate of approximately 5%. Renal
disease and arthralgias may accompany the high fever and
mucocutaneous lesions. Hair and nails may be shed and rarely
blindness develops. These two variants are particularly likely to
occur as a result of hydantoin and sulfa type drug reactions. Toxic
epidermal necrolysis must be differentiated from staphylococcal
scalded skin syndrome. (See "bullous impetigo" below).

COURSE AND PROGNOSIS

Bullous erythema multiforme is a more severe disease than the
nonbullous variety. However, in most instances the disease will run
its course in 10 to 15 days and then subside spontaneously. Lesions
in general heal without evidence of scarring. When oral mucous

membranes are involved patients may not be able to eat or drink; hospitalization is then required for intravenous therapy. Recurrent episodes of erythema multiforme bullosum are possible particularly in those instances where the disease is associated with recurrent herpes simplex infections.

PATHOGENESIS

In most instances no etiology can be identified. However, medication reactions, infections, collagen vascular disease, dysproteinemia, and systemic malignancy should be considered (see Chapter 14). Circulating immune complexes may be present but there is little evidence that their deposition is important in pathogenesis.

THERAPY

Most patients with erythema multiforme bullosum will require no specific therapy. Patients with mucous membrane involvement, Stevens-Johnson syndrome, and toxic epidermal necrolysis will usually require hospitalization for intravenous fluids and evaluation of possible systemic involvement. Such patients are almost always given prednisone in a dosage of 60 to 80 mg per day but proof that such treatment modifies the course of the disease is lacking. Oral analgesics such as elixir of Benadryl, Xylocaine Viscous, or Dyclone solution may be helpful. Topical steroids are not indicated but soaks may be useful if there is an appreciable amount of weeping and crusting.

SELECTED READING

(See references for erythema multiforme in Chapter 14.)

POISON-IVY-TYPE CONTACT DERMATITIS

DIAGNOSTIC HALLMARKS

1. Distribution: exposed areas; asymmetrical locations
2. Angular and linear lesions
3. History of exposure

CLINICAL PRESENTATION

The antigens responsible for the development of allergic contact dermatitis due to poison ivy, poison oak, or poison sumac are, for all practical purposes, identical. In a sensitized patient, direct skin contact with the resin from any of these plants results in an inflammatory, blistering eruption which develops 24 to 48 hours

later. The eruption consist of bright red, edematous papules and
plaques. Some evidence of weeping and crusting is usually
observed. Vesicles and bullae are frequently present and are
surmounted on the inflammatory lesions. Reflecting external
causation, there is usually a unilateral or asymmetrical
distribution pattern. Linear and angular shapes, which occur as a
result of antigen deposition in scratch marks, are highly
distinctive for this disease. Lesions can also occur on nonexposed
areas. Hands can carry antigen to other parts of the body,
especially the genitalia. The antigen penetrates wet, sweaty
clothing surprisingly well in which case edematous plaques may be
found in areas such as the buttocks and knees. Palms and soles are
usually spared because of the protective effect of their thick
stratum corneum. Pruritus is intense and some evidence of
excoriation is often present.

Allergic contact dermatitis to substances other than poison ivy
rarely results in vesiculobullous reactions. The more common
patterns of allergic contact dermatitis are covered with the
eczematous diseases in Chapter 16.

Poison Ivy Variants. When the leaves of poison ivy are burned
small particles of resin are carried with the smoke. Sensitized
individuals will develop marked erythema and edema of the face but
there is little or no evidence of vesiculation. Poison ivy contact
dermatitis is occasionally seen in circumstances where there has
been no recent exposure to the plants. Such cases may be due to
contact with contaminated firewood or with clothing that was
previously contaminated and was then stored without washing.

COURSE AND PROGNOSIS

Individuals previously sensitized to poison ivy develop lesions
only after a latent period of 24 to 48 hours. Lesions appear first
at the site of heaviest antigen deposition but new lesions can
continue to develop for an additional 3 or 4 days at sites where
antigen concentration was less intense. Spontaneous healing begins
within a week and is usually complete by the end of two weeks.
Allergy to poison ivy is maintained for long periods of time and
thus subsequent exposure, even years later, regularly leads to
redevelopment of the eruption.

PATHOGENESIS

The specific antigen responsible for the reaction is found in
the resin of poison ivy, poison oak, and poison sumac. Its chemical
structure is that of a pentadecylcatechol. Substances chemically
related to this compound can be found in cashew oil and in some oils
used for lacquers. The antigen is extraordinarily potent; nearly
every individual given sufficient exposure will become sensitized.

Probably 30 to 50% of the American population has developed allergy
as the result of sporadic natural contact. The resin is not found
on the exterior surface of the plants and thus development of a
chemical reaction requires breakage of leaves or stems. Within 30
minutes of contact the resin has bound sufficiently well to the skin
such that washing will not prevent the appearance of the rash.
However, enough unbound resin remains on the fingernails and
clothing to cause additional lesions when it is transferred
elsewhere. Washing with soap and water does remove and inactivate
this resin. On the other hand the fluid within blisters does not
contain resin and contact of this fluid with areas of uninvolved
skin does not result in the development of new lesions.

The immunologic aspects of poison ivy contact dermatitis are
similar to those of other types of allergic contact dermatitis;
these are discussed in Chapter 16.

THERAPY

Mild attacks of poison ivy contact dermatitis can be treated
with high potency topical steroids. Patients with more severe
involvement and those with lesions on the face are better treated
with a "burst" of prednisone given in a dosage of 60 to 80 mg per
day. Itching, redness, and swelling are much improved by the second
day but treatment must be continued for 7 to 10 days lest the
lesions rapidly reappear when the steroids are stopped. Soaks and
antihistamines, as needed, can be added to this program. All
exposed clothing, including shoes, should be washed with soap and
water to remove any remaining resin. Pets who have been exposed to
the plants should likewise be shampooed.

It is theoretically possible to hyposensitize patients through
long term, oral administration of antigen. However, at the
practical level this cannot reliably be carried out.

SELECTED READING

Stoner JG, Rasmussen JE: Plant dermatitis.   J Am Acad Dermatol 9:1,
    1983.

BULLOUS IMPETIGO

DIAGNOSTIC HALLMARKS

    1. Distribution: face, hands, intertriginous areas, elbows,
        and knees
    2. Evidence of contagion
    3. Bacterial culture
    4. Response to antibiotic therapy

CLINICAL PRESENTATION

The diagnosis of bullous impetigo is easily missed because patients lack the clinical symptoms and signs usually associated with bacterial infection. There is no rubor, color, tumor, or dolor. The blisters of bullous impetigo generally arise from normal appearing skin and the fluid contained within them is clear or at most only slightly cloudy. Frank pus is never present in the early stages. The blisters, which range in size from 1 to 3 cm, are quite fragile. Within a day or so of onset they break, leaving a crusted, erythematous erosion. Pus may, at this point, accumulate underneath the crusts. Individual lesions heal rapidly but even as this is occurring new blisters often appear on nearby normal skin. In children impetigo is most commonly found on the face around the nose and mouth. Lesions also occur in intertriginous areas and on the hands, arms, and legs. Fever and regional lymphadenopathy are seldom found.

A clinical diagnosis must be confirmed through bacterial culture. This can be accomplished through needle aspiration of an intact blister or by way of a swab applied to the purulent material under a crust. Gram stain done on the blister fluid is rarely helpful because of the high dilution factor.

Impetigo Variants. Staphylococcal scalded skin syndrome (sometimes called toxic epidermal necrolysis of the Ritter type) can be viewed as a variant of bullous impetigo. In this condition certain phage types of Staphylococcus aureus release an exotoxin which causes disruption of epithelial cell cohesion at the mid epidermal level. Large blisters may form but more often sheets of epidermis peel off such as occurs following thermal burns. The initial lesions usually start in intertriginous areas particularly around the neck or in the groin. Cultures from the skin lesions are not necessarily positive since the bacterial toxin can be spread hematogenously as a result of infection elsewhere. Staphylococcal scalded skin syndrome is most often seen in small children but occasional cases have been reported in adults.

Toxic shock syndrome is another rarely encountered staphylococcal infection in which epithelium desquamates secondary to toxin production. Actual blisters, however, are not encountered. The initial flat, red skin lesions occur in association with fever, hypotension, and gastrointestinal disturbances. The infection is particularly likely to occur during menstruation in women who are using tampons. The mortality rate is approximately 10%. Toxic shock syndrome should be differentiated from mucocutaneous lymph node syndrome (Kawasaki disease) and from staphylococcal and streptococcal scarlet fever.

COURSE AND PROGNOSIS

Bullous impetigo left untreated is a chronic, smouldering
problem. New lesions appear as fast as old lesions heal. Contagion
to others often occurs. The disease does, however, respond quickly
and completely to systemically administered antibiotics. On the
other hand, the two variants staphylococcal scalded skin syndrome
and toxic shock are associated with significant morbidity. Such
patients generally require hospitalization and treatment with
parenterally administered antibiotics.

PATHOGENESIS

Bullous impetigo is caused by S. aureus bacterial infection.
Streptococci, when recovered, are usually secondary colonizers. The
blisters of bullous impetigo presumably develop as a result of the
elaboration of an epidermolytic staphylococcal toxin.

THERAPY

Bullous impetigo should be treated with orally administered
antibiotics resistant to degradation by penicillinase. Either
erythromycin or the semisynthetic penicillins (see Chapter 4) can be
administered. Topically applied antibiotics are of very limited
usefulness. Soaks may be used to remove crusts but scrubbing with
antibacterial soaps is contraindicated because of tissue trauma
which usually accompanies this therapeutic approach.

SELECTED READING

Dillon HC Jr: Topical and systemic therapy for pyodermas.   Int J
    Dermatol 19:443, 1980.
Lyell A: The staphylococcal scalded skin syndrome in historical
    perspective: Emergency of dermopathic strains of Staphylococcus
    aureus and discovery of the epidermolytic toxin.   J Am Acad
    Dermatol 9:285, 1983.
Wikas SM, Tomecki KJ: Staphylococcal scalded-skin syndrome.   The
    Cleveland Clinic experience.   Cleve Clin Q 50:141, 1983.

MISCELLANEOUS BULLOUS ERUPTIONS

Traumatic blisters can arise under a variety of circumstances
such as friction, thermal burns, and ischemia due to pressure during
coma.
Patients with porphyria cutanea tarda generally present with
bullae and erosions on the dorsal surface of the hands. There is no
inflammation surrounding the lesions. Blisters on the hands
identical with these (but without the accompanying porphyria)
occasionally occur in patients taking tetracycline, nalidixic acid

(NegGram), and furosemide (Lasix). Similar bullae have been reported in patients with renal failure who are receiving dialysis. An idiopathic, immunobullous disease known as epidermolysis bullosa aquisita also is associated with the appearance of bullae on the dorsal surface of the hands.

Bullae may occur as a part of the condition known as fixed drug eruption. Patients with this problem develop one or more clustered bullae each time they take certain medications such as sulfa type drugs, phenophthalein laxatives, and tetracycline derivatives. The blisters, which occur on an erythematous base, recur in exactly the same location during each episode and are most commonly found on the genitalia.

Trauma induced blisters are encountered in the several genetically determined diseases of the epidermolysis bullosa group. These bullae arise from normal appearing skin and develop following surprising modest degrees of friction. The diseases in this group are separately identified on the basis of inheritance pattern, histologic site of the blister, and the presence or absence of scarring at the time of healing.

Diabetics occasionally develop blisters on the otherwise normal skin of the lower legs and feet. Such blisters seem unrelated to trauma, ischemia, or infection.

SELECTED READING

Chan HL: Fixed drug eruptions. A study of 20 occurrences in Singapore. Int J Dermatol 23:607, 1984.

Harber LC, Bickers DR: Porphyria and pseudoporphyria. J Invest Dermatol 82:207, 1984.

Wintroub BU, Stern R: Cutaneous drug reactions: Pathogenesis and clinical classification. J Am Acad Dermatol 13:167, 1985.

Haber RM, Hanna W, Ramsay CA, Boxall LBH: Hereditary epidermolysis bullosa. J Am Acad Dermatol 13:252, 1985.

Grossman ME, Poh-Fitzpatrick MB: Porphyria cutanea tarda. Diagnosis, management, and differentiation from other hepatic porphyrias. Dermatol Clinics 4:297, 1986.

Kero M, Niemi K-M: Epidermolysis bullosa. Int J Dermatol 25:75, 1986.

Sehgal VH, Gangwani OP: Genital fixed drug eruptions. Genitourin Med 62:56, 1986.

Group 2:
The Pustular Diseases

GROUP IDENTIFICATION

The recognition of pustules is ordinarily quite easy. They appear as white or yellow-white fluid filled vesicles 1 to 4 mm in diameter. Since they are composed of densely packed neutrophils, themselves a hallmark of an inflammatory response, it is perhaps not surprising that pustules almost always arise on an erythematous base. Pustules must be distinguished from cloudy vesicles. Nearly all vesicles accumulate a few inflammatory cells as they age and thus lose their translucency while gradually taking on a cloudy appearance. Such lesions remain classified as vesicles; pustules must have been completely white from their inception. Pustules must also be distinguished from pseudopustules. The latter are small white papules in which the white color is due to compacted keratin. Such lesions are solid in consistency and for this reason incision with a blade or needle readily separates them from the fluid filled, true pustules.

ACNE VULGARIS

DIAGNOSTIC HALLMARKS

1. Distribution: face and shoulders
2. Pustules are intermingled with comedones and inflammatory papules.

CLINICAL PRESENTATION

A wide variety of lesions are found in acne, only a portion of which are pustules. Open comedones (blackheads) consist of a pigmented keratinous plug firmly situated at the orifice of a sebaceous follicle. The reason for the black color is not fully understood but most likely it occurs because of the deposition of melanin granules in the multiple layers of compacted keratinocytes which make up the plug.

Closed comedones are dome shaped 1- to 2-mm papules. They are skin colored rather than black. These, too, occur because of a keratinous plug in the outlet of a sebaceous follicle but in these lesions the plug lies below the surface of the skin at a point too deep to pick up color from the surface melanocytes.

Pustules situated on an inflammatory base occur when the plugged duct of an androgen-driven sebaceous follicle ruptures with extrusion of the keratin plug and retained bacterial and sebaceous materials into the surrounding dermis. This extrusion causes a brisk local neutrophilic inflammatory response. Thus acne pustules contain both a solid white keratin core and accompanying pus cells.

Inflammatory papules without a surmounted pustule occur when the follicular rupture and induced inflammatory response occur at a level too deep to result in a visible pustule. Inflammatory cysts and pseudocysts, 1 to 2 cm in diameter, develop when the process described above is unusually intense and occurs even deeper at the level of the sebaceous gland itself. Such cystic lesions are often fluctuant and painful. Moreover, as opposed to the other lesions of acne, they heal with scar formation.

Most instances of pustular acne begin at puberty. The initial lesions generally consist of comedones and small pustules and these are usually found on the forehead and upper cheeks. During the late teen years the mix of lesions shifts toward larger, more inflammatory pustules and papules. These lesions generally occur on the lower cheeks, chin, and jawline. Inflammatory lesions may also develop over the shoulders and upper arms. The diagnosis of acne is made on the basis of history and clinical examination.

Atypical Presentations. Acne conglobata is the name used for the presence of multiple, deep, cystic, scarring lesions over the face and upper trunk. It occurs predominantly in individuals with genetically malformed sebaceous follicles. One indication of these structural abnormalities is the presence of multiple, closely spaced twin comedones in the skin adjacent to cysts. Some individuals with severe acne conglobata have associated fever, leukocytosis, and arthralgia.

The administration of phenytoin (Dilantin) to individuals already prone to acne has an adverse effect on the severity and duration of what is otherwise typical appearing acne vulgaris. Administration of corticosteroids can cause an acne-like folliculitis in which small pustules without keratin plugs develop in considerable profusion on the chest, back, and shoulders. Comedones and cysts are not found. Ingestion of large amounts of iodine also leads to the presence of an acneiform eruption.

Acneiform lesions are sometimes induced through occupational exposure to tars, cutting oils, and chlorinated hydrocarbons and through the use of petrolatum pomades as hair dressings. The use of

the herbicide Agent Orange in Viet Nam led to the development of
such "chloracne" in many soldiers. Babies occasionally develop a
few acne lesions during the first month or so of life presumably as
a result of maternal hormonal stimulation.

Acne excoriee des jeunes filles occurs when individuals
neurotically pick at acne lesions. Because of this chronic picking
minor acne lesions are kept inflamed and active for weeks or even
months at a time. The excoriated papules eventually heal with
hypopigmentation and, sometimes, frank scarring.

COURSE AND PROGNOSIS

Generally the peak activity of acne is in the mid to late teen
years with steady improvement then beginning around age 20.
However, occasionally disease activity continues into the fourth
decade. Women seem particularly prone to this long lasting form of
acne.

Hormonal factors play an important role in the course of acne:
acne in general seems to be more severe in men and cystic lesions,
which are common in men, are only rarely found in women. In women a
monthly peak of acne activity often occurs during the week prior to
their menses. Acne tends to improve during the third to ninth month
of pregnancy but rebound worsening sometimes occurs following
parturition and cessation of lactation.

It is difficult to predict the future severity of acne at the
time a young patient is first seen. The presence of cysts and a
family history of scarring acne are, however, bad prognostic signs.

When acne is untreated, individual small papules and pustules
resolve spontaneously in 7 to 10 days. Resolution of these lesions
does not result in scarring even when some relatively modest degree
of picking is carried out. Large papules and cysts require several
weeks to resolve and subsequent postinflammatory color changes may
persist for months. Scarring is occasionally found at the site of
deep seated papules and is almost invariably present following
resolution of fluctuant cysts.

PATHOGENESIS

Acne is a disease of complex genetic and hormonal factors.
Identical twins tend to have acne which is of equal severity and
similar type. Parents who have had troublesome acne tend to have
children with a similar problem. However, differences in severity
of acne among siblings from one generation to the next suggest that
genetics simply provides a permissive setting for other, acquired
factors. Some of these are discussed in the paragraphs below.

Stimulation of the sebaceous glands by way of androgenic
hormones appears to be a necessary factor for induction of acne in
both men and women. Acne does not occur until puberty when such

hormonal stimulation first begins to develop. Castrated men and oophorectomized women do not develop acne. Serum androgen levels may be slightly elevated in men and women with cystic acne but in addition it is likely that there is some degree of end organ hyper-responsiveness at the level of the sebaceous gland. The importance of androgenic factors in women is underscored by the regular presence of acne in patients with polycystic ovarian disease and in those with sterol hydroxylase deficiencies.

Hormonal stimulation as described above leads to increased sebaceous gland size and to increased sebum output. The presence and severity of acne correlate in a general sort of way with production levels of sebum; but high sebum flow rates alone, in the absence of follicular plugs, do not cause acne.

The presence of a follicular plug is an important and necessary factor for the development of an acne lesion in any given follicle. Such blockages are caused by the accumulation of compacted, dead, cornified cells within the orifice of the follicle itself. Several hypotheses exist to explain the formation of these plugs: genetic malformation of the follicle; stimulation of follicular keratinization by bacteria present in the follicle; or hormonal effects on the follicle wall. Such information as is available favors the first of these.

Once a blockage is present in a follicle, bacteria, such as the omnipresent Propionibacterium acnes, causes lipolysis of the sebum with consequent formation of free fatty acids. It is hypothesized that these free fatty acids, bits of keratin, and bacterial proteins are then extruded through the distended and subsequently disrupted follicular wall into the dermis where they call forth an intense neutrophilic inflammatory infiltrate.

The various therapeutic modalities discussed below attempt to address the roles played by these factors of hormonal stimulation, follicle plugging, and bacterial induction of inflammation.

THERAPY

Mild acne (comedones and small pustules) can be treated with topical preparations which, by way of their peeling effect, unplug the blocked follicles. Benzoyl peroxide lotion, gel, or cream in a 5% concentration can be applied once nightly after normal facial washing. If at the end of the first week no peeling effect is noted, the frequency of application is increased to twice daily or the strength of the benzoyl peroxide is increased to 10%. Mild redness and chapping is an expected effect of this therapy during the first few weeks of application. This reaction becomes less troublesome during the second month of treatment even though the therapeutic effect continues in an undiminished manner. Benzoyl peroxide not only unplugs follicles by way of the induction of peeling but also reduces the number of P. acnes through oxidative destruction of the organisms.

If the use of benzoyl peroxide has not resulted in satisfactory improvement by the end of 2 months an attempt may be made to use topically applied retinoic acid (Retin-A). The gel in a 0.025% concentration or the cream in a 0.05% concentration is applied once daily. The strength and frequency of applications can be modified as described above for the use of benzoyl peroxide. The effect of Retin-A on follicular plugs is twofold: it removes plugs through the induction of postinflammatory peeling and also "dissolves" the plugs by way of its disruptive effect on the cement-like substance which binds the keratinized cells together. Some clinicians believe that a synergistic effect can be obtained if benzoyl peroxide is used in the morning and retinoic acid is used at night.

A number of alternate approaches for the induction of peeling exist. These include 1) the application of sulfur, salicylic acid, and resorcinol in an alcohol vehicle; 2) natural or artificially administered ultraviolet light; 3) mechanical scrubbing of the face with various abrasive products; and 4) the use of cryotherapy in the form of liquid nitrogen spray or carbon dioxide slush. All of these methods result in peeling and thus help to free plugged follicles. No one of them is superior to benzoyl peroxide or retinoic acid.

Patients with more severe acne (inflammatory papules, large pustules and cysts) almost always require the addition of antibiotics either applied topically or administered systemically. Orally administered tetracycline in a dosage of 500 to 1000 mg daily has historically been the antibiotic of choice. This approach has an excellent record of safety and efficacy. Recently it has been shown that topically applied 1.5 to 2.0% erythromycin or 1% clindamycin can result in a degree of improvement roughly equal to that obtained with 500 mg of tetracycline given in a daily, oral dose. With any one of these three preparations 75% of patients will be substantially improved by the end of 6 weeks of treatment. For the remaining 25% of patients other orally administered antibiotics are usually substituted. Erythromycin, because of its low cost and freedom from side effects, is usually tried first. The dosage used is 1.0 gram per day. Tetracycline derivatives are the subsequent drugs of choice. Minocycline (Minocin) and doxycycline (Vibramycin) given as 100 mg once or twice daily are equally efficacious. The former occasionally causes disturbance in vestibular function and cutaneous discoloration; both are very expensive.

Mechanical extrusion (acne surgery) of the follicular keratinous plugs is carried out by many physicians. Such manipulation can be temporarily helpful but its usefulness in the long run is much less clear. Patients often object to this manipulation because of discomfort and the unsightly appearance which remains for hours after the procedure. I do relatively little acne surgery and instead allow patients to open and squeeze out the plugs themselves

at home. Chronic picking and squeezing is, however, discouraged
since repeated manipulation creates additional inflammation and
prolonged healing times. Neither acne surgery by the physician nor
gentle extrusion by the patient causes scarring; scarring is
directly related to the depth and severity of the inflammation in
the acne lesion itself.

Dietary therapy is sometimes advised. Anecdotal reports of its
usefulness are numerous but the few controlled studies available
suggest that it is of little help. In women, oil based cosmetics
should be used as little as possible. Animal studies suggest that
these products have some propensity for the induction of comedone
formation.

Many acne patients, particularly those over the age of 20,
experience a flare of their acne during periods of stress. Usually
little can be done to lessen this problem, but occasionally
counseling, tranquilizers, or antidepressants are indicated.

Blockage of the androgen effect on the sebaceous glands can be
achieved through the use of estrogens. The estrogens are usually
administered in the form of birth control pills. Oral
contraceptives used for the control of acne probably need to contain
50 to 80 micrograms of estrogen. Brands such as Ortho-Novum,
Norinyl, and Enovid would be good choices to minimize the sebotropic
effects of the progestational agents found in some pills.

Patients with severe acne unresponsive to the therapeutic
regimens described above deserve a trial of orally administered
13-cis-retinoic acid (Accutane). Use of this retinoid in a dose of
40 to 80 mg per day for a 4-month period leads to very impressive
improvement. Unfortunately, the side effects are troublesome (see
Chapter 4) and the cost is high. Nevertheless, this approach leads
to a virtual guarantee of satisfaction in 95% of patients.
Moreover, for most patients, no further treatment is likely to be
necessary for at least the subsequent 12 months.

SELECTED READING

Goldstein JA, Comite H, Mescon H, Pochi PE: Isotretinoin in the
    treatment of acne. Histologic changes, sebum production, and
    clinical observations. Arch Dermatol 118:555, 1982.
Gratton D, Raymond CP, Guertin-Larochelle S, et al: Topical
    clindamycin versus systemic tetracycline in the treatment of
    acne. J Am Acad Dermatol 7:50, 1982.
Burke B, Eady EA, Cunliffe WJ: Benzoyl peroxide versus topical
    erythromycin in the treatment of acne vulgaris. Br J Dermatol
    108:199, 1983.
Levine RM, Rasmussen JE: Intralesional corticosteroids in the
    treatment of nodulocystic acne. Arch Dermatol 119:480, 1983.
Rasmussen JE: What causes acne? Pediatr Clin North Am 30:511, 1983.

114   DERMATOLOGY FOR THE HOUSE OFFICER

Shalita AR, Smith EB, Bauer E: Topical erythromycin vs. clindamycin
    therapy for acne. A multicenter, double-blind comparison. Arch
    Dermatol 120:351, 1984.
Tucker SB, Tausend R, Cochran R, Flannigan SA: Comparison of
    topical clindamycin phosphate, benzoyl peroxide, and a
    combination of the two for the treatment of acne vulgaris. Br J
    Dermatol 110:487, 1984.
Parish LC, Witkowski JA: Bacteriology and acne. Int J Dermatol
    23:36, 1984.
Darley CR: Recent advances in hormonal aspects of acne vulgaris.
    Int J Dermatol 23:539, 1984.
Esterly NB, Koransky JS, Furey NL, Trevisan M: Neutrophil
    chemotaxis in patients with acne receiving oral tetracycline
    therapy. Arch Dermatol 120:1308, 1984.
Lookingbill DP, Horton R, Demers LM, et al: Tissue production of
    androgens in women with acne. J Am Acad Dermatol 12:481, 1985.
Greenwood R, Burke B, Cunliffe WJ: Evaluation of a therapeutic
    strategy for the treatment of acne vulgaris with conventional
    therapy. Br J Dermatol 114:353, 1986.
Gammon WR, Meyer C, Lantis S, Shenefelt P, et al: Comparative
    efficacy of oral erythromycin versus oral tetracycline in the
    treatment of acne vulgaris. J Am Acad Dermatol 14:183, 1986.

ROSACEA (ACNE ROSACEA)

DIAGNOSTIC HALLMARKS

1.   Distribution: vertical, central third of the face
2.   Pustules and papules against a background of erythema
     and telangiectasia

CLINICAL PRESENTATION

    Rosacea is characterized by the presence of dusky erythema and
telangiectasia over the nose and cheeks. Often the glabella and
chin are involved such that the eruption forms a vertical line down
the central third of the face. In the more severe cases pustules
and inflammatory papules are superimposed against this erythematous
background. Comedones do not occur. Men with longstanding rosacea
sometimes develop a distinctive connective tissue overgrowth of the
nose known as rhinophyma. This condition is colloquially referred
to as potato nose. Rosacea is seen primarily in middle aged or
older individuals. Those of Celtic and northern European background
seem particularly predisposed to the disease. The diagnosis of
rosacea is made on a clinical basis.

COURSE AND PROGNOSIS

Rosacea is a chronic disease characterized by periodic exacerbations and remissions. Gradual worsening with more permanent redness and telangiectasia occurs in some patients whereas in others the disease gradually fades out over a period of many years. Men with rosacea, as noted above, may eventually develop rhinophyma. Conjunctivitis, blepharitis, and keratitis accompany the disease in isolated instances. Treatment leads to considerable cosmetic improvement but probably is only suppressive with little change in the ultimate course of the disease.

PATHOGENESIS

The cause of rosacea is unknown. Familial predisposition for the disease and the remarkable tendency for those of Celtic background to develop the problem suggest that genetic factors are important. Ingestants such as spicy foods, alcohol, and beverages drunk at hot temperatures are widely believed to worsen the disease. Certainly they temporarily increase the background redness and the prominence of the telangiectasia but it is not clear that they permanently alter the eventual course of the disease. Contrary to folklore, rosacea is not a sign of excess alcoholic intake. The pustules of rosacea appear to be follicular abscesses; they lack the component of keratinous plugging found in the pustules of acne vulgaris.

THERAPY

Tetracycline administered orally in dose of 500 to 1000 mg per day is extremely effective in suppressing the occurrence of papules and pustules. It has a useful but less dramatic effect on the underlying redness and telangiectasia. Topically applied steroids will reduce the redness but their prolonged use is contraindicated since rebound flaring and eventual worsening of the process is quite likely. The application of preparations containing sulfur such as Liquimat, Fostril, Rezamid, and Sulfacet are believed to be helpful by some clinicians. Oil based makeups are avoided when possible since they often seem to worsen the process. Nervousness and stress temporarily worsen the appearance of the disease but of course they are difficult to control. In the most severe cases a 4-month course of orally administered 13-cis-retinoic acid is warranted.

SELECTED READING
Wilkin JK: Rosacea. Int J Dermatol 22:393, 1983
Marsden JR, Shuster S, Neugebauer M: Response of rosacea to
    isotretinoin. Clin Exp Dermatol 9:484, 1984.

Blom I, Nornmark A-M: Topical treatment with sulfur 10 per cent for
    rosacea. Acta Derm Venereol 64:358, 1984.
Schmidt JB, Gebhart W, Raff M, Spona J: 13-cis-retinoic acid in
    rosacea. Acta Derm Venereol 64:15, 1984.

BACTERIAL FOLLICULITIS

DIAGNOSTIC HALLMARKS

1. Distribution: the groin and exposed areas of the arms and
    legs
2. Bacterial culture
3. Response to therapy

CLINICAL PRESENTATION

The small 1- to 2-mm pustules of bacterial folliculitis are
yellow-white in color and are surrounded by a narrow ring of
erythema. Those that are not pierced by a hair are dome shaped;
those that are pierced by a hair are acuminate (pointed). Only a
few pustules are present at any one time and there is relatively
little tendency for clustering. Fever and lymphadenopathy are not
seen. The diagnosis of bacterial folliculitis is usually made on a
clinical basis but confirmation can be obtained by Gram stain and
bacterial culture.

COURSE AND PROGNOSIS

Individual untreated pustules resolve spontaneously in about a
week but often as quickly as one heals one or more new pustules
appear elsewhere on the body. This spread develops as the result of
external inoculation via the fingernails. Hematogenous spread does
not occur. On rare occasions bacterial folliculitis leads to deeper
infection such as cellulitis or furunculosis.

PATHOGENESIS

Bacterial folliculitis usually represents infection of the upper
hair follicle with Staphylococcus aureus. Streptococci are also
occasionally found but they rarely if ever are the inciting
organism. A few cases of Pseudomonas sp. folliculitis have been
reported. These occurred during the use of contaminated hot tubs.
Minor skin trauma of various sorts probably plays a role in the
development of bacterial folliculitis.

THERAPY

Topical antibiotics may be used if only one or two pustules are present. Systemic antibiotics are preferred for patients who have a large number of lesions or who have problems with recurrent lesions. Some of these latter patients will be found to be staphylococcal carriers.

SELECTED READING

Sheagren JN: Staphylococcus aureus. The persistent pathogen. N Engl J Med 310:1368, 1984.
Fox AB, Hambrick GW Jr: Recreationally associated Pseudomonas aeruginosa folliculitis. Report of an epidemic. Arch Dermatol 120:1304, 1984.
Kosatsky T, Kleeman J: Superficial and systemic illness related to a hot tub. Am J Med 79:10, 1985.

FUNGAL FOLLICULITIS

DIAGNOSTIC HALLMARKS

   1.   Distribution: hands, arms, legs, scalp
   2.   Marked tendency for clustering
   3.   Lack of response to antibacterial therapy
   4.   KOH preparation and fungal culture

CLINICAL PRESENTATION

The dermatophyte fungi Microsporum canis, Trichophyton rubrum, T. mentagrophytes, and T. verrucosum may cause a perifollicular abscess which is clinically characterized by the presence of follicular pustules. All of these organisms except T. rubrum cause sharply marginated, markedly inflammatory plaques upon which the pustules are situated. These pustule-studded plaques are rather easily recognized as the zoophilic, inflammatory forms of tinea capitis, tinea barbae, or tinea corporis.

Perifollicular pustules due to T. rubrum infection are somewhat harder to recognize. They occur in two settings. First, women with tinea pedis may, in the course of shaving their legs, implant T. rubrum into traumatized follicles. This results in the appearance of scattered but grouped pustules on the lower legs. Second, the erroneous use of topical steroids on plaques of ordinary tinea corporis results in the development of grouped follicular pustules even while the erythema which ordinarily accompanies such lesions is minimized by the anti-inflammatory effect of the steroids. Such lesions are most often encountered on the face and dorsal surface of the hands where they are misdiagnosed at first as being of bacterial

origin. Their fungal etiology is often not suspected until they
fail to respond to antibacterial treatment.

A clinical diagnosis of fungal folliculitis should be confirmed
by KOH preparations or by fungal culture (see Chapter 5). Fungal
hyphae may be recognized on regular biopsy specimens but for good
reliable visualization special stains must be ordered.

COURSE AND PROGNOSIS

Folliculitis due to T. rubrum continues its chronic low grade
course indefinitely unless treated. Slow peripheral extension
occurs even while the central area heals. Fungal folliculitis due
to the other, zoophilic organisms eventually resolves spontaneously.

PATHOGENESIS

Fungal folliculitis is caused by the dermatophyte organisms
listed in the paragraph on clinical presentation. Implantation is
usually preceded by minor trauma to the skin.

THERAPY

Griseofulvin or, possibly, ketoconazole (see Chapter 4) should
be used in the treatment of fungal folliculitis. There is some
response to the use of topical antifungal agents but complete
clearing does not reliably occur. During the course of therapy,
trauma to the infected skin should be avoided. Women who shave
their legs should be advised to use a chemical depilatory during
treatment.

CANDIDIASIS (MONILIASIS) OF INTERTRIGINOUS SKIN

DIAGNOSTIC HALLMARKS

1.   Distribution: groin and other intertriginous areas
2.   Satellite papules and pustules
3.   KOH preparation and fungal culture

CLINICAL PRESENTATION

Candidiasis of intertriginous skin occurs as poorly marginated,
bright red plaques with satellite papules and pustules scattered
around the periphery of the main lesion. In some cases pustules may
also be found studded over the surface of the main plaque. The
satellite pustules are 2 to 4 mm in diameter whereas those
superimposed over the main plaque are usually less than 1 mm in
diameter. The inflammatory plaques have a moist, slightly crusted
surface and thus appear eczematous (see Chapter 16). Candidiasis is

seen most commonly in the groin but also occasionally occurs in the
axillary folds, inframammary folds, and interdigital web spaces.

In men the initial lesions appear in the inguinal-scrotal fold
with later involvement of the inner thighs, gluteal cleft, and
scrotum. In women, candida vaginitis usually precedes the
development of vulvar disease. As might be expected visible lesions
appear first in the vestibule and on the labia. Spread subsequently
occurs to the inner thighs and gluteal cleft.

Pruritus is generally present. When itching is followed by
excoriation pustules are disrupted and the entire process takes on
the morphology of an eczematous disease.

A clinical diagnosis should be confirmed by way of KOH
preparations or cultures. These studies are more likely to be
positive if they are performed on material recovered from intact
pustules. Positive cultures in the absence of a positive KOH test
must be interpreted with care since Candida sp. may colonize other
inflammatory diseases occurring in intertriginous areas.

Atypical Presentations. Candidiasis of mucous membranes can
appear either as white plaques or as inflammatory erosive disease.
The former are frequently found in the mouth (Chapter 21) and vagina
whereas the latter is the typical appearance of Candida balanitis
(Chapter 20). Candida paronychia is described in Chapter 19.

Chronic mucocutaneous candidiasis is a rare disease of
immunodeficiency characterized by widespread candidiasis of the skin
and mucous membranes. Congenital and acquired forms exist. In both
types the cutaneous lesions are particularly notable on the hands
and feet where they simulate the papulosquamous appearance of
chronic dermatophyte infection. The scalp is covered with thick
yellow crusts. Pustules may be present on the scalp, face, and
intertriginous skin.

PATHOGENESIS

Candidiasis is a yeast infection due to Candida sp. Of these,
Candida albicans accounts for the vast majority of the infections.
The clinical picture is the same regardless of which species is
responsible.

C. albicans in its spore form is a normal inhabitant of the
entire gastrointestinal tract. The vagina in women may be similarly
colonized. Disease, in contradistinction to colonization, due to C.
albicans is not said to be present unless the organism has converted
to the mycelial growth phase. This change is easily recognized on
KOH preparations, but the distinction cannot, of course, be made on
the basis of culture.

Development of clinical disease usually requires both the
presence of damaged skin for implantation and the presence of a warm
moist environment. Once C. albicans has invaded the stratum corneum
it activates complement and acts as a chemotactic stimulus for

polymorphonuclear leukocytes. Thus pustules are likely to develop.
Antibiotics (by enchancing multiplication of Candida sp. in the gut)
and systemically administered steroids (by reducing immunologic
defense) increase the likelihood of developing candidiasis.

THERAPY

Nystatin (Mycostatin), haloprogin (Halotex), miconazole
(Micatin), and clotrimazole (Lotrimin) applied twice a day are
effective in the treatment of candidiasis. In those patients for
whom inflammation is prominent or where pruritus is severe, the
addition of a topically applied steroid such as hydrocortisone
reduces the discomfort and shortens the time for healing.
Alternatively the combination of an antifungal agent and topical
steroid packaged together as Lotrisone cream would also be
appropriate. Orally administered ketoconazole is only rarely
indicated in uncomplicated cases. Attention should be given to
environmental factors in the treatment program. Specifically the
skin should be kept cool, dry, and free from trauma. In women with
involvement of the groin, concomitant treatment of the vagina with
nystatin, miconazole, or clotrimazole is also necessary. In both
men and women with recurrent infections, orally administered
ketoconazole in a dose of 200 mg per day (see Chapter 4) for 2 weeks
may reduce the number of organisms in the gut and vagina and thus
decrease reseeding onto adjacent skin.

SELECTED READING
Odds FC: Genital candidosis. St. John's Hospital Dermatological
    Society: Symposium on Genital Infections 1981. Clin Exp
    Dermatol 7:345, 1982.
Felman YM, Nikitas JA: Sexually transmitted diseases. Genital
    candidiasis. Cutis 31:369, 1983.
Vulvovaginal candidiasis -- what we do and do not know. Ann
    Intern Med 101:390, 1984.

MISCELLANEOUS PUSTULAR DISEASES

Acne necrotica miliaris is a pustular scalp disease which occurs
predominantly in men. It is characterized by the presence of
pruritic, inflammatory papules surmounted by a small pustule.
Because of the pruritus, many patients present with excoriated
papules rather than with intact pustules. The cause of the disease
is unknown but it frequently occurs in anxious, stressed
individuals. Cultures reveal only the presence of Propionibacterium
acnes. Orally administered tetracycline as used in the treatment of
acne vulgaris is reasonably effective.
    An acne-like folliculitis of the skin develops in some
individuals following exposure to halogenated hydrocarbons and some

other chemicals. This reaction is known as <u>chloracne</u>. Interest in this condition has increased because of its recent recognition as a reaction to Agent Orange.

Perioral <u>dermatitis</u> generally presents as an eczematous disease (see Chapter 16) but occasionally the process is predominated by the presence of pinpoint pustules. Avoidance of topically applied steroids and the administration of tetracycline is quite helpful.

<u>Gonococcemia</u> may result in the development of arthritis, tenosynovitis, and the appearance of cutaneous cloudy or hemorrhagic vesicles. Some of these vesicles are opaque enough to be considered as pustules. Such lesions are generally few in number and are usually located on the hands and feet or are scattered in proximity to the large joints. Organisms cannot be cultured from the skin lesions but are recoverable from such sites as the cervix, rectum, or pharynx. Penicillin is curative.

Clustered minute pustules on the fingers, toes, palms, and soles occur in several diseases grouped under the title <u>acral pustular dermatoses</u>. The cause is unknown, but some of the patients have, or will develop, more typical lesions of psoriasis elsewhere on the body.

A few patients with widespread inflammatory psoriasis develop thousands of minute pustules superimposed on their cutaneous plaques. This condition, known as <u>pustular psoriasis</u> of Von Zumbusch, requires hospitalization, intensive topical therapy, and systemically administered agents such as Accutane or methotrexate.

SELECTED READING

Sanchez NP, Perry HO, Muller SA, Winkelmann RK: Subcorneal pustular dermatosis and pustular psoriasis. <u>Arch Dermatol</u> <u>119</u>:715, 1983.
O'Brien JP, Goldenberg DL, Rice PA: Disseminated gonococcal infection: A prospective analysis of 49 patients and a review of pathophysiology and immune mechanisms. <u>Medicine</u> <u>62</u>:395, 1983.
Tindall JP: Chloracne and chloracnegens. <u>J Am Acad Dermatol</u> <u>13</u>:539, 1985.
Hook EW III, Holmes KK: Gonococcal infections. <u>Ann Intern Med</u> <u>102</u>:229, 1985.
Piamphongsant T, Nimsuwan P, Gritiyarangsan P: Treatment of generalized pustular psoriasis -- Clinical trials using different therapeutic modalities. <u>Clin Exp Dermatol</u> <u>10</u>:552, 1985.
Lassus A, Lauharanta J, Eskelinen A: The effect of etretinate compared with different regimens of PUVA in the treatment of persistent palmoplantar pustulosis. <u>Br J Dermatol</u> <u>112</u>:455, 1985.

PSEUDOPUSTULES

The small, white, keratotic papules of keratosis pilaris and milia are frequently mistakenly identified as pustules. They are classified with the white lesions of Group 4 and are discussed in Chapter 10.

Group 3: The Skin Colored Papules and Nodules

GROUP IDENTIFICATION

The skin colored papules and nodules are usually easy to identify. Two general rules, however, should be kept in mind. First, a skin colored lesion is the same color as the surrounding skin. Thus a dark skinned person would have skin colored lesions which are brown in color whereas a light skinned person would have skin colored lesions which are nearly white in color. Second, a lesion which appears to be made up of nothing but scale, that is, a lesion with no color or substance other than scale, is classified as a skin colored lesion. This occurs with particular frequency in the case of actinic keratoses.

ROUGH SURFACED WARTS (VERRUCA VULGARIS, PARONYCHIAL WARTS, AND PLANTAR WARTS)

DIAGNOSTIC HALLMARKS

1. Distribution: hands and feet
2. Tendency for clustering when more than one is present
3. Verrucous surface
4. Paring reveals black dots or pinpoint bleeding

CLINICAL PRESENTATION

Warts can occur at any age but are most commonly seen in children and young adults. They begin as pinhead sized papules which grow quickly to a stable, final size of 5 to 10 mm in diameter. Shedding, and subsequent implantation, of wart virus into surrounding skin results in the development of new warts in a cluster around the original "mother" wart. Tightly clustered warts may merge as they enlarge, forming mosaic warts 1 to 3 cm in diameter.

Verruca vulgaris is the name used for warts which develop on "nonpressure" dry surfaces of the skin. They are most commonly found on the dorsal surface of the fingers, hands, arms, and toes, but in adults they may be encountered on the face, neck, or upper trunk. These warts extend 2 to 8 mm above the surrounding skin surface and are approximately as wide as they are tall. Their margination is extremely sharp; in cross section they are square shouldered. The surface is verrucous; that is, rough on palpation and somewhat saw-toothed or jagged in appearance. Verruca vulgaris are usually skin colored but sometimes they are slightly hyperpigmented compared to surrounding normal skin.

Paronychial warts are verruca vulgaris that grow in the skin folds which surrounds the nails. There is a marked tendency for confluent growth such that these warts are regularly wider than they are tall. Otherwise, their appearance is similar to conventional verruca vulgaris.

Plantar warts occur on the plantar surface of the feet. Constant pressure from walking affects the appearance of these warts in two ways. First, the mass of the wart is indented into the underlying soft tissue; these warts do not seem greatly raised above the surface of the surrounding normal skin. Second, the surface of the wart becomes heavily callused and thus is less verrucous on appearance and palpation than is true for the other warts discussed above. Paring of the callused surface reveals an underlying translucent core peppered with black dots. These black dots represent thromboses in the vertically oriented capillaries which provide nutrition for the warts. Calluses and corns unassociated with warts lack these black dots. Single plantar warts may be only 2 or 3 mm in diameter but there is a marked tendency for enlargement and confluent growth such that mosaic patterns 2 or more cm in diameter are frequently found. Most warts are asymptomatic but plantar warts may be painful on walking because of compression against the underlying tissue.

The diagnosis of keratotic warts is made on the basis of clinical history and examination. Recognition of thrombosed or bleeding capillaries following paring is especially helpful. Biopsy is occasionally indicated to separate warts from other tumors. Electron microscopy will show, if enough fields are examined, the distinctive viral particles.

COURSE AND PROGNOSIS

In children untreated warts almost always disappear
spontaneously. Twenty percent of warts disappear in as little as 1
month and in the majority of children all warts will be gone within
2 or 3 years. Spontaneous resolution may also occur in adults but
the average time to disappearance is longer.

Left untreated, warts tend to spread through a process of
autoinoculation. Viral particles which are shed from the surface of
the skin are implanted into small cuts and scratches elsewhere on
the body. Warts appear to be spread from person to person as a
result of direct contact.

The human papilloma virus has the potential for oncogenic
behavior. Fortunately, this is expressed only rarely and seems to
be of clinical importance only in the case of genital wart virus
infection.

PATHOGENESIS

Warts are caused by the human papilloma virus. More than 35
subtypes of this spherical DNA virus have been identified and some
of these subtypes appear to cause clinically specific types of
warts. These wart virus subtypes are morphologically identical but
differ immunogenetically and can be individually identified on the
basis of hybridization studies. Several types of human papilloma
virus have been cloned but none has as yet been cultured and thus
Koch's postulates have not been fulfilled.

Human wart viruses have specific affinity for epidermal cells
and they cannot replicate in dermal connective tissue cells or other
types of nonepithelial tissue. After implantation into the
epidermis, the viruses enter the nuclei of lower and mid epidermal
cells. There they take over the machinery of cell reproduction and,
while replicating themselves, they induce a rapid proliferation of
epithelial cells. On electron microscopy viral particles are most
numerous between 6 and 12 months of growth of an individual wart.
Thereafter the number of visible particles decreases to the point
where, after 2 to 3 years of growth, they become difficult if not
impossible to find.

Like other viral infections the presence of the wart virus in
human skin incites an immunologic response. In the early months of
wart growth, IgM antibodies predominate. Later these are replaced
with IgG antibodies. Antibody measurements suggest that infection
with the wart virus is almost universal. By late adult life, most
of the population have developed antibodies, suggesting previous
infection. Resolution of warts depends on cell mediated immune
responsiveness rather than on antibody production. The importance
of the cell mediated response is reflected by the frequency and
severity of wart virus infections in renal transplant patients and

individuals with Hodgkin's disease. In all individuals the immune
response which leads to spontaneous clearing of the warts is not
long lasting. Reinfection can occur within months.

THERAPY

The contagious nature of warts suggests that they should be
treated in spite of their tendency for spontaneous resolution.
Verruca vulgaris in young children can be treated with the
application of mild keratolytics such as salicylic acid (Occlusal or
Duofilm) on a twice daily basis. Such applications, continued for 4
to 6 weeks, result in a cure rate of approximately 70%. Older
children and adults can be treated with cryotherapy (see Chapter
4). Three to five freezes at weekly intervals results in an 80%
cure rate. The efficacy of these two methods probably depends in
part on the induction of inflammation and the subsequent "turning
on" of cell mediated immune responsiveness. Electrosurgical
destruction can also be used. This has the advantage of requiring
only one office visit, but this advantage is balanced by a prolonged
healing time, a tendency for bacterial infection, and scarring at
the site of treatment.

Paronychial warts can be treated with liquid nitrogen or by the
weekly application of trichloracetic acid (see Chapter 5) or
cantharidin (Cantharone). The latter preparation, made from
extracts of the blister beetle, results in the formation of a
subepidermal blister. Since the wart virus is confined to the
epidermis, repeated application of this fluid results in removal of
virally infected tissue without any destruction of the underlying
dermis. Unfortunately, its use is followed by frequent seeding of
virus into the blister edge with the resultant formation of a
recurrent "doughnut" wart.

Plantar warts are difficult to treat because the constant
pressure on the wart drives the expanding compartment of epithelial
cells into the underlying dermis rather than allowing for outward
growth. Surgical, electrosurgical, and cryosurgical attempts to get
at these inwardly proliferating epithelial cells result in
appreciable discomfort and some risk of dermal destruction and
scarring. Plantar warts are better treated by the repeated
application of chemical caustics. To achieve effective application
overlying callus must be removed by paring. The exposed translucent
wart core can then be periodically treated with trichloracetic acid,
10 to 20% salicylic acid, or 20% Formalin. Alternately, once the
wart has been pared, a lesion sized piece of 40% salicylic acid
plaster can be taped in place. Forty-eight hours later the patient
removes the plaster and repeats the process. The interval between
the reapplication of the plaster can be varied such that discomfort
need not be great. The patient is then seen at biweekly intervals
for paring and re-evaluation of the treatment. All of these

approaches to the treatment of plantar warts require 6 to 10 weeks
of faithful compliance by the patient.

Several specialized therapies for recalcitrant warts also are
available. These include laser therapy, dinitrochlorobenzene (DNCB)
sensitization, and injection with bleomycin or interferon. For the
most part these should be considered as experimental approaches
which are not applicable for use by the generalist.

Placebo therapy (folk cures, hypnosis, over-the-counter
medications, etc.) can be used for all types of warts. The placebo
cure rate for warts is about 30%.

(See also the section on condyloma acuminatum and flat warts.)

SELECTED READING

Lutzner MA: The human papillomaviruses. A review. Arch Dermatol
    119:631, 1983.
Bender ME, Ostrow RS, Watts S, et al: Immunology of human
    papillomavirus: warts. Pediatr Dermatol 1:121, 1983.
Pfister H: Biology and biochemistry of papillomaviruses. Rev
    Physiol Biochem Pharmacol 99:111, 1984.

ACTINIC KERATOSES

DIAGNOSTIC HALLMARKS

1. Sun exposed surfaces of the face, bald scalp, hands,
    and arms
2. Lesions occur on visibly sun damaged skin
3. Lesions occur primarily in fair skinned individuals who
    tan poorly

CLINICAL PRESENTATION

Except for the scale which overlies them, actinic keratoses have
very little apparent substance. Small lesions are often more
apparent on palpation than they are on visualization. They are
barely elevated and feel like slightly roughened spots of skin.
More advanced keratoses appear as small flecks of gray, white, or
slightly yellow scale which seems to be "stuck on" the underlying
skin. Early lesions may be as little as 2 to 4 mm in diameter;
older lesions are 5 to 15 mm in diameter. In both cases they are
wider than they are tall. Actinic keratoses occur against a
background of freckled, atrophic, reddened, telangiectatic, sun
damaged skin. Thus they are found primarily on the face, bald
scalp, and dorsal surface of the hands and arms. Occasionally the
shoulders and back are involved. The development of carcinomatous
proliferation in an advanced actinic keratosis is recognized by the
presence of an underlying nonkeratotic firm papule or a shallow
erosion.

The diagnosis of an actinic keratosis is generally made on a clinical basis. Confirmation, if desired, can easily be obtained by shave biopsy. Lesions which have a papular or an eroded base require biopsy so that the presence of carcinomatous change can be recognized.

COURSE AND PROGNOSIS

Most clinicians believe that actinic keratoses left untreated will eventually transform into squamous cell carcinomas. That potential no doubt exists but it often remains unexpressed. Small actinic keratoses can be left untreated for years at a time without exposing the patient to undue risk. Nevertheless, their premalignant nature should be appreciated by both clinician and patient lest a cavalier attitude lead to the development of an otherwise easily preventable, serious problem. Recurrences at the margins of treated actinic keratoses are frequently seen. These are expected and simply reflect the fact that surrounding skin has shared in significant sun damage. Such lesions should be evaluated on their own merits; the fact of recurrence itself carries no particular implication of malignancy.

PATHOGENESIS

Actinic keratoses consist of localized areas of epithelial cells which are undergoing dysplastic change. These changes are induced by long term exposure to sunlight. The wavelengths of sunlight responsible for carcinogenesis appear to be in the 280- to 310-nm UVB (sunburn) spectrum. Longer wavelengths in the UVA spectrum (310 to 400 nm) may play a synergistic role through the process of photoaugmentation. Oncogenic damage to the skin is not instantaneous. It requires both years of cumulative exposure and a long latent period. Thus patients, often to their considerable surprise, develop their first lesions years after their most intense outdoor exposure. In addition to the quantity of sunlight received, oncogenic risk factors include the quality of the sunlight and the ability of the individual to mount a protective, tanning response. Thus sunlight exposure occurring in equatorial latitudes and at high elevations contains a higher proportion of UVB wavelengths and is proportionally more carcinogenic. Light skinned individuals, particularly those of Celtic origin, who tan poorly are at additional risk. Animal studies show that other environmental effects such as heat, humidity, and wind augment the carcinogenic effect of sunlight.

THERAPY

Individual keratoses which are sharply demarcated are best treated with liquid nitrogen cryotherapy (see Chapter 4). Patients with more diffusely damaged skin can be treated with topically applied fluorouracil (see Chapter 4) if they are willing to accept the unsightly appearance and considerable discomfort which accompanies the use of this agent. Unfortunately, fluorouracil treatment of the hands and arms is considerably less effective than that carried out for the face and bald scalp.

Biopsy is not necessary prior to treating actinic keratoses with either cryotherapy or fluorouracil unless there is clinical evidence of carcinomatous change (see above). However, all treated patients should be re-examined at regular intervals so that new lesions (whether keratoses or carcinomas) can be recognized in their earliest stages.

Patients with actinic keratoses should be taught sun protective techniques. Outdoor work and hobbies should be transferred to the early morning or late afternoon. When midday exposure is necessary protective clothing and hats should be worn. Most important of all, patients should be instructed in the daily use of topically applied sunscreens (see Chapter 4). But even if all of these measures are taken, patients will continue to develop new lesions for many additional years based on the latent damage of previous exposure. Patients should be forewarned of this eventuality so that they do not become discouraged over what appears to be a lack of efficacy of their sun protective efforts.

SELECTED READING

Vitaliano PP, Urbach F: The relative importance of risk factors in nonmelanoma carcinoma. Arch Dermatol 116:454, 1980.
Wulf HC, Poulsen T, Brodthagen H, Hou-Jensen K: Sunscreens for delay of ultraviolet induction of skin tumors. J Am Acad Dermatol 7:194, 1982.
Schreiber MM, Moon TE, Meyskens FL, Murdon JA: Solar ultraviolet radiation and skin cancer. A public education program. Cutis 30:516, 1982.
Lubritz RR, Smolewski SA: Cryosurgery cure rate of actinic keratoses. J Am Acad Dermatol 7:631, 1982.
Abo-Darub JM, MacKie R, Pitts JD: DNA repair in cells from patients with actinic keratoses. J Invest Dermatol 80:241, 1983.
Epstein JH: Photocarinogenesis, skin cancer, and aging. J Am Acad Dermatol 9:487, 1983.
Marks R, Selwood TS: Solar keratoses. The association with erythemal ultraviolet radiation in Australia. Cancer 56:2332, 1985.
Fitzpatrick TB, Sober AJ: Sunlight and skin cancer. N Engl J Med 313:818, 1985.

CORNS AND CALLUSES

DIAGNOSTIC HALLMARKS

1. Distribution: bony prominences of the feet
2. Absence of black dots and pinpoint bleeding when lesions are pared

CLINICAL PRESENTATION

The volar epithelium of the palms, soles, and digits is embryologically designed to undergo a proliferative and hyperkeratotic response as a protective reaction against chronic trauma. Repeated irritation to these tissues results in acanthosis and massive thickening of the stratum corneum. These histologic changes are reflected clinically by the presence of corns or calluses.

Corns appear as sharply marginated, square shouldered, firm papules 3 to 10 mm in diameter. They have a slightly roughened surface and are skin colored to yellow in appearance. They are classically found overlying the interphalangeal joints of the toes especially on the dorsi-lateral surface of the fifth toe but they also occur on the lateral aspect of the fourth toe. These latter lesions are sometimes called "soft" corns. A translucent core lacking blood vessels will be visible if the top of any corn is pared with a scalpel blade.

Calluses are larger lesions with more diffuse, slope shouldered margins. They, too, are skin colored or slightly yellow in appearance and have a slightly roughened surface. Calluses are most commonly found on the medial side of the great toe, around the edges of the heel, and over the plantar surface of the metatarsal heads. Calluses may, of course, occur on the hand if sufficient, chronic trauma is experienced. Calluses, when pared, also generally reveal a translucent central core, but in any event no black dots (thrombosed capillaries) or pinpoint bleeding spots such as are seen in warts are present. Small corns and calluses may be asymptomatic but larger ones are quite painful.

COURSE AND PROGNOSIS

Corns and calluses remain in place as long as the trauma which initiated their presence continues. They disappear spontaneously if and when this trauma can be removed. Pain caused by the thickness and firmness of these lesions sometimes leads to improper foot position while walking. This in turn can cause chronic pain in the foot, knee, or hip. Deformity of the toes is sometimes noted.

PATHOGENESIS

Corns and calluses occur when chronic rubbing or pressure compresses volar epithelium against a firm bony surface. This irritation causes an increased mitotic rate in the epithelium which in turn leads to massive production and retention of stratum corneum cells. It is the widened stratum corneum layer which primarily accounts for the bulkiness of the lesions.

There is no inherent biologic difference between corns and calluses. Corns occur when sharply localized pressure develops over the narrow radius of the heads of the phalanges. More diffuse pressure, especially when it occurs over bone surfaces with less curvature or surfaces better protected by a connective tissue cushion, results in the formation of calluses.

THERAPY

The first step in the treatment of corns and calluses is an attempt to remove the source of chronic trauma. For instance, ill fitting shoes can be discarded, arch supports can be inserted, or metatarsal bars can be added to the sole of the shoes. Second, the thickened, hyperkeratotic portion of the corn or callus can be removed by paring. Third, the remainder of the lesion can be softened by the daily application of a 5 to 10% salicylic acid ointment. The second and third steps can be continued indefinitely if the causative trauma cannot be modified.

On rare occasions orthopedic procedures are required in order to repair underlying bony abnormalities. Surgical excision of corns and calluses is best avoided since it does not get at the cause of the disease and the resultant scarring may only complicate it.

SMOOTH SURFACED WARTS (CONDYLOMA ACUMINATA AND FLAT WARTS)

DIAGNOSTIC HALLMARKS

1. Distribution: face and legs (flat warts); genitalia and
    perirectal area (condyloma acuminata)
2. Tendency for clustering or confluent growth when more than
    one is present

CLINICAL PRESENTATION

Condyloma acuminata and flat warts lack visible or palpable surface keratin and both demonstrate a marked tendency for clustering and a lesser tendency for confluent growth. They are otherwise quite different in appearance.

Condyloma acuminata (venereal warts) appear as thin, flexible, stalk-like papules. They are taller than they are wide. The distal

tip of these warts sometimes has a fine filiform appearance.
Multiple adjacent lesions may develop a confluent growth pattern
forming a large cauliflower-like nodule. On rare occasions dense
mats of the warts can grow over large surface areas so as to almost
occlude the vaginal or rectal orifices. Condyloma acuminata can
grow on any moist surface, but they are most commonly found on the
glans penis, at the vaginal introitis, and at the anal orifice.
Since they are transferred through sexual activity, they are found
most often in young and middle aged sexually active adults.
Condyloma acuminata are asymptomatic. Other morphologic types of
warts may also occur in and around the genitalia. These include
warts with the morphology of verruca vulgaris, large globular
nodules (Buschke-Lowenstein tumors), small rounded papules
(cobblestone warts), and flat warts. The diagnosis is made on a
clinical basis.

Flat warts (verruca plana) appear as barely elevated, square
shouldered, flattopped papules 1 to 3 mm in diameter. These lesions
may be almost inapparent on visual examination. New flat warts
appear rapidly and by the time patients are first examined dense
clusters of the lesions are usually present. Linear arrangements
are sometimes seen because of implantation of viral particles into
scratch marks. Flat warts are generally skin colored but some may
be lightly hyperpigmented compared to adjacent skin. In children
flat warts are most commonly found on the face or on traumatized
surfaces of the arms and legs. In adults the distribution assumed
is often related to shaving. Thus men frequently develop flat warts
on the face whereas they are found on the lower legs in women. As
noted above they may also be located on the genitalia. Flat warts
are asymptomatic. The diagnosis is made on a clinical basis.

COURSE AND PROGNOSIS

Condyloma acuminata appear to be more contagious than other
types of warts. They are not only spread easily on the patient's
own skin through autoinoculation but they also can be passed on to
sexual partners. Left untreated there is the same tendency for
eventual, spontaneous disappearance as is found in verruca
vulgaris. However, evidence is currently accumulating to suggest
that under certain circumstances the papillomaviruses affecting the
genitalia may play a role in the development of genital malignancy.
This evidence is particularly strong in the case of HPV 16 and 18
induced flat warts involving the cervix and in the condition known
as Bowenoid papulosis.

Flat warts, when they occur in children, go through a short
phase of very rapid growth and spread. This is followed by a
plateau period involving little change in growth. The plateau
period is, in turn, succeeded by a phase of steady, rapid,
spontaneous resolution. Flat warts when they occur in adults are

much more stubborn and when left untreated they tend to persist for years. Flat warts occurring on nongenital surfaces are considered as totally benign lesions, but here, too, evidence is accumulating to suggest that at least one subtype of flat wart virus has some oncogenic potential. That potential is now recognized only in the very rare syndrome of epidermodysplasia verruciformis. Overall the oncogenic potential of the human wart viruses seems to depend on the specific subtype of virus involved, the presence of depressed cell mediated immune responsiveness, and probably on the exposure to certain tumor promoters.

PATHOGENESIS

Condyloma acuminata and flat warts appear to be primarily caused by HPV 6 and 11 subtypes of the human papilloma virus. Less commonly HPV 16 and 18 infections are encountered. These latter infections appear to have some oncogenic potential but unfortunately they cannot be separately identified on a clinical basis. Implantation and growth of these viruses seems to require some degree of preceding minor skin trauma.

THERAPY

Filiform condyloma acuminata are best treated with 20 to 25% podophyllin in tincture of benzoin. This compound is applied to the entire surface of the wart; care is taken to avoid contact with normal surrounding skin. Generally instructions are given to wash the painted area 4 to 8 hours later but I do not personally find that this reduces the degree of inflammation and discomfort. Weekly applications for a month will clear 60 to 80% of these lesions. Podophyllin is, however, a very toxic product; only small amounts should be applied on each visit and its use should be avoided during pregnancy. The flatter types of venereal warts are better treated with weekly applications of trichloracetic acid or liquid nitrogen. Large cauliflower-like lesions should be either excised or destroyed with electrosurgical or laser therapy. Anoscopy and speculum examination of the vagina are generally desirable and must be carried out if warts are visible at the rectal or vaginal orifice. Intrarectal and intravaginal warts can be treated with podophyllin, cryotherapy, or laser therapy.

Flat warts on nongenital surfaces are best treated with peeling agents such as Retin-A or benzoyl peroxide. These products are applied once or twice daily just as in acne therapy. Most patients will require 4 to 6 weeks of continuous therapy. Individual lesions can also be treated with daily applications of 16% salicylic acid (Duofilm or Occlusal). Cryotherapy, trichloracetic acid, light electrosurgery, and curettage without electrosurgery are also effective but must be used very carefully.

(See also the section on verruca vulgaris, plantar warts, and paronychial warts.)

SELECTED READING

Margolis S: Therapy for condyloma acuminatum: A review. Rev
    Infect Dis 4:S829, 1982.
Levine RU, Crum CP, Herman E, et al: Cervical papillomavirus
    infection and intraepithelial neoplasia: A study of male sexual
    partners. Obstet Gynecol 64:16, 1984.
Gissmann L, Boshart M, Durst M, et al: Presence of human
    papillomavirus in genital tumors. J Invest Dermatol 83:26S,
    1984.
Lynch PJ: Condyloma acuminata (anogenital warts). Clin Obstet
    Gynecol 28:142, 1985.
Ferenczy A, Mitao M, Nagai N, et al: Latent papillomavirus and
    recurring genital warts. N Engl J Med 313:784, 1985.
Smith KT, Campo MS: The biology of papillomaviruses and their role
    in oncogenesis. Anticancer Res 5:31, 1985.
Obalek S, Jablonska S, Beaudenon S, et al: Bowenoid papulosis of the
    male and female genitalia: Risk of cervical neoplasia. J Am
    Acad Dermatol 14:433, 1986.
Mitchell H, Drake M, Medley G: Prospective evaluation of risk of
    cervical cancer after cytological evidence of human
    papillomavirus infection. Lancet 1:573, 1986
Patterson JW, Kao GF, Graham JH, Helwig EB: Bowenoid papulosis.
    A clinicopathologic study with ultrastructural observations.
    Cancer 57:823, 1986.

BASAL CELL CARCINOMA

DIAGNOSTIC HALLMARKS

1. Distribution: sun exposed portions of the face and
    ears
2. Occurrence against a background of sun damaged skin
3. Rolled, translucent border

CLINICAL PRESENTATION

Basal cell carcinomas appear as smooth surfaced, skin colored, somewhat translucent ("pearly") papules. Lesions 4 to 6 mm in size are flattopped with rounded or rolled shoulders. Those 6 to 8 mm in diameter usually show a central dimpling. Larger lesions frequently have a central ulceration. Telangiectatic vessels are sometimes found on the shoulders of the lesion. The papules are firm on palpation but bleed easily following even minor trauma. They are otherwise asymptomatic. Basal cell carcinomas grow very slowly and patients will sometimes claim that they have been present unchanged

for a year or more. Nearly all basal cell carcinomas are found on
the sun exposed surfaces of the face and ears. An occasional lesion
develops on sun damaged skin of the hands, arms, and shoulders.
They are rarely seen before age 40.

Clinically suspicious lesions should be positively identified by
biopsy.

Uncommon Clinical Presentations. The nevoid basal cell
carcinoma syndrome (also known as the basal cell nevus syndrome) is
a familial syndrome consisting of multiple basal cell carcinomas,
keratotic pits on the palms, keratinous cysts of the jaw, skeletal
abnormalities, cerebral calcification, and a variety of soft tissue
tumors. The development of multiple basal cell carcinomas prior to
the age of 50 or a family history of basal cell carcinomas should
alert the clinician to the possibility of this syndrome.

Superficial basal cell carcinomas are clinically quite distinct
from the papular and nodular lesions described above. They are very
similar to the sharply marginated, red plaques of Bowen's disease.
Both of these in situ carcinomas are listed with the papulosquamous
diseases.

COURSE AND PROGNOSIS

Basal cell carcinomas, left untreated, inexorably enlarge.
Centrifugal growth is accompanied by deep invasion of the dermis
and, eventually, subcutaneous structures. Response to early
treatment is excellent. Five year cure rates of 95 to 100% are
obtainable. Metastases to regional lymph nodes, bone, and lungs
occur in considerably less than 1% of cases.

PATHOGENESIS

Basal cell carcinomas arise from relatively nondifferentiated
epithelial cells of the basal layer of skin and skin appendages.
The induction of this proliferative response seems to depend
primarily on damage done by long term ultraviolet light exposure.
In fact, the factors responsible for the appearance of basal cell
carcinoma are almost identical with those responsible for the
development of actinic keratoses (see above).

THERAPY

Basal cell carcinomas less than 2 cm in diameter can be
successfully treated in several ways: excisional surgery, curettage
and electrosurgery, radiation therapy, and cryosurgery. All four
approaches result in initial cure rates of better than 90% and, when
retreatment for recurrence is added, ultimate cure rates of 98% or
better can be obtained. Excisional surgery has the advantage of
furnishing a complete specimen which may be histologically checked

for adequacy of removal. Cryosurgery and curettage with electrosurgery offer simplicity, speed, and low cost. Radiation therapy results in the least tissue destruction. The choice of modality used depends on the size and location of the lesion, the age of the patient, patient preference, and skills of the operator.

Recurrent lesions and initial lesions larger than 2 cm in diameter are perhaps best treated by the use of microscopically controlled surgery. This approach, often termed the Mohs surgery, results in maximum conservation of tissue and extraordinarily high cure rates (see Chapter 5).

SELECTED READING

O'Dell BL, Jessen RT, Becker LE, et al: Diminished immune response in sun damaged skin. Arch Dermatol 116:559, 1980.

Totten JR: The multiple nevoid basal cell carcinoma syndrome. Cancer 46:1456, 1980.

Vitaliano PP, Urbach F: The relative importance of risk factors in non-melanoma carcinoma. Arch Dermatol 1:454, 1980.

Weiman VM, Ceilley RI, Goeken JA: Cell-mediated immunity in patients with basal and squamous cell skin cancer. J Am Acad Dermatol 2:143, 1980.

Jacobs GH, Rippey JJ, Altini M: Prediction of aggressive behavior in basal cell carcinoma. Cancer 49:533, 1982.

Pollack SV, Goslen JB, Sherertz EF, Jegasothy BV: The biology of basal cell carcinoma: A review. J Am Acad Dermatol 7:569, 1982.

Wilkinson JD: Current treatment of epitheliomas of the skin. Special Symposium on Dermatological Therapy: IV. Treatment of skin tumours. Clin Exp Dermatol 7:75, 1982.

Spiller WF, Spiller RF: Treatment of basal cell epithelioma by curettage and electrodesiccation. J Am Acad Dermatol 11:808, 1984.

Domarus HV, Stevens PJ: Metastatic basal cell carcinoma. Report of five cases and review of 170 cases in the literature. J Am Acad Dermatol 10:1043, 1984.

SQUAMOUS CELL CARCINOMA

DIAGNOSTIC HALLMARKS

1. Distribution: sun exposed surfaces of the face, ears, arms, and hands
2. Association with an actinic keratosis
3. Erosion or ulcer lacking a defined, translucent border

CLINICAL PRESENTATION

Squamous cell carcinoma of the skin is more than a single type
of tumor. At least five clinical variants are recognized. Each of
these has a different appearance and a different prognosis.

By far the most common type of cutaneous squamous cell carcinoma
is that which arises on chronically sun damaged skin in association
with an actinic keratosis. These lesions are called actinically
induced squamous cell carcinomas. Early tumors look much like
ordinary actinic keratoses except that the scale, instead of
appearing flush with the skin, is situated at the summit of a small
skin colored papule. Larger lesions of this type ulcerate and at
that point scale is mixed with, or is replaced by, crust. These
ulcerated lesions resemble basal cell carcinomas, but they usually
lack the sharply defined, rolled translucent border. Not
surprisingly these actinically induced squamous cell carcinomas
occur only against a background of atrophic, telangiectatic, sun
damaged skin.

The second type, known as nodular squamous cell carcinoma,
consists of a dome shaped, skin colored papule or nodule which is
usually ulcerated at the summit. These lesions differ from
actinically induced squamous cell carcinoma by virtue of their
marked outward growth pattern, their hemispherical shape, and their
sharp margination. They may or may not occur on sun damaged skin
and are most commonly located on the lower lip, the ears, and the
dorsal surface of the hands.

The third type of squamous cell carcinoma is the lesion known as
a keratoacanthoma. This lesion, because of its tendency for
spontaneous resolution, is not accepted by all authorities as a true
carcinoma. However, both its histological and clinical appearance
are very similar to the nodular squamous cell carcinoma described
above. Keratoacanthomas are dome shaped, skin colored nodules which
have a distinctive keratin filled, cup shaped crater at the summit.
At first glance this crater is mistaken for an ulceration filled
with crust but closer inspection reveals that the plug is primarily
keratinous.

The fourth type of squamous cell carcinoma arises as a nodular,
ulcerated growth in the margin of a chronic ulcer. These lesions
often are not clearly distinguishable from the edge of the ulcer
itself and thus multiple biopsies should be taken from the margin of
any chronic ulcer which has been present for 5 or more years.

The fifth type of squamous cell carcinoma occurs as a firm,
poorly marginated ulcer at the site of previously administered X-ray
therapy. Such lesions are very slow to develop. They generally
appear 15 or more years after the radiation has been given. This
type of squamous cell carcinoma is identified by the characteristic
pattern of radiation induced atrophy and telangiectasia which
surrounds the ulcerated area.

Uncommon Clinical Presentations. Patients with the recessively
inherited disease xeroderma pigmentosum lack the enzymatic ability
to repair ultraviolet light induced radiation damage to their
deoxyribonucleic acid. These individuals develop large numbers of
cutaneous carcinomas at an early age. They inevitably die as a
result of metastases from these carcinomas.

COURSE AND PROGNOSIS

Left untreated, all squamous cell carcinomas destroy and invade
surrounding tissue in a relentless fashion. The metastatic rate,
however, varies by type. Actinically induced squamous cell
carcinomas have a metastatic rate of 1 to 2%. Nodular squamous cell
carcinomas have a metastatic rate of about 10% and the rate of those
carcinomas arising in radiation damaged skin and in old ulcers is
even higher. Keratoacanthomas for all practical purposes do not
metastasize.

With treatment, actinically induced squamous cell carcinomas
less than 2 cm in size have an excellent prognosis. There is a 10%
recurrence rate following initial treatment but retreatment leads to
an ultimate cure rate of 98% or better. Lesions larger than 2 cm do
less well; 5 year cure rates are about 90 to 95%. Keratoacanthomas
behave benignly but do have a rather high local recurrence rate.

PATHOGENESIS

All types of squamous cell carcinoma appear to arise from
moderately well differentiated epithelial cells. Low grade squamous
cell carcinomas show considerable evidence of keratinization and
have relatively few mitoses per high powered field. More aggressive
squamous cell carcinomas show less evidence of keratinization and
have greatly increased mitotic rates. Actinically induced squamous
cell carcinomas arise as the result of chronic sun damage. These
factors are discussed in greater detail in the section on actinic
keratoses and basal cell carcinomas. Squamous cell carcinomas which
arise in X-ray damaged skin develop because of radiation damage to
deoxyribonucleic acid. The mechanism through which squamous cell
carcinomas arise in chronic ulcers is not known.

THERAPY

The four treatment modalities described for the therapy of basal
cell carcinomas can be used for small actinically induced squamous
cell carcinomas. The other four types of squamous cell carcinomas
and actinically induced lesions larger than 2 cm in diameter are
probably best treated with excisional surgery. Radiation therapy
might be appropriate in older individuals who could not tolerate the
rigors of extensive surgery. Microscopically controlled surgery

(Mohs technique) is usually the treatment of choice for recurrent
lesions.

SELECTED READING

Dzubow LM, Rigel DS, Robins P: Risk factors for local recurrence of
    primary cutaneous squamous cell carcinomas. Treatment by
    microscopically controlled excision. Arch Dermatol 118:900,
    1982.
Immerman SC, Scanlon EF, Christ M, Knox KL: Recurrent squamous cell
    carcinoma of the skin. Cancer 51:1537, 1983.
Barr LH, Menard JW: Marjolin's ulcer. The LSU experience. Cancer
    52:173, 1983.
Lifeso RM, Bull CA: Squamous cell carcinoma of the extremities.
    Cancer 55:2862, 1985.
(See also references for basal cell carcinoma and actinic keratoses.)

EPIDERMOID CYSTS ("SEBACEOUS" CYSTS)

DIAGNOSTIC HALLMARKS

1. Distribution: trunk, face, ears, neck, and scalp
2. Palpable as an encapsulated dermal lesion

CLINICAL PRESENTATION

   Epidermoid cysts are slope shouldered or dome shaped nodules 1
to 4 cm in diameter. They have a smooth surface. Lesions which
have not been traumatized are skin colored or slightly white in
hue. Traumatized lesions may become inflamed and tender (see
Chapter 13). A central pore is occasionally visible at the summit
of the nodule. Palpation reveals a well defined (encapsulated)
spherical nodule which feels deep to the examining finger. Small
lesions have a very firm feel whereas large ones may be slightly
fluctuant. Epidermoid cysts may be confused with lipomas but the
latter feel softer and more lobular. Epidermoid cysts are most
commonly found on the trunk, neck, face, and scalp. Those which
occur on the scalp (trichilemmal or pilar cysts) are colloquially
known as "wens."
   Milia represent a subtype of epidermoid cyst. They are very
small (less than 3 mm in diameter) and are bright white in color.
They are discussed with the white lesions in Chapter 10.
   Confirmation of a clinical diagnosis is occasionally desirable.
Expression of semisolid white material through a stab incision is
pathognomonic. They may also, of course, be excised for biopsy.
   Uncommon Clinical Presentations. True sebaceous cysts (those
filled with sebum rather than keratin) are seen only in the rare
familial syndrome of steatocystoma multiplex. Epidermoid cysts

represent one of the cutaneous components in the nevoid basal cell carcinoma syndrome and in Gardner's syndrome. On very rare occasions microscopic evidence of basal or squamous cell carcinoma may be found on histologic examination of the lining of otherwise typical epidermoid cysts.

COURSE AND PROGNOSIS

Epidermoid cysts, when they first appear, enlarge over weeks or months to a given size and thereafter, unless rupture occurs, remain unchanged and asymptomatic. Chronic irritation or direct trauma occasionally leads to rupture and a resultant marked inflammatory response (see Chapter 13).

PATHOGENESIS

Epidermoid cysts probably arise from embryologic remnants of malformed hair follicles. At some point in adult life the epithelial cells of these remnants begin making keratin. The signal which triggers this activity is unknown but trauma and hormonal stimulation are possible factors. Some cysts open to the surface through a thin follicular orifice but most have no continuity with the surface. A small minority of epidermoid cysts occur as the result of traumatic implantation of epithelial fragments. These buried bits of epithelium then "round up" and begin producing keratin. Such cysts are termed inclusion cysts.

As is probably evident at this point, the old terminology of "sebaceous" cysts is nearly always in error since the cells which line epidermoid cysts produced semisolid white keratin rather than colorless, oily sebum.

THERAPY

Asymptomatic cysts require no medical attention. Those that are cosmetically unacceptable and those that are repeatedly traumatized can be treated in a variety of ways. For small lesions, elliptical excision with suture closure is appropriate and definitive. Some cysts, particularly those on the scalp, can be "delivered" through a simple incision but cyst rupture and resultant incomplete removal of the wall sometimes complicate the procedure. For large cysts it is perhaps best to incise the cyst and extrude the contents in an initial procedure. Over the next several weeks the cyst shrinks considerably in size. A subsequent, excisional removal can then be carried out. The treatment of inflamed cysts is discussed in Chapter 13.

LIPOMAS

DIAGNOSTIC HALLMARKS

1. Distribution: trunk, neck, and proximal extremities
2. Palpable as soft, multilobular masses
3. Long history of stable size

CLINICAL PRESENTATION

Lipomas are slope shouldered or dome shaped nodules 2 to 10 cm in diameter. They have a smooth surface on visual inspection. Lipomas most often occur as isolated lesions but some 5% of patients have multiple lesions. On palpation, lipomas feel soft and somewhat "doughy." They are also multilobular or "lumpy." The spherical, encapsulated feel of epidermoid cysts is lacking. These fatty tumors are most often located on the trunk, neck, and proximal extremities. Lipomas develop during adult life and are ordinarily asymptomatic. The diagnosis is made on a clinical basis. Confirmation if desired can be obtained by biopsy.

COURSE AND PROGNOSIS

Lipomas, when first recognized, have generally reached their final size. They then remain unchanged indefinitely. Lipomas are almost always asymptomatic. Pain and tenderness are sometimes present in the multiple trunk lesions of obese women with Dercum's disease (adiposis dolorosa). Lipomas occur as minor cutaneous components of neurofibromatosis and Gardner's syndrome.

PATHOGENESIS

Lipomas are benign tumors of fat cells. The reason for their occurrence is unknown but genetic factors may be important since familial patterns are sometimes found.

THERAPY

No therapy is indicated for lesions that are stable in size. Excision can be carried out if the patient desires removal.

MOLLUSCUM CONTAGIOSUM

DIAGNOSTIC HALLMARKS

1. Distribution: face and extremities (children); groin and genitalia (adults)

2.   Tendency for clustered formation
3.   Central umbilication

CLINICAL PRESENTATION

Molluscum contagiosum occur as skin colored or white papules 2
to 10 mm in diameter. They are smooth surfaced and dome shaped.
Occasionally lesions are translucent enough to erroneously suggest
vesicle formation. They are, however, firm on palpation. A central
umbilication is present in about 25% of lesions and is a
pathognomonic sign if visible. Molluscum contagiosum may develop
anywhere. In children they are most often found on the face, arms,
and trunk, whereas in adults they are usually present on the inner
thighs, lower abdomen, or genitalia. When multiple lesions are
present there is almost always some evidence of clustering.
Molluscum contagiosum are almost always asymptomatic.
    Clinical diagnosis can be confirmed by biopsy or by the
extrusion of a characteristic white globule of viral protein through
a central incision.

COURSE AND PROGNOSIS

As befits their name and viral origin, molluscum contagiosum are
capable of spreading both on the patient through autoinoculation and
to others through close personal contact. Left untreated, the
number of molluscum lesions generally increases. In children this
increase may be explosive with 20 to 50 lesions occurring in a
matter of several weeks. The growth phase is followed by a period
of relative stability and this in turn is succeeded by a final phase
of spontaneous resolution such that all lesions have usually
disappeared within 12 to 24 months of first appearance. Subsequent
reinfection does not commonly occur. Traumatic extrusion of viral
protein into the surrounding dermis sometimes develops in one or
more lesions. This leads to an inflammatory response which
occasionally is brisk enough to simulate furunculosis.

PATHOGENESIS

The lesions of molluscum contagiosum are caused by a DNA virus
of the Poxvirus group. Viral particles are inoculated into the
epidermis through small cuts and scratches during close personal
contact. After an incubation period which averages about 1 to 2
months, viral replication begins within the cytoplasm of the mid
epidermal keratinocytes. This leads to epithelial cell
proliferation and the development of a visible papule. The
parasitized epidermal cells are recognized as a central white
globule of viral protein which can sometimes be extruded through the
characteristic umbilication. Presumably spontaneous release of

these cells accounts for spread of virus to other areas of skin or
to other individuals.

The molluscum contagiosum virus cannot be cultured and thus
Koch's postulates have not been fulfilled. Antibody response to
molluscum contagiosum virus infection does occur but resolution of
the lesions probably depends on the triggering of a cell mediated
immune response.

THERAPY

Molluscum contagiosum should be treated because of their
potential for spread. In very young children the application of
cantharidin (Cantherone) results in the formation of a subepidermal
blister containing the wart in its roof. Spontaneous sloughing of
the roof and contained wart occurs 7 to 10 days later. The whole
process is essentially painless. In older children and adults,
cryotherapy with liquid nitrogen, application of trichloracetic
acid, or incision followed by curettage work equally well.
Electrosurgery and excision should be avoided as they may result in
unnecessary scarring.

SELECTED READING

Brown ST, Nalley JF, Kraus SJ: Molluscum contagiosum. Sex Transm
     Dis 8:227, 1981.
Pierard-Franchimont C, Legrain A, Pierard GE: Growth and regression
     of molluscum contagiosum. J Am Acad Dermatol 9:669, 1983.
Felman YM: Molluscum contagiosum. Cutis 33:113, 1984.
Niizeki K, Kano O, Kondo Y: An epidemic study of molluscum
     contagiosum. Relationship to swimming. Dermatologica 169:197,
     1984.

MISCELLANEOUS SKIN COLORED PAPULES

Skin tags (acrochordon) are extraordinarily common. They occur
as tiny soft pedunculated papules in the axillae and around the
neck. Occasionally they are somewhat hyperpigmented compared to
surrounding skin. Multiple lesions, sometimes 50 or more in number,
are always present. Skin tags occur primarily in women, especially
those who are obese. Recent controversial studies have suggested
that patients with colonic polyps have an unexpectedly high
frequency of skin tags. Skin tags may be clipped at the base with a
small scissors; anesthesia is not required for this procedure.

Pigmented intradermal nevi become lighter colored as they age.
Some of these may lose all of their pigment and become totally skin
colored. These hypopigmented nevi are found in older adults in whom
they appear as soft dome shaped papules, 4 to 8 mm in diameter.
Occasionally one or more coarse hairs will be observed as growing
from the papule. They are most commonly located on the face and

upper trunk. Softness on palpation and long history of stable size are important diagnostic clues. No treatment is necessary but cosmetically objectionable lesions can be removed by shave excision.

Ganglion cysts are really subcutaneous lesions. They represent outpouchings of synovial sheath between the bones of the hand. They appear as dome shaped or slope shouldered nodules 1 to 3 cm in diameter. They are most often found on the dorsal surface of the wrist or hands. They are asymptomatic and are best left untreated. Their colloquial name "Bible tumor" arises from the fact that temporary resolution sometimes follows a sharp blow with a heavy object.

Mucinous cysts are sometimes encountered on the dorsal surface of distal fingers. These lesions may be skin colored or slightly translucent. They are dome shaped and are medium soft to firm on palpation. When incised, a viscous gel-like material can, with pressure, be extruded. Treatment is best carried out with intralesional steroid injections.

Closed comedones are minute, 2- to 3-mm, dome shaped firm papules occurring on the face. Sometimes a tiny pore is visible at the summit. Open comedones and other lesions of acne may or may not be located on surrounding facial skin. These lesions form as a result of deep keratinous plugging of a pilosebaceous unit. Treatment is not necessary but if desired usually requires incision followed by extrusion of the entrapped keratin through the use of a comedone extractor.

During mid to late adult life individual sebaceous glands on the face can undergo substantial enlargement. These hypertrophic sebaceous glands appear as skin colored or white papules 2 to 4 mm in diameter. The ostia of the follicle is usually visible as a central pore and the whole papule may be somewhat lobulated. No treatment is necessary.

Individual sebaceous glands similar to, but smaller than, those described above can occur ectopically on the lip or buccal mucous membrane. This process is known as Fordyce's condition. It has no medical meaning and requires no treatment.

SELECTED READING

Beitler M, Eng A, Kilgour M, Lebwohl M: Association between acrochordons and colonic polyps. J Am Acad Dermatol 14:1042, 1986.
Sonnex TS: Digital myxoid cysts: A review. Cutis 37:89, 1986.

Group 4:
The White Lesions

GROUP IDENTIFICATION

Lesions must not only be white but must be lighter than the surrounding skin to be classified in this group. For this reason, in very light skinned individuals, it is sometimes difficult to decide whether a lesion should be classified with the skin colored or with the white lesions. When in doubt the list of differential diagnoses should be made up from diseases in both groups.

PITYRIASIS ALBA

DIAGNOSTIC HALLMARKS

1. Distribution: cheeks and lateral arms
2. Children and young adults
3. Lesions lack sharp margins

CLINICAL PRESENTATION

Pityriasis alba consists of poorly marginated, small white patches occurring on the cheeks or lateral arms of children. Anywhere from one to a dozen or more patches may be present. Some lesions, particularly those on the arms, will be studded with pinpoint white papules. These minute papules represent accentuation and keratinization of the follicular orifices. Scale, if visible at all, is fine and light, thus explaining the term "pityriasis" in the name of the disease. On palpation the lesions feel smooth or slightly roughened. Generally the skin in patients with pityriasis alba is quite xerotic. Lesions are most commonly seen in children 3 to 10 years of age. They are rarely present after age 25.

The disease appears to be more common in dark skinned individuals because of the considerable contrast between involved and uninvolved areas. In light skinned individuals the disease is most apparent in the summer time when tanning of surrounding normal skin heightens the contrast. Most lesions are asymptomatic but moderate pruritus is occasionally present. Patients who experience pruritus sometimes scratch and develop lesions of atopic dermatitis within the patches of pityriasis alba.

COURSE AND PROGNOSIS

Pityriasis alba is a chronic disease characterized by periodic exacerbations and remissions. Lesions are almost always less apparent in the winter as surrounding skin fades in color. The lesions do not tan and during the summer they may become reddened with even modest amounts of sunlight exposure. Permanent resolution of the disease slowly occurs during the second or third decade.

PATHOGENESIS

The cause of pityriasis alba is unknown. The condition is primarily seen in those who have a genetic predisposition for the atopic diseases. This fact, together with the frequent presence of xerosis and follicular keratinization, suggests that pityriasis alba is itself a part of the atopic diathesis. The white color is due at least in part to the presence of scale which blocks the effect of ultraviolet light but other defects in melanin production or transfer might also be present.

THERAPY

No effective therapy is available. The application of lubricating cream improves roughness or dryness but it does not improve the color. The use of mild coal tar preparations (see Chapter 4) may be somewhat helpful. Topical application of steroids reduces redness due to sunburn or spontaneous inflammation, but here, too, the pigmentation is not changed.

PITYRIASIS (TINEA) VERSICOLOR

DIAGNOSTIC HALLMARKS

1.   Distribution: chest, back, and shoulders
2.   Sharp margination
3.   Central confluence, peripheral satellite macules
4.   Fine scale, visible only with scraping
5.   Positive KOH preparations

CLINICAL PRESENTATION

The word "versicolor" means various colors. On sun exposed surfaces the lesions are usually white but on covered areas they are often brown or brown-red in color. The initial lesions of tinea versicolor are sharply marginated macules 3 or 4 mm in diameter. Centrifugal growth leads to enlargement and subsequent coalescence of adjacent lesions. Rather large patches may be formed. Small, isolated satellite macules are characteristically found at the periphery of the large patches. Scale is neither visible nor palpable, but when the lesions are scraped with the edge of a scalpel blade, plentiful fine (pityriasis-type) scale can be demonstrated.

Lesions are most commonly found on the central area of the upper chest and back, but where the disease is extensive lesions can also occur on the upper arms, antecubital fossae, lower trunk, and groin. The face is almost always spared. This distribution pattern together with the sharp margination of the lesions helps to clinically distinguish pityriasis versicolor from pityriasis alba.

A clinical diagnosis should be confirmed by way of a KOH preparation. The microscopic appearance of the KOH preparation in pityriasis versicolor is described in Chapter 5. Culture of the organism in ordinary clinical laboratories is not possible.

COURSE AND PROGNOSIS

Pityriasis versicolor occurs at any age but it is found most commonly in teenagers and young adults. Left untreated, the infection persists indefinitely with varying degrees of exacerbation and remission. When the lesions are treated, scale formation stops and the KOH becomes negative. However, the white color present at the site of the lesions remains for several months before normal skin color gradually returns. Patients should be forewarned that this persistence of hypopigmentation is not necessarily an indication of treatment failure. The disease has a marked tendency for recurrence even after adequate treatment has been administered.

PATHOGENESIS

Pityriasis versicolor is caused by the mycelial form of the yeast Pityrosporum orbiculare. This organism, in its spore phase, is a normal inhabitant of the stratum corneum of human skin. The trigger which converts the spore phase to mycelial growth is unknown but environmental factors are probably important. For instance, the prevalence of the disease correlates well with climatic conditions of high heat and high humidity and also correlates with work environments which favor the production of copious sweating. Other factors such as pH and variations in skin lipid formation may also play a role. Treatment presumably reconverts growth of the organism to the spore phase without eradicating it completely from the skin. This hypothesis, if true, would explain the great predilection for periodic recrudescence of the disease. The cause of the hypopigmentation in this disease is not known but the presence of fungal products such as dicarboxylic acids which influence melanin production has been postulated.

THERAPY

Pityriasis versicolor responds to a variety of different treatment programs. Selenium sulfide shampoo (Exsel and Selsun), used as a soap daily for 3 weeks, is the most commonly prescribed medication. Imadazole preparations such as clotrimazole (Lotrimin) or miconazole (Micatin, Monistat), although more expensive, are also quite effective when they are applied twice daily for several weeks. As mentioned above, patients should be forewarned that the whiteness will remain for months following treatment. Orally administered griseofulvin and topically applied tolnaftate (Tinactin, Aftate) are not effective in the treatment of this disease. Ketoconazole in a dose of 200 mg per day for 5 to 10 days does seem to be remarkably efficacious. Since the recurrence rate is very high, patients are well advised to retreat themselves each spring prior to the "tanning season."

SELECTED READING

Faergemann J, Fredriksson T: Tinea versicolor: Some new aspects on etiology, pathogenesis, and treatment. Int J Dermatol 21:8, 1982.
Tanenbaum L, Anderson C, Rosenberg MH, Akers W: 1% sulconazole cream vs. 2% miconazole cream in the treatment of tinea versicolor. Arch Dermatol 120:216, 1984.
Sanches JL, Torres VM: Double-blind efficacy study of selenium sulfide in tinea versicolor. J Am Acad Dermatol 11:235, 1984.
Rausch LJ, Jacobs PH: Tinea versicolor: Treatment and prophylaxis with monthly administration of ketoconazole. Cutis 34:470, 1984.
Dotz WI, Henrikson DM, Yu GSM, Galey CI: Tinea versicolor: A light and electron microscopic study of hyperpigmented skin. J Am Acad Dermatol 12:37, 1985.

VITILIGO

DIAGNOSTIC HALLMARKS

1. Distribution: face, axillae, and dorsal surface of the hands
2. Sharp margination
3. No scale

CLINICAL PRESENTATION

Vitiligo consists of variously sized, white, sharply marginated macules and patches. Centrifugal growth with coalescence of adjacent lesions often results in the formation of large, irregularly shaped areas of depigmentation. The gyrate configuration of such patches is quite distinctive. No scale is present visually or on scraping. The lesions are asymptomatic. Vitiligo can occur at any age but the peak incidence occurs from late childhood to mid adult life.

The lesions of vitiligo are most commonly found on the dorsal surface of the hands, periorificial areas of the face, and in the axillae. Patients with extensive disease may have lesions anywhere. In most instances the distribution pattern is bilateral and fairly symmetrical. However, unilateral, segmental patterns are occasionally seen. In those with very fair skin, lack of contrast between normal and diseased skin makes recognition of the lesions difficult. In such a situation, examination with a Wood's lamp (see Chapter 5) may be helpful.

The diagnosis is made on a clinical basis.

Uncommon Clinical Presentations. Piebaldism, the congenital appearance of a white patch of skin or hair, can be considered as a variant of vitiligo. The white patch remains stable in size and there is little or no likelihood of later extension. Vitiligo occurs along with uveitis in the Vogt-Koyanagi syndrome.

Chronic exposure to certain phenolic compounds found in industrial cleaning solvents occasionally causes areas of hypopigmentation indistinguishable from those seen in vitiligo. In this situation the initial lesions occur on the hands but with the passage of time scattered lesions may appear elsewhere.

COURSE AND PROGNOSIS

Vitiligo usually develops in a few small patches and slowly extends to new areas over succeeding months and years. Then, at some point which cannot be predicted in advance, extension of the disease stops and the process stabilizes. Small areas of repigmentation may develop within the lesions but complete repigmentation is practically never seen. Patients whose initial lesions occur in a segmental distribution have a slightly better chance for early stabilization and even pigment return. Lesions of vitiligo occurring in sun exposed areas sunburn very easily and sometimes present as reddened patches.

At least 10% of patients with vitiligo will have serologic or clinical evidence of one or more associated autoimmune diseases. These include conditions such as autoimmune thyroid disease, Addison's disease, type 1 diabetes mellitus, pernicious anemia, alopecia areata, and uveitis. The conditions may either precede or follow the development of pigment loss.

PATHOGENESIS

Vitiligo may well be an autoimmune process. Evidence for this explanation includes the frequent association with other autoimmune diseases and the recent but unsubstantiated discovery of antibodies directed toward the patient's own melanocytes. As might be expected in an autoimmune disease, genetic factors are also important. Nearly half of all patients with vitiligo will have one or more family members with the same process and the frequency of HLA-D4 seems to be double that of the normal population.

The proximate cause for melanocyte dysfunction and destruction is unknown. Production and retention of toxic intermediates during the formation of melanin are currently under consideration as possible mechanisms.

THERAPY

The treatment of vitiligo is not very satisfactory. The skin in most patients can be induced to regain some color but complete and permanent repigmentation is rarely achieved. Treatment depends on the injestion or application of various psoralen compounds which, because of their photosensitizing properties, stimulate viable but resting melanocytes in the deeper portions of the adnexal structures. The actual treatment program is very similar to that used in psoralen ultraviolet light (PUVA) treatment of psoriasis (see Chapter 4). During treatment the dosage of both the psoralens and the ultraviolet light is manipulated such that mild pinkness is maintained in the depigmented skin. Evidence of response is first recognized by the appearance of brown dots at individual hair follicles within the depigmented area. In about 50% of patients these islands of pigment gradually spread and become coalescent. Unfortunately, much of the regained pigmentation is lost when psoralen therapy is discontinued. It is not possible to predict for a given patient what degree of improvement will occur, although younger individuals and those who have had their disease for only a short time generally respond the best.

Recent reports suggest that there is considerable potential for the therapy of vitiligo with grafts from uninvolved skin containing viable melanocytes. The long term usefulness of this approach remains to be determined.

Rarely, in cases of very extensive vitiligo, it is more practical to lighten the surrounding skin with repeated applications of quinone-type bleaches. If patients choose not to undergo therapy of if therapy is unsuccessful, waterproof opaque makeup such as Lydia O'Leary's Covermark can be used to mask the lesions. If

cosmetic coverup is not carried out sunscreens should be applied to
prevent the occurrence of sun damage.

SELECTED READING

Grimes PE, Minus HR, Chakrabarti SG: Determination of optimal
    topical photochemotherapy for vitiligo. J Am Acad Dermatol
    7:771, 1982.
Naughton GK, Eisinger M, Bystryn J-C: Detection of antibodies to
    melanocytes in vitiligo by specific immunoprecipitation. J
    Invest Dermatol 81:540, 1983.
Foley LM, Lowe NJ, Misheloff E, Tiwari JL: Association of HLA-DR4
    with vitiligo. J Am Acad Dermatol 8:39, 1983.
Grimes PE, Halder RB, Jones C, et al: Autoantibodies and their
    clinical significance in a black vitiligo population. Arch
    Dermatol 119:300, 1983.
Sharquie KE: Vitiligo. Clin Exp Dermatol 9:117, 1984.
Klaus S, Lerner AB: Vitiligo. J Am Acad Dermatol 11:997, 1984.
Suvanprakorn P, Dee-Ananlap S, Pongsomboon C, Klaus SN: Melanocyte
    autologous grafting for treatment of leukoderma. J Am Acad
    Dermatol 13:968, 1985.

MISCELLANEOUS WHITE PATCHES AND PLAQUES

The presence of any inflammatory disease sufficiently severe to
damage melanocytes results in postinflammatory hypopigmentation.
The localization and configuration of the hypopigmentation should
match the historical description of the original reddened area.
Patches of postinflammatory hypopigmentation are often encircled by
a narrow ring of postinflammatory hyperpigmentation.
Postinflammatory hypopigmentation is rather commonly seen following
diaper dermatitis, in the antecubital fossae of individuals with
atopic dermatitis, and on the legs of patients with stasis
dermatitis. Hypopigmentation is also, of course, seen in scarring
processes such as discoid lupus erythematosus, thermal burns, and
other destructive conditions. In these latter situations the
pigment loss is permanent, whereas in the former repigmentation can
be expected within a matter of months.

Morphea is a localized condition characterized by the presence
of scleroderma-like thickening and hardening of connective tissue.
These plaques may be ivory white or waxy colored. The diagnosis is
unmistakable once the lesions are palpated. It is possible for
morphea to occur at any age but most cases begin in childhood. Both
round plaques and linear forms occur.

Lichen sclerosus et atrophicus occurs in two forms. The most
common of these affects the genitalia. In women the lesions appear
as a flat, white, nonscaling patch which surrounds and involves the
vulva. Some cases in adults go on to vaginal stenosis and
effacement of the labia minora. The same condition occurring on the

glans penis is known as <u>balanitis</u> <u>xerotica</u> <u>obliterans</u>. The second
type of lichen sclerosus et atrophicus occurs on the trunk in the
form of small, shiny, flattopped, white papules. In some areas
these will coalesce to form plaques. Later in the course of the
disease the lesions will appear atrophic and wrinkled. Biopsy is
definitive in both types of disease.

The earliest clue to the existence of <u>tuberous</u> <u>sclerosis</u> is
often the presence of small, elliptically shaped, white patches.
These so called "ash leaf" spots are generally no larger than 2 or 3
cm in their long diameter. They may be present at birth or may
develop during the first few years of life. As for almost all white
lesions they are best recognized when the patient is examined in a
dark room with a Wood's lamp (see Chapter 5).

Scaling white patches are sometimes encountered in patients with
sarcoid and leprosy. Individuals with scleroderma occasionally have
small white patches intermingled with hyperpigmented skin on the
chest and arms.

SELECTED READING

Thomas RHM, Ridley CM, Black MM: The association of lichen
    sclerosus et atrophicus and autoimmune-related disease in
    males. <u>Br</u> <u>J</u> <u>Dermatol</u> <u>109</u>:661, 1983.
Serup J: Clinical appearance of skin lesions and disturbances of
    pigmentation in localized scleroderma. <u>Acta</u> <u>Derm</u> <u>Venereol</u>
    <u>64</u>:485, 1984.
Friedrich EG Jr, Kalra PS: Serum levels of sex hormones in vulvar
    lichen sclerosus, and the effect of topical testosterone. <u>N</u>
    <u>Engl</u> <u>J</u> <u>Med</u> <u>310</u>:488, 1984.
Woo TY, Rasmussen JE: Juvenile linear scleroderma associated with
    serologic abnormalities. <u>Arch</u> <u>Dermatol</u> <u>121</u>:1403, 1985.
Piette WW, Dorsey JK, Foucar E: Clinical and serologic expression
    of localized scleroderma. <u>J</u> <u>Am</u> <u>Acad</u> <u>Dermatol</u> <u>13</u>:342, 1985.

MILIA

DIAGNOSTIC HALLMARKS

1.   Distribution: face and dorsal surface of the hands
2.   Size: 2 mm or less in diameter
3.   Firm; filled with white solid material

CLINICAL PRESENTATION

Milia are most often found on the face where they occur as dome
shaped, smooth surfaced white papules 1 to 2 mm in diameter. They
are firm on palpation. No symptoms are associated with their
presence. Similar lesions develop occasionally on the dorsal
surface of the hands and over the knees. In these latter two

locations there is often a history of preceding trauma or bulla
formation.

COURSE AND PROGNOSIS

Once present milia remain indefinitely. The lesions do not
enlarge with the passage of time.

PATHOGENESIS

No cause is known for the development of those lesions which
appear on the face. Those that occur following trauma and blister
formation in diseases such as porphyria cutanea tarda and
epidermolysis bullosa may be due to the implantation of tiny bits of
epithelium. Histologically milia are filled with keratin. They
differ only in size from the epidermoid cysts discussed in Chapter 9.

THERAPY

A No. 11 scalpel blade is used to nick the lesion, after which
the small white keratin plug can be extruded by squeezing or with
compression from a comedone extractor.

KERATOSIS PILARIS

DIAGNOSTIC HALLMARKS

1.   Distribution: lateral arms, anterior thighs, and buttocks
2.   Size: less than 2 mm in diameter
3.   Firm, filled with semisolid white material
4.   Formed at a follicular orifice
5.   Sandpaper feel on palpation

CLINICAL PRESENTATION

Keratosis pilaris is a common condition of children and young
adults. It consists of clustered, firm, white papules approximately
1 mm in diameter. They are most often found on the lateral upper
arms and on the anterior thighs. The buttocks are occasionally
involved. Their presence causes the skin to have a sandpaper-like
feeling. Occasionally an inflammatory halo surrounds the white
papule. The lesions are located at follicular orifices and often
can be scooped out with a fingernail or dermal curet. When this is
done a coiled hair is sometimes found within the white semisolid
material. The lesions are usually asymptomatic though sometimes
mild pruritus is present.

COURSE AND PROGNOSIS

Individual papules come and go over a matter or weeks but the overall course of the process is chronic. The condition gradually disappears during the third decade.

PATHOGENESIS

The lesions of keratosis pilaris occur as keratin plugs at the ostia of hair follicles. The cause of this follicular keratinization is unknown, but since it commonly occurs in association with atopic disorders and several types of ichthyosis, genetic factors are probably important. Lesions similar to keratosis pilaris can be found in patients with hypovitaminosis A.

THERAPY

There is no good treatment for the idiopathic type of keratosis pilaris. Prolonged bathtub soaks followed by mild scrubbing with a stiff brush temporarily remove the plugs but they quickly reform. Lubricants, especially those with lactic acid, may soften the dry skin which usually accompanies the condition. The application of peeling agents such as Retin-A can be tried but the irritation they cause may be more troublesome than any mild benefit which is obtained.

MISCELLANEOUS WHITE PAPULES

The small dome shaped (and sometimes umbilicated) papules of molluscum contagiosum may be white instead of skin colored. Likewise, the facial papules of sebaceous gland hyperplasia which occur in mid or late adult life may appear white (or yellow-white) when the skin around them is stretched. These two diseases are also considered in Chapter 9.

Group 5:
The Brown-Black Lesions

GROUP IDENTIFICATION

Lesions assigned to this group must be darker than the surrounding, normal skin. Colors appropriately considered for the lesions in this group include tan, brown, and black hues. In the case of red-brown colors one might also have to consider the red lesions (Groups 7-10) in forming a list of differential diagnoses.

FRECKLES

DIAGNOSTIC HALLMARKS

     1.   Distribution: sun exposed surfaces
     2.   Fade in winter, darken in summer
     3.   Size: smaller than 4 mm
     4.   Occurrence primarily in children

CLINICAL PRESENTATION

Freckles are light brown macules 1 to 3 mm in diameter. They occur as closely set but not confluent lesions on sun exposed skin. They occur primarily in fair skinned individuals and are particularly prominent in those of Celtic background. Freckles appear in early childhood and may slowly increase in number thereafter. There is a marked tendency for seasonal variation in color: they are darker in the summer and lighter in the winter.

Lentigines and freckles are somewhat similar in clinical appearance but do have different clinical implications. Lentigines are discussed in the section which follows.

COURSE AND PROGNOSIS

Freckles are more or less permanent lesions. However, gradual fading does occur if sunlight stimulation is not maintained year after year. They have no malignant potential, but they do represent sun damage and as such should be viewed as a signal of caution regarding more significant problems in the future. Basically freckles indicate that the individual in question is never going to tan well and that if the present level of sun exposure is continued over a lifetime malignant skin lesions are essentially certain to develop.

PATHOGENESIS

Freckles represent an uneven response of the melanocytes to ultraviolet light exposure in individuals who do not tan well. Histologically there is no increase in the number of melanocytes but individual melanocytes show evidence of increased stimulation: the cells are more prominent, they are filled with more melanosomes, and their dendritic processes are longer and more numerous.

THERAPY

No therapy is necessary. Some bleaching effect can be obtained through long term application of hydroquinone (Eldoquin Forte, Melanex) and regular application of sunscreens.

LENTIGINES

DIAGNOSTIC HALLMARKS

1. Distribution: sun exposed surfaces of the face, hands, and shoulders
2. No seasonal variation in pigment density
3. Size: 5 to 20 mm
4. Occurrence in adults

CLINICAL PRESENTATION

Lentigines (singular: lentigo) are light brown to dark brown macules 5 to 20 mm in diameter. They occur singularly or as multiple, closely set (but not confluent) lesions on chronically sun exposed skin. They are particularly common on the cheeks, dorsal surface of the hands, and top portion of the shoulders. Unlike freckles, lentigines do not appear until mid adult life and their pigmentation is constant without seasonal variation. They are also darker in color, larger in diameter, and more irregularly shaped. Lentigines are most commonly found on fair skinned individuals but they can also develop on more darkly pigmented patients.

COURSE AND PROGNOSIS

Lentigines are permanent lesions. Continued sunlight exposure is not necessary to maintain their activity. Those occurring on the hands, arms, and shoulders can be considered as having no malignant potential. For the most part this is also true for those that occur on the face. However, a small proportion of these latter lesions develop into lentigo maligna or lentigo maligna melanoma.

Atypical Manifestations. Sometimes one or more lentigines on the face will develop small speckles of dark pigmentation superimposed on the lighter brown background color of the original lesion. Biopsy of these brown-black speckles reveals appreciable dysplasia of individual melanocytes situated in the basal layer of the epidermis. Such lesions are called lentigo maligna (Hutchinson's freckle) and they should be considered as obligate precursors for invasive melanomas (see section on melanomas). The lesions of lentigo maligna should be removed by way of surgical excision with narrow (2- to 5-mm) margins.

A lesion known as lentigo simplex can be differentiated from the actinically induced lentigines discussed above. Lentigo simplex occurs as scattered black macules no larger than 3 mm in diameter. They occur at any time from the teen years to late adult life, but based on their randomly scattered distribution pattern, their development seems to be unrelated to sunlight exposure. Histologically they are similar to actinically induced lentigines except there is less elongation of the rete ridges and there is more evidence of incontinent melanin in dermal melanophages. Occasionally a few nests of junctional nevus cells will also be present. The lesions of lentigo simplex are particularly likely to be seen in individuals with the dysplastic nevus syndrome.

PATHOGENESIS

Lentigines for the most part arise because of chronic ultraviolet light exposure. Histologically there is hyperpigmentation due both to increased activity and increased numbers of individual melanocytes. There is, however, no clustering of melanocytes (nest formation) such as seen in nevi. The keratinocytic compartment of the epidermis is also enlarged by way of finger-like elongation of the rete ridges.

THERAPY

Those lentigines which are evenly colored throughout require no
therapy. They are best left untreated but some bleaching can be
obtained through long term application of hydroquinone (Eldoquin
Forte, Melanex) and sunscreens. Some lentigines develop black
speckling with the passage of time. In these instances an area of
the lentigo containing prominent speckling should be biopsied. If
the changes of lentigo maligna are present the entire lesions ought
to be surgically excised. Lesions containing areas of black
speckling which are palpable should be excised with a presumptive
diagnosis of lentigo maligna melanoma.

SELECTED READING

Clemmensen O: Hutchinson's freckle. Am J Dermatopathol 4:425, 1982.
Green A, Little JH, Weedon D: The diagnosis of Hutchinson's
    melanotic freckle (lentigo maligna) in Queensland. Pathology
    15:33, 1983.

JUNCTIONAL, COMPOUND, AND INTRADERMAL NEVI

DIAGNOSTIC HALLMARKS

1.   Distribution: random; but some predilection for sun
      exposed skin
2.   Size: 3 to 7 mm
3.   Round and evenly pigmented
4.   Long history of unchanged appearance

CLINICAL PRESENTATION

Nevi are pigmented lesions which may be flat (junctional) or
elevated (compound and intradermal). They generally vary in color
from light brown to dark black but some intradermal nevi in older
adults are so lightly pigmented as to appear skin colored. They
range in size from 2 to 10 mm but most are 3 to 7 mm in diameter.
For the most part nevi are remarkably round, evenly pigmented, and
soft on palpation.

Nevi may be found anywhere on the body including the scalp,
palms, soles, mucous membranes, and nail matrix. They are, however,
more numerous on sun exposed surfaces. Everyone except true albinos
have one or more nevi and in some individuals hundreds may be
present. Junctional nevi, because of their flatness, may be
confused with freckles and lentigines, but the junctional nevus
tends to be larger, darker, and more perfectly round. A few nevi
may be present at birth but most develop during the childhood
years. The development of new nevi in mid and late adult life is

uncommon. Nevi in children are predominantly junctional whereas in adults they are usually compound or intradermal.

The diagnosis of a nevus is generally made on a clinical basis. Pigmented lesions which cannot be reliably recognized as benign nevi should be biopsied. Discussion of the clinical differences between nevi and melanomas is found in Chapter 23.

COURSE AND PROGNOSIS

Nevi are very stable lesions. Once present they change very little in size or color. However, over a lifetime nevi may pass through successive stages of junctional, compound, and intradermal development. Evidence that this occurs is based primarily on the predominance of junctional nevi in children and of intradermal nevi in older adults. Longitudinal studies showing such transitions have not, however, been carried out.

The overwhelming majority of nevi are, and will remain, benign lesions. The odds that any one nevus will undergo malignant degeneration are probably on the order of 1 in 100,000. Unfortunately, except for dysplastic nevi, there is no way to identify prospectively which nevi will evolve into melanomas. There are some theoretical reasons to believe that chronic trauma might increase the risk of melanoma development and for this reason some physicians in the past recommended the prophylactic removal of nevi from palms, soles, genitalia, and belt lines. However, at the practical level there is no evidence to support this belief and since 10% of the population have nevi in such locations it is clear that removal of all such lesions would be quite impractical.

PATHOGENESIS

The cells which make up pigmented nevi are called nevus cells. Nevus cells are almost certainly derived from melanocytes which had migrated to the epidermis from the neural crest during early fetal development. The transition from melanocytes to nevus cells appears to involve a "rounding-up" and loss of dendritic processes as the cells proliferate in a clustered, or nest-like, pattern. Pigment production in nevus cells appears identical with that of melanocytes.

In junctional nevi the clusters of nevus cells are found solely at the dermal-epidermal junction. In compound nevi the clusters of nevus cells are located both at the dermal-epidermal junction and within the upper portions of the dermis. In intradermal nevi the nests of nevus cells appear solely within the dermis.

The significance of nevi and the reasons for their development are unknown. Since everyone has them and since some of them develop during fetal life, it is tempting to consider them as normal components of human skin. On the other hand, there are also several reasons to consider them as pathologic processes. First, they continue to develop in postfetal life. Second, their distribution seems greatly influenced by patterns of ultraviolet light exposure. Third, from time to time the body mounts a lymphocytic, destructive attack against them in the process clinically recognized as halo nevus formation. Finally, some of the large congenital nevi (see below) have an unusually high rate of malignant transformation.

THERAPY

Normal nevi need not be removed regardless of their location. However, lesions which demonstrate one or more atypical characteristics (see below and Chapter 23) and those which are cosmetically unacceptable can be removed in a variety of ways. Most dermatologists favor the use of shave biopsy for reasons of simplicity and freedom from scarring. This approach works well for middle aged and older adults. However, in younger individuals, shave biopsy is followed by a very high recurrence rate of speckled pigmentation. This is a development which is disturbing to doctor and patient alike. For this reason I prefer the use of elliptical excision with suture closure in patients under the age of 30. I believe that all nevi should be histologically examined at the time of removal and thus am opposed to the destruction of such lesions with electrosurgery, cryosurgery, or chemocautery.

SELECTED READING

Mackie RM, English J, Aitchison TC, Fitzsimons CP, Wilson P: The number of distribution of benign pigmented moles (melanocytic naevi) in a healthy British population. Br J Dermatol 113:167, 1985.

Green A, MacLennan R, Siskind V: Common acquired naevi and the risk of malignant melanoma. Int J Cancer 35:297, 1985.

DYSPLASTIC NEVI

DIAGNOSTIC HALLMARKS

1. Distribution: back, chest
2. Color variation within and among the nevi
3. Red-brown hues

CLINICAL PRESENTATION

Some pigmented nevi have clinical features which make them suspect as possible precursors of melanomas. These include: 1) lesions with red or red-brown hues; 2) lesions larger than 7 mm (lead pencil eraser size) in diameter; 3) irregular, rather than perfectly round, shapes; and 4) speckled, rather than evenly spread, pigmentation. Lesions possessing these features clinically are also noted to have certain histologic features (see below) which confirm their nature as dysplastic nevi.

Dysplastic nevi occur in two major settings. The first is that of individuals of northern European (usally Celtic) background with light hair color and freckled complexion. It would appear that such individuals are poorly able to protect their skin from ultraviolet light damage through tanning and that their dysplastic nevi generally arise as a result of chronic sunlight exposure. The second is that of a familial setting in which other family members also have dysplastic nevi and in which there may be a history of one or more melanomas in the patient or in the family. Such individuals are said to have the familial dysplastic nevus syndrome.

COURSE AND PROGNOSIS

Individuals with the familial dysplastic nevus syndrome are almost certain to develop one or more melanomas with the passage of time. Some authorities believe these individuals are also at risk for the development of nonmelanomatous malignancy as part of a "cancer prone family" syndrome.

Patients with acquired dysplastic nevi are also at increased risk for the development of cutaneous melanomas though no consensus regarding the degree of risk as of yet exists.

In either case individual lesions can undergo malignant change within a matter of months and all patients with dysplastic nevi deserve extraordinarily close and careful follow-up.

PATHOGENESIS

A definite histologic pattern is correlated with the clinical appearance of dysplastic nevi. Some of the microscopic features include individual cell atypia, bridging of adjacent rete ridges with enlarged nests of nevus cells, and the presence of a lymphocytic, inflammatory dermal infiltrate. The reasons for the development of these clinical and histologic changes are not understood. As indicated above, genetic aspects (both in the sense of individual families and from a standpoint of certain nationalities) are undoubtedly important. Sunlight damage also plays a role based on distribution patterns, history of undue exposure (especially in the form of sunburn), and the presence of associated, nonmelanocytic evidence of sun damage. However, sun damage is not absolutely necessary as evidenced by the not infrequent presence of dysplastic nevi on the buttocks, scalp, and female breasts.

THERAPY

No consensus exists as to how these patients should be cared
for. First, of course, the diagnosis must be established. This
requires the biopsy of one or more clinically suspicious lesions.
Once a diagnosis has been confirmed patients should be followed at
6-month intervals. Some authorities believe that all the nevi
should be photographed so that on subsequent visits those lesions
which on comparison show even minor degrees of change can be
surgically removed. Others recommend surgical removal of all
lesions demonstrating any clinically suspicious features regardless
of whether or not change can be demonstrated. Still others rely on
clinical judgment regarding change with isolated removal of only
those lesions which have changed grossly. In any event when removal
is to be carried out nearly all recommend that this be done by total
excision rather than by shave technique.

SELECTED READING

Sagebiel RC, Banda PW, Schneider JS, Crutcher WA: Age distribution
    and histologic patterns of dysplastic nevi. J Am Acad Dermatol
    13:975, 1985.
Kopf AW, Lindsay AC, Rogers GS, et al: Relationship of nevocytic
    nevi to sun exposure in dysplastic nevus syndrome. J Am Acad
    Dermatol 12:656, 1985.
Rigel DS, Friedman RJ, Kopf AW, et al: Precursors of malignant
    melanoma. Problems in computing the risk of malignant melanoma
    arising in dysplastic and congenital nevocytic nevi. Dermatol
    Clinics 3:361, 1985.
Rigel DS, Friedman RJ; The management of patients with dysplastic
    and congenital nevi. Dermatol Clinics 3:251, 1985.
Greene MH, Clark WH Jr, Tucker MA, et al: High risk of malignant
    melanoma in melanoma-prone families with dysplastic nevi. Ann
    Intern Med 102:458, 1985.
Friedman RJ, Heilman ER, Rigel DS, Kopf AW: The dysplastic nevus.
    Clinical and pathologic features. Dermatol Clinics 3:239, 1985.
Greene MH, Clark WH Jr, Tucker MA, Elder DE: Acquired precursors of
    cutaneous malignant melanoma. The familial dysplastic nevus
    syndrome. N Engl J Med 312:91, 1985. (color photos)

MELANOMA

Malignant melanoma occurs in several distinct clinical
settings. In each of these settings the melanoma has a different
clinical appearance, histologic pattern, and prognosis. These
various types of melanoma are grouped together because they share
common color changes, a common cell of origin, and the important
biologic trait of progressive, inexorable growth.

DIAGNOSTIC HALLMARKS (see also Chapter 23)

1.   Distribution: pattern variable with type of melanoma
2.   Irregular shape
3.   Irregular pigmentation
4.   History of change in size or color

CLINICAL PRESENTATION

    Superficial Spreading Melanoma. This tumor, the most common of melanomas, presents as a relatively flattopped, slowly growing, pigmented papule or plaque. It is characterized by the following features. First, the lesion generally has an irregular rather than round configuration. This irregularity in shape occurs because of a differential growth rate in one or more portions of the lesion. Second, the lesion is usually irregularly pigmented. Most commonly this takes the form of black speckling, but in larger, more advanced lesions there are often distinct areas of red, white, or blue color. Third, the lesion is almost always wider than it is tall. This occurs because there is a long period of horizontal (centrifugal) growth before appreciable vertical growth (invasion) begins. Fourth, in larger, more advanced lesions the surface has a somewhat "bumpy" or lobulated appearance due to the same differential growth rates which resulted in the development of an irregular configuration. Finally, there may be pigment spread ("bleeding of pigment") from the periphery of the lesion onto the normal adjacent skin.
    Superficial spreading melanomas are most commonly found on sun exposed areas of skin. In men the back is the area most frequently involved whereas in women the legs are the most common site. Because they grow so slowly and are asymptomatic, superficial spreading melanomas are often serendipitously identified during routine examination for other medical reasons.
    Nodular Melanoma. Nodular melanomas appear as dome shaped, darkly pigmented papules or nodules. They grow considerably faster and develop a deeper color than superficial spreading melanomas. These two traits are likely to bring them to the attention of patients. Nodular melanomas, in contrast to superficial spreading melanomas, are also more evenly pigmented, are as tall as they are wide, and tend to have a smooth rather than lobulated surface. Changes which occur in well advanced lesions include the spread of pigment onto surrounding skin, the presence of satellite papules, and the development of an erosion or ulcer on the surface of the tumor.
    Amelanotic variants of nodular melanoma can occur but are rarely seen. Such lesions simulate the appearance of pyogenic granulomas because of their reddish color but are otherwise clinically similar to the pigmented variety described above.

Nodular melanomas are unrelated to chronic sunlight damage and thus may be seen on any portion of the body. In darkly pigmented individuals they are particularly common on the soles of the feet.

Lentigo Maligna Melanoma. These lesions are found almost exclusively on the face of elderly adults. They arise from a pre-existing lentigo (lentigo maligna) and thus appear as one or more small darkly pigmented papules superimposed on a flat, light brown patch. The black, smooth surfaced papule has all the physical characteristics of a nodular melanoma except those of smaller size and slower growth rate. Here again the very slow growth rate fails to disturb the patient and these lesions are often first recognized during the course of a routine examination.

Acrolentiginous Melanoma. This variant has only recently been recognized as a separate type of melanoma. It consists of one or more dark, smooth papules appearing against a background of gray or black macular, unevenly speckled pigmentation. It is the most common type of melanoma occurring on the digits and on the palms and soles. Although it shares some clinical features with lentigo maligna melanoma, its growth characteristics are those of nodular melanoma.

For all practical purposes the melanomas described above occur only after the age of puberty. A rapidly growing pigmented papule in a child will, on biopsy, usually turn out to be a benign spindle and epitheloid cell nevus (Spitz nevus).

COURSE AND PROGNOSIS

The outlook for patients with melanoma depends on several interrelated factors such as the clinical type of lesion, the presence or absence of lymphadenopathy, and the histologic level of dermal invasion. Thus patients with a lentigo maligna melanoma present with a 5- to 10-year history of slow growth and are unlikely to have palpable regional nodes. Histologically the lesion is likely to be quite superficial. On the other hand, superficial spreading melanomas when first recognized have usually been present for 2 to 5 years. Lymphadenopathy is only occasionally present and histologically the lesions are either superficial or intermediate in depth. Finally, nodular melanomas are usually noted by the patient within the first 6 to 12 months of appearance. Lymphadenopathy is frequently present and histologically the lesions are often deeply invasive.

Among the factors discussed above, the one which most closely correlates with prognosis is the histologic depth of invasion. This is best determined by micrometer measurement of the thickness of the tumor (Breslow technique). Thus 5-year survival rates for patients with tumors less than 0.75 mm in thickness are nearly 100%. Rates for those with tumors 0.75 to 1.5 mm in thickness and for those with tumors thicker than 1.5 mm are approximately 85% and 60%,

respectively. The prognosis for patients in these last two groups
can be further refined based on the status of their regional lymph
nodes. The presence of microscopic metastases in more than one or
two nonpalpable nodes reduces the survival rate by at least 20%.
The presence of clinically evident, palpable nodes, regardless of
the depth of the primary lesion, reduces the eventual survival rate
to only a few percent.

Nevertheless, in spite of the figures given above, it should be
recognized that melanoma can at times be very slow growing and that
it is the malignancy with the highest rate of spontaneous
regression. Moreover, there have been many individual case reports
of patients who have lived with metastatic disease for exceptionally
long periods of time.

PATHOGENESIS

During the last 30 years the incidence of melanoma has
approximately doubled each decade. Most of this increase has been
due to larger numbers of superficial spreading melanomas. This type
of melanoma occurs primarily on the sun exposed skin of individuals
who tan poorly. However, in contrast to the situation with other
types of skin cancer where total lifetime exposure appears critical,
the risk in melanoma may be more closely related to the number and
severity of individual episodes of sunburn.

Genetic factors may also play a role in the pathogenesis of
melanomas. About 10% of patients have a positive family history for
melanoma. This genetic predisposition is most marked in the
dysplastic nevus syndrome where an astonishingly large proportion of
family members develop multiple primary melanomas.

A third predisposing factor revolves around the presence of
certain congenital nevi. Thus a patient with a giant hairy
congenital nevus (see below) has a risk of developing a melanoma
which may be 100 times greater than the risk of those with ordinary
acquired nevi.

A fourth factor relates to the presence of immune
responsiveness. Individuals with either innate or iatrogenic
reduction in immune responsiveness appear to be at increased risk
for the development of melanomas even as they are for the
development of other types of malignancy.

Finally hormonal factors may also be important. Men have an
increased incidence of melanomas and also have a considerably poorer
prognosis when compared to women having similar types of lesions.

THERAPY

Therapy is based primarily on tumor thickness. Lesions thinner
than 0.75 mm require only wide local resection. Historically
margins of 3 to 5 cm have been obtained but recent reports suggest

that 1.5- to 2.0-cm margins are entirely adequate. In fact, it is
appropriate to suggest that such thin lesions be removed with the
widest margins that can be obtained without necessitating the
placement of a graft. Lymph node metastases rarely occur in these
thin lesions and thus lymphadenectomy is not routinely carried out.

Lesions with a thickness of 0.75 to 1.5 mm are handled more
aggressively. Local recurrences are relatively common and thus
margins wide enough to require grafting may be necessary. Palpably
enlarged lymph nodes are removed; an en bloc excision is done where
feasible. No consensus is available regarding the necessity of
regional lymphadenectomy in tumors of this thickness when nodes are
not palpable. Microscopic metastases are found about 20% of the
time when nonpalpable nodes are removed but patients having only one
or two nodes with involvement seem to have a prognosis as good as
that for those without microscopic metastases.

The treatment of melanomas thicker than 1.5 mm falls outside the
scope of this book. Interested readers are referred to the current
literature and to standard textbooks in oncology and surgery.

SELECTED READING

Beral V, Evans S, Shaw H, Milton G: Cutaneous factors related to
    the risk of malignant melanoma. Br J Dermatol 109:165, 1983.
Trau H, Rigel DS, Harris MN, et al: Metastases of thin melanomas.
    Cancer 51:553, 1983.
Balch CM, Soong S-J, Milton GW, et al: Changing trends in cutaneous
    melanoma over a quarter century in Alabama, USA, and New South
    Wales, Australia. Cancer 52:1748, 1983.
Reintgen DS, Cox EB, McCarty KS Jr, et al: Positive efficacy of
    elective lymph node dissection in patients with intermediate
    thickness primary melanoma. Ann Surg 198:379, 1983.
Adam YG, Efron G: Cutaneous malignant melanoma: Current views on
    pathogenesis, diagnosis, and surgical management. Surgery
    93:481, 1983.
Kopf AW, Kripke ML, Stern RS: Sun and malignant melanoma. J Am
    Acad Dermatol 11:674, 1984.
Aitken DR, James AG, Carey LC: Local cutaneous recurrence after
    conservative exvision of malignant melanoma. Arch Surg 119:643,
    1984.
Cosimi AB, Sober AJ, Mihm MC, Fitzpatrick TB: Conservative surgical
    management of superficially invasive cutaneous melanoma. Cancer
    53:1256, 1984.
Balch CM, Karakousis C, Mettlin C, et al: Management of cutaneous
    melanoma in the United States. Surg Gynecol Obstet 158:311,
    1984.
MacKie RM, Young D: Human malignant melanoma. Int J Dermatol
    23:433, 1984.
Roses DF, Harris MN, Gumport SL: Surgery for primary cutaneous
    malignant melanoma. Dermatol Clinics 3:315, 1985.

Rigel DS, Rogers GS, Friedman RJ: Prognosis of malignant melanoma.
    Dermatol Clinics 3:309, 1985.
Lew RA, Kohn HK, Sober AJ: Epidemiology of cutaneous melanoma.
    Dermatol Clinics 3:257, 1985.
Friedman RJ, Rigel DS: The clinical features of malignant
    melanoma. Dermatol Clinics 3:271, 1985.
Metcalf JS, Maize JC: Melanocytic nevi and malignant melanoma.
    Dermatol Clinics 3:217, 1985.
Elder DE, Guerry D, VanHorn M, et al: The role of lymph node
    dissection for clinical stage I malignant melanoma of
    intermediate thickness (1.51-3.99 mm). Cancer 56:413, 1985.
Urist MM, Balch CM, Soong S-J, et al: The influence of surgical
    margins and prognostic factors predicting the risk of local
    recurrence in 3445 patients with primary cutaneous melanoma.
    Cancer 55:1398, 1985.
Naruns PL, Nizze JA, Cochran AJ, et al: Recurrence potential of
    thin primary melanomas. Cancer 57:545, 1986.

SEBORRHEIC KERATOSES

DIAGNOSTIC HALLMARKS

1. Distribution: chest, back, and face
2. Square shouldered, sharp margination
3. "Stuck on" appearance

CLINICAL PRESENTATION

Seborrheic keratoses are flattopped, brown papules 5 to 20 mm in diameter. They are sharply marginated and square shouldered in cross section. They are always wider than they are tall and their superficial, exophytic growth pattern gives them a "stuck on" appearance. Early, relatively flat lesions are generally light brown in color whereas more advanced, elevated lesions are dark brown or even black. Visible scale is often lacking on early lesions but may be quite apparent on older, larger lesions. Scraping with the edge of a scalpel blade will reveal the presence of scale on lesions of all stages.

Seborrheic keratoses are most commonly found on the chest and back but they may also occur on the face and arms. Those that occur around the folds of the neck and near the axillae are often only 2 or 3 mm in diameter and may closely resemble skin tags. Seborrheic keratoses begin to develop in mid adult life and they are universally present by age 60. The number of lesions found on patients varies greatly. Some individuals will have only one or two whereas in others as many as 50 to 100 may be present.

The diagnosis of seborrheic keratoses is established clinically. They are usually easy to recognize but sometimes they

are confused with actinic keratoses. This problem in differential
diagnosis is covered in Chapter 22. Confirmation of a clinical
diagnosis can easily be obtained by way of shave biopsy.

COURSE AND PROGNOSIS

The number of seborrheic keratoses present on an individual
gradually increases over a period of years. They are permanent
lesions. Once an individual lesion has fully matured it remains in
place, unchanged, indefinitely. The number of lesions and the age
at which they develop seem to be at least partially dependent on
genetic, familial patterns.

Seborrheic keratoses are benign lesions which have no malignant
potential. However, the explosive development of hundreds of
lesions sometimes serves as a clue to the presence of an internal
malignancy. This rarely seen phenomenon is known as the sign of
Leser-Trelat.

PATHOGENESIS

Seborrheic keratoses represent the proliferation of moderately
well differentiated cells from the basal layer area of the
epidermis. However, unlike the situation in basal cell carcinomas,
these cells do show evidence of keratinization. Moreover, the cells
of a seborrheic keratosis never proliferate in an uncontrolled
fashion nor do they invade the dermis by breaking through the
basement membrane zone.

The reason for the development of these benign tumors is
unknown. Their appearance in late adult life suggests that they may
be part of the aging process. Genetic factors may also be important
since familial patterns in terms of numbers of lesions and age of
onset are often seen. Chronic sunlight exposure seems to play no
role in their development.

THERAPY

Seborrheic keratoses require no therapy. Nevertheless, patients
sometimes wish to have them removed because of their unsightliness
and their tendency to catch on clothing. This can be accomplished
in a number of ways. Their superficial location allows for easy
destruction with cryosurgery or chemocauterants (see Chapter 5).
Alternatively they can be destroyed with light electrosurgery or can
be removed by shave biopsy. Because of their pigmented nature the
latter method, which results in a suitable specimen for histologic
examination, is preferable for less experienced clinicians. All of
these methods result in rather superficial destruction and their use
is occasionally followed by partial regrowth. These recurrent
lesions can simply be retreated as necessary.

DERMATOFIBROMAS

DIAGNOSTIC HALLMARKS

1. Distribution: legs and shoulders
2. Invagination when squeezed from sides

CLINICAL PRESENTATION

Dermatofibromas are firm, slope shouldered or dome shaped papules 10 to 15 mm in diameter. The summit of the lesion is often skin colored or only light brown in color whereas the lower portion and immediately adjacent normal skin are usually quite a bit darker in pigmentation. When these papules are compressed between the thumb and forefinger they tend to invaginate rather than "pop up." This "pucker" sign is surprisingly reliable in distinguishing dermatofibromas from other pigmented papules. Dermatofibromas are common lesions. They can be found in 20% of women and 5% of men. The most common location is that of the lower leg but thigh and shoulder lesions are also frequently encountered. Most often only a single lesion is present.

COURSE AND PROGNOSIS

Dermatofibromas are benign lesions with no malignant potential. They, like other pigmented lesions, darken during pregnancy and in this setting are occasionally suspected clinically of being melanomas. Unsubstantiated reports suggest that multiple dermatofibromas develop with unexpected frequency in patients with lupus erythematosus.

PATHOGENESIS

As the name implies, the histology of dermatofibromas is that of a localized area of connective tissue overgrowth. Occasionally there is a significant component of histiocytic cells or vascular tissue. The cause for the appearance of this hamartoma is completely unknown.

THERAPY

No therapy is necessary. Occasionally lesions will need to be removed in order to histologically rule out the presence of a melanoma. Partial removal, such as occurs with shave biopsy, is followed by regrowth to the original size. Thus, excision is favored when removal is necessary. Some authorities believe that appreciable improvement in size and consistency of lesions occur when they are treated with cryotherapy.

MISCELLANEOUS BROWN PAPULES AND NODULES

Skin tags (see Chapter 9) are occasionally hyperpigmented. These lesions do not otherwise differ from their skin colored counterparts.

Flat warts (see Chapter 9) are also occasionally hyperpigmented. Here, too, the prognosis and therapy are no different than for skin colored lesions.

Open comedones are occluded hair follicles in which the keratin plug is visible within the ostium as a black, partially depressed dot. Confirmation of a diagnosis is obtained by compression of the lesion which results in extrusion of the plug. Similar black plugs sometimes occur at the outlet of epidermoid cysts.

Actinic keratoses sometimes present as small, brown, rough surfaced papules. The color may be related to melanin granule retention in the multiple layers of the hyperkeratotic stratum corneum which histologically characterize this lesion. Brown actinic keratoses have no particular clinical significance.

CAFE-AU-LAIT PATCHES

DIAGNOSTIC HALLMARKS

1.   Distribution: random
2.   Flat, nonpalpable
3.   Homogeneous, light brown color

CLINICAL PRESENTATION

Individual cafe-au-lait patches are flat, light brown, evenly pigmented patches 1 to 10 cm in diameter. Most lesions are round but irregular and angular shapes are also seen. Cafe-au-lait patches may be present at birth but sometimes they do not develop until childhood. Clinically, it is not possible to distinguish a solitary cafe-au-lait patch from the flat, brown birthmarks which occur in about 10% of the population.

COURSE AND PROGNOSIS

Individuals with more than four or five pigmented patches greater than 1 cm in diameter are rather likely to develop associated features of neurofibromatosis. Lesions somewhat similar in appearance to cafe-au-lait patches are also found in Albright's syndrome.

Cafe-au-lait patches are permanent. Once present they remain stable in size and color indefinitely. There is no predisposition to melanoma formation in these pigmented lesions.

PATHOGENESIS

The cause of cafe-au-lait patches is unknown. Electron
microscopy reveals the presence of larger then normal melanin
granules within the melanosomes of the melanocytes.

THERAPY

No therapy is available or necessary.

GIANT PIGMENTED CONGENITAL NEVI

DIAGNOSTIC HALLMARKS

    1.   Distribution: random
    2.   Present at birth
    3.   Variegate color

CLINICAL PRESENTATION

Giant congenital nevi, which generally are covered with hair,
represent another type of pigmented birthmark. These lesions differ
from cafe-au-lait lesions by being darker in color and palpably
thickened. The pigmentation in these lesions is often speckled and
occasionally dark brown or black papules stud the surface. Lesions
2 to 10 cm in diameter are relatively common; larger lesions occur
but are fortunately very rare. Giant congenital nevi are present at
birth. Once present, they do not enlarge except in proportion to
body growth. A thinner variant of these lesions, lacking hair, is
known as nevus spilus.

COURSE AND PROGNOSIS

Garment sized congenital nevi have a considerably increased risk
of melanoma transformation. Data concerning the magnitude of this
risk are confusing but a reasonable consensus would suggest that 10%
of the affected individuals will develop one or more melanomas.
Small lesions of this type have not been adequately studied but
linear extrapolation would suggest that the likelihood of melanoma
development in palm sized and smaller lesions is about 0.1 to 1.0%.
Melanomas, when they do develop, can occur at any age. Such lesions
probably account for the majority of melanomas which occur in
children. Moreover, they are always nodular in type and thus are
associated with an extremely poor prognosis.

PATHOGENESIS

Nothing is known about the cause and pathogenesis of these lesions. They do differ histologically from small acquired nevi in that nevus cells extend deeper into the dermis and neural elements are present. The significance of these observations is unknown.

THERAPY

Considerable controversy exists regarding the need for prophylactic excision of congenital giant nevi. Problems in decision making are compounded by the fact that the most dangerous nevi (those that are the largest) are obviously the ones for which surgery is the most difficult. Moreover, surgery, if it is to be carried out, must be done early in life because the melanomas which arise in these nevi can develop at any age. Dermatologists generally favor removal but that is to be expected since they are not the ones who have to carry out the complicated surgery! A decision regarding surgery should be reached only after all interested parties -- surgeon, pediatrician, dermatologist, and parents -- have had a chance to discuss the problem. Obviously, if surgery is not carried out, extraordinarily careful follow-up will be required.

SELECTED READING

Solomon LM: The management of congenital melanocytic nevi. Arch Dermatol 116:1017, 1980.

Rhodes AR: Pigmented birthmarks and precursor melanocytic lesions of cutaneous melanoma identifiable in childhood. Pediatr Clin North Am 30:435, 1983.

Zitelli JA, Grant MG, Abell E, Boyd JB: Histologic patterns of congenital nevocytic nevi and implications for treatment. J Am Acad Dermatol 11:402, 1984.

Sweren RJ: Management of congenital nevocytic nevi: A survey of current practices. J Am Acad Dermatol 11:629, 1984.

Illig L, Weidner F, Hundeiker M, et al: Congenital nevi less than or equal to 10 cm as precursors to melanoma. Arch Dermatol 121:1274, 1985.

Kopf AW, Levine LJ, Rigel DS, et al: Prevalence of congenital-nevus-like nevi, nevi spili, and cafe au lait spots. Arch Dermatol 121:766, 1985.

Backman ME, Kopf AW: Iatrogenic effects of general anesthesia in children: Considerations in treating large congenital nevocytic nevi. J Dermatol Surg Oncol 12:4, 1986.

MISCELLANEOUS BROWN PATCHES AND PLAQUES

The macules and patches of <u>pityriasis (tinea) versicolor</u> often
assume a brown or brown-red color on areas of the body that receive
little or no sunlight. This condition is covered more fully in
Chapter 10.

Hyperpigmentation frequently follows the presence of cutaneous
inflammation. This <u>postinflammatory darkening</u> is particularly
common in lichen planus, psoriasis, and many of the eczematous
diseases. Tanning after sunburn perhaps can be viewed as a variant
of this process. Postinflammatory hyperpigmentation gradually fades
to normal skin color after a period of several months.

<u>Chloasma</u>, also known as melasma, is the term used for the
patches of pigmentation which are found on the forehead, malar
prominences, and zygomatic areas of the face. It is mostly seen in
women where it occurs during pregnancy and in association with the
use of birth control pills. Idiopathic cases, unassociated with
hormonal changes, are occasionally seen in both men and women. The
use of bleaches together with sunscreens as described for lentigines
(see above) may be helpful if treatment is desired.

GENERALIZED HYPERPIGMENTATION

The conditions associated with the development of generalized
hyperpigmentation are discussed in Chapter 26.

Group 6:
The Yellow Lesions

GROUP IDENTIFICATION

The yellow lesions are the easiest of the ten groups to recognize. The yellow color is readily apparent in the smooth surfaced subgroup but some problems may arise in classification of lesions with yellow crust or yellow scale. Generally other features of these latter lesions should be used for assignment to either the vesiculobullous group (Group 1) or the eczematous group (Group 10).

XANTHELASMA

DIAGNOSTIC HALLMARKS

1. Distribution: eyelids
2. Sharp margination

CLINICAL PRESENTATION

Xanthelasma presents as soft, sharply marginated, slightly elevated flattopped papules and plaques 0.5 to 2.0 cm in diameter. These lesions are confined to the eyelids. The first lesions to appear are usually found near the inner canthus of the upper eyelid. Slow enlargement occurs but eventually a stable size is reached. They are asymptomatic. Primary amyloidosis involving the skin of the eyelid has a somewhat similar morphology but the lesions almost always demonstrate some element of purpura.

COURSE AND PROGNOSIS

Once present, the lesions remain in place indefinitely. Approximately 40% of patients with xanthelasma have elevated serum lipids.

PATHOGENESIS

The lesions result from the accumulation of lipids in the macrophages of the connective tissue. The source of the lipid may be the plasma but it is also possible that the lipids are synthesized locally.

THERAPY

Reduction in plasma lipids rarely affects the appearance of xanthelasma. Destruction or excision of the lesions can be carried out but the improvement is temporary. New lesions quickly reform.

NECROBIOSIS LIPOIDICA DIABETICORUM

DIAGNOSTIC HALLMARKS

1. Distribution: anterior shins
2. Violaceous border
3. Central atrophy or ulceration

CLINICAL PRESENTATION

Necrobiosis lipoidica diabeticorum (NLD) occurs as one or more yellow plaques on the anterior lower legs. Rarely lesions may be found on the arms, face, and dorsal surface of the feet. Most of the plaques are 2 to 10 cm in diameter. The center of the plaque has a yellow, waxy appearance; the borders of the plaques are dusky red or violaceous in color. Atrophy is present and for this reason underlying veins are easily visible. Occasionally the atrophic areas break down and ulcerate. The lesions are asymptomatic. Sometimes there is overlap between the clinical appearance of granuloma annulare and NLD.

COURSE AND PROGNOSIS

The lesions of NLD remain present for long periods of time. Usually there is some element of slow centrifugal expansion. Approximately 60% of the patients with necrobiosis lipoidica diabeticorum have overt diabetes mellitus. Conversely only about 0.5% of patients with diabetes develop these lesions.

PATHOGENESIS

The cause of NLD is unknown although some clinicians believe that the plaques occur as the result of the same microangiopathy that is responsible for other complications of diabetes. There is an amazing histologic similarity between NLD and the lesions of granuloma annulare and rheumatoid nodules.   The significance of this observation is unknown.

THERAPY

Therapy is not very effective. Some improvement is occasionally seen following the use of topical steroids when they are used under occlusion. Intralesionally injected steroids are more effective but there is some risk that the injected steroids will create more atrophy and increase the likelihood of ulceration. There has been some recent enthusiasm for the use of oral agents which interfere with platelet aggregation and activation but proof of efficacy has not been shown.

SELECTED READING

Huntley AC: The cutaneous manifestations of diabetes mellitus. J Am Acad Dermatol 7:427, 1982.
Sibbald RG, Schachter RK: The skin and diabetes mellitus. Int J Dermatol 23:567, 1984.

MISCELLANEOUS SMOOTH YELLOW LESIONS

Patients with primary amyloidosis sometimes develop flat yellow patches on the skin. The eyelids are the areas most prominently involved. The yellow color occurs because the amyloid which is densely deposited in the papillary dermis offers very poor support for the small blood vessels of the skin; their frequent rupture with even minor trauma results in the intermittent presence of purpura. In fact, "pinch" purpura is used as a very effective clinical clue to the presence of cutaneous amyloidosis.

Increased levels of carotene are seen in some diabetic patients, in some individuals who rapidly lose weight while exercising, and in those who ingest large amounts of yellow and green vegetables. The skin of patients with carotenemia becomes diffusely yellow but the sclerae remain normal in color. This observation rules out the presence of jaundice as an explanation for the yellow skin color.

Cutaneous mastocytomas occur in infancy and usually present as one or more dome shaped, yellow papules or nodules. Rubbing these lesions results in wheal formation (Darier's sign). Bulla formation is occasionally seen on the surface of lesions. Spontaneous resolution occurs after several years.

Xanthomas, other than xanthelasma, occasionally are found on the palms, around tendons, and in the skin overlying joints. These appear as smooth surfaced yellow papules and nodules of varying size. All such patients have associated hyperlipidemia.

Jaundice occurs as diffuse yellow pigmentation throughout the skin; the sclerae are also involved. The color is due to elevated levels of bilirubin. Most often jaundice is an indicator of hepatic disease but occasionally it develops after massive hemolysis.

The small, umbilicated facial papules of <u>sebaceous gland hyperplasia</u> may appear yellow or yellow-white in color (see also Chapters 9 and 10).

MISCELLANEOUS CRUSTED YELLOW LESIONS

Any significant accumulation of serum on the surface of the skin results in the formation of yellow crusts or, if scale is present, in the formation of yellow colored scale. Thus any disease listed in the vesiculobullous or eczematous group may assume a yellow color. This phenomenon is particularly prominent in impetigo and seborrheic dermatitis. Yellow crusts, yellow scale, or both are also seen occasionally with <u>actinic keratoses</u> and small actinically induced squamous cell carcinomas. Corns and calluses are often slightly more yellow than the surrounding normal skin.

Group 7:
The Red Papules and Nodules

GROUP IDENTIFICATION

The red papules and nodules are characterized by the presence of smooth surfaced, nonscaling erythematous papules and nodules. Since these characteristics are shared by the diseases of Group 8 (the vascular reactions) some rules of thumb are necessary to help separate the two groups. First, the cross-sectional profiles of lesions in Group 7 are dome shaped whereas the lesions of Group 8 are generally flattopped. Second, solitary lesions, no matter what their morphology, are almost always assigned to Group 7. Third, purpuric lesions are always assigned to Group 8. Fourth, confluence of lesions, when present, favors assignment to Group 8. One exception to this rule occurs in the case of granuloma annulare wherein individual papules may partially coalesce to form annular lesions.

In spite of these rules there will be instances in which assignment to one of the two groups cannot be made with certainty. In such cases the list of differential diagnoses may need to contain diseases from both groups.

INSECT BITES

DIAGNOSTIC HALLMARKS

1.   Distribution: pattern depends on the insect
2.   Sudden onset
3.   Spontaneous resolution in several days

CLINICAL PRESENTATION

Most insect bites result in the development of nonscaling, dome shaped, red papules 4 to 8 mm in size. A central punctum, if present, is diagnostic. Itching is usually, but not invariably, present. The papules often appear within minutes of the bite but some reactions are delayed and are not apparent until 6 to 12 hours later. In the case of these delayed reactions patients are often totally unaware that they have been bitten. In such instances the number and distribution of the papules may offer considerable diagnostic help. For instance, bed bug bites are characterized by the clustering of several bites on the trunk, flea bites are most often found on the lower legs, and chigger bites are clustered where clothing binds. Those bites and stings of ants, spiders, and bees usually do not cause much diagnostic difficulty since the lesions are clinically apparent immediately after the insult.

Most bites and stings resolve spontaneously over several days, but occasionally, in an unusually reactive patient, an urticarial response may be perpetuated for weeks by repeated scratching. Such lesions, known as papular urticaria, are particularly common in children. Anaphylaxis (see Chapter 14) is an uncommon but potentially fatal complication of some insect bites and stings.

PATHOGENESIS

Bites fall into three categories from a standpoint of pathogenesis: 1) toxic reactions which cause pain (bee stings), 2) toxic reactions which cause itching due to pharmacologic release of histamine (mosquito bites), and 3) allergic reactions which cause itching due to antigen deposition and immunologic release of inflammatory mediators (flea bites). These allergic reactions can be particularly troublesome from a diagnostic standpoint since the reaction does not occur in everyone who is exposed. Thus most patients will be surprised and somewhat unwilling to consider insect bites when only one member of an exposed family develops lesions.

THERAPY

Most bites require no specific therapy. Soaks and topically applied steroids may offer symptomatic improvement for those with unusually severe reactions. For the most part, identification of the cause allows the patient to take appropriate steps (such as personal application of repellents and in some cases treatment of animal hosts) to avoid future problems. Those insect repellents with high concentrations of diethyltoluamide (DEET) such as Cutter's and Off seem to work best. Some interesting studies testing the use of orally ingested vitamins as insect repellents are promising but proof of efficacy is lacking.

SELECTED READING

Golden DBK, Valentine MD: Insect sting allergy. Ann Allergy 53:444, 1984.
Heng MCY, Kloss SG, Haberfelde GC: Pathogenesis of papular urticaria. J Am Acad Dermatol 10:1030, 1984.

CHERRY ANGIOMAS

DIAGNOSTIC HALLMARKS

1.   Distribution: chest and back
2.   Occurrence in mid to late adult life
3.   Long history of unchanged appearance

CLINICAL PRESENTATION

Cherry angiomas (also known as Campbell de Morgan spots or senile angiomas) are dusky red or violaceous, dome shaped papules 2 to 8 mm in diameter. They are most often found on the upper trunk in middle aged and older adults. In a given patient there may be considerable variation in the size and color of adjacent lesions. They are asymptomatic and do not blanch easily with pressure.

PATHOGENESIS

The cause of these lesions is unknown. They seem to be a part of the aging process.

THERAPY

No therapy is needed. Cosmetically objectionable lesions can be treated with light electrosurgery or can be removed by punch biopsy. Lesions dark enough in color to simulate the appearance of a melanoma should be biopsied.

PYOGENIC GRANULOMAS

DIAGNOSTIC HALLMARKS

1.   Distribution: face, hands, feet, and upper trunk
2.   Size: 5 to 15 mm
3.   Rapid growth
4.   Occurrence in children and teenagers
5.   Occurrence during pregnancy

CLINICAL PRESENTATION

Pyogenic granulomas are smooth surfaced, red papules 5 to 15 mm in diameter. Most lesions are dome shaped but some are pedunculated. They may occur anywhere on the body but are most commonly seen over the shoulders and the face. Lesions on the hands and feet are also seen from time to time. Most pyogenic granulomas are found in children aged 5 to 15. Pregnant women are also at risk. They are asymptomatic but the larger ones bleed easily following trauma. Such lesions will have a partially crusted surface.

COURSE AND PROGNOSIS

Pyogenic granulomas first appear as pinhead sized papules but they grow rapidly within weeks to their final size. Left untreated pyogenic granulomas eventually undergo spontaneous resolution. They have no malignant potential but their rapid growth and occasional dusky color sometimes simulate the appearance of melanoma. Such lesions should obviously be biopsied. Recurrence after treatment (occasionally with the presence of new satellite lesions) is not uncommon.

PATHOGENESIS

The cause of pyogenic granulomas is unknown. In spite of their name they are not granulomas and they are not caused by an infectious process. Histologically they appear to be true hemangiomas. Their occurrence in late childhood and in pregnant women suggests that hormonal factors may play a role in their development. Satellite recurrence in some patients after removal seems to indicate that a field defect involving the surrounding vascular bed may be present.

THERAPY

Lesions may be removed by elliptical excision or, after shave removal, the base may be destroyed with electrosurgery. Cryotherapy is sometimes successful especially if it is repeated on several occasions. Recurrences are frequently observed if the original therapy was insufficiently aggressive.

GRANULOMA ANNULARE

DIAGNOSTIC HALLMARKS

1.   Distribution: dorsal feet and hands; elbows and ankles
2.   Annular configuration

3.   Slowly evolving shapes and sizes
4.   Violaceous color

CLINICAL PRESENTATION

The primary lesion of granuloma annulare is a nonscaling, dome shaped or slightly flattened papule 3 to 6 mm in diameter. These papules may be skin colored, pink, or violaceous. Lesions on the lower extremities are more darkly colored than are those located elsewhere. The multiple papules of granuloma annulare are typically arranged in the form of a ring. The size of these rings ranges from 1 to 8 cm in diameter. The individual papules which make up the border are closely set but are not usually completely confluent. This gives a "beaded" appearance to the border. The depressed center of the ring is sometimes darker than the papular edge. Multiple rings are present in about half of the patients. Adjacent rings may grow together, forming a single larger lesion with a polycyclic configuration.

Lesions are most commonly found on the dorsal surface of the feet and on the dorsal surface of the hands and fingers. The extensor surfaces of the arms and legs (to include the elbows and knees) are also fairly frequently involved. Granuloma annulare occurs at any age but the peak incidence occurs in children aged 4 to 12. Lesions are asymptomatic. A clinical diagnosis can be confirmed by biopsy.

Atypical Clinical Presentations. Occasionally adults will develop a disseminated pattern consisting of hundreds of small rings. The entire body may be involved but there may be some predilection for sun exposed surfaces. Subcutaneous lesions resembling rheumatoid nodules are occasionally seen in children. Very rarely, papules and nodules of granuloma annulare undergo ulceration (perforating granuloma annulare). On some occasions granuloma annulare simulates the appearance of necrobiosis lipoidica diabeticorum to the point where the two diseases cannot be distinguished.

COURSE AND PROGNOSIS

Individual ringed lesions grow in size and change shapes over a period of weeks to months. The disease is, however, self-limiting and within a year or two usually all trace of the lesions has disappeared.

Controversy exists as to whether or not there is a relationship between granuloma annulare and diabetes mellitus. Suffice it to say that such a correlation, if it exists, is of no clinical importance in children. Adults, especially those who develop disseminated lesions, probably warrant a determination of blood sugar levels.

PATHOGENESIS

The cause of granuloma annulare is unknown. The lesions are histologically similar to those of necrobiosis lipoidica diabeticorum and rheumatoid nodules. Moreover, there is some clinical overlap among these diseases as well. The significance of these observations is unknown. Genetic factors may play some role in the development of the generalized form of the disease since a large proportion of such patients have the HLA BW35 antigen.

The location of granuloma annulare on the hands and feet and an occasional distribution on sun exposed skin suggest that trauma of some sort plays an etiologic role. However, new lesions cannot experimentally be induced in this way. In fact, nonspecific trauma, such as saline injections, sometimes causes resolution in established lesions. A role for immune complex formation and cell mediated immune response in the pathogenesis of granuloma annulare has been suggested but the importance of these findings remains moot.

THERAPY

There is no established treatment for granuloma annulare. Lesions occasionally respond to topically applied steroids when they are used with occlusion. Intralesionally injected steroids are somewhat more effective. However, discomfort during injection and the development of postinjection atrophy limit the usefulness of this approach. A number of other approaches including the use of systemically administered chlorambucil and dapsone have been suggested but proof of efficacy has not been established.

SELECTED READING
Muhlbauer JE: Granuloma annulare. J Am Acad Dermatol 3:217, 1980.

MISCELLANEOUS ERYTHEMATOUS PAPULES

The lesions of pityriasis rosea (see Chapter 15) are occasionally devoid of visible scale. The possibility of pityriasis rosea should be considered in any patient that has 30 or more inflammatory papules located mainly on the trunk. A careful search usually reveals a few typical oval lesions but if such are not present secondary syphilis and pityriasis lichenoides should also be considered.

Pityriasis lichenoides is a rare disease in which patients develop crops of dome shaped, red papules 2 to 6 mm in size. As the name implies, very fine scale may be present, but often no scale can be appreciated clinically. Ten to fifty individual papules may be present at any one time. No oral lesions are present and the extremities as well as the trunk are usually involved. The

condition is chronic and lasts for months to years. In the acute
type of pityriasis lichenoides (Mucha-Habermann disease) the papules
may appear somewhat vesicular or eroded and some may heal with
scarring.

A considerable proportion of the patients with secondary
syphilis (see Chapter 15) will have inflammatory papules 2 to 4 mm
in diameter which are clinically devoid of scale. Such eruptions
can easily be mistaken for insect bites, pityriasis rosea, and
pityriasis lichenoides. Patients with lesions such as these should
be examined carefully for condyloma lata, mucous patches, hair loss,
lymphadenopathy, and papular lesions of the palms and soles. A
serologic test for syphilis (see Chapter 16) should, of course, also
be obtained.

SELECTED READING
LeVine MJ: Phototherapy of pityriasis lichenoides.   Arch Dermatol
119:378, 1983.

FURUNCLES

DIAGNOSTIC HALLMARKS

    1.   Distribution: no characteristic pattern
    2.   Sudden onset
    3.   Pain and tenderness
    4.   Response to therapy

CLINICAL PRESENTATION

    Furuncles are dome shaped or slope shouldered, bright red,
painful nodules 1.5 to 3 cm in diameter. Usually only a single
furuncle is present; multiple lesions, if closely grouped, may
coalesce to form a carbuncle. The classic signs of inflammation
(rubor, dolor, color, and tumor) are all present. The development
of a furuncle is an acute event. From the point of onset to full
development requires only 24 to 48 hours. Early lesions are firm on
palpation but older lesions may develop a central area of
fluctuance. Lesions which become fluctuant may "point" with a small
pustule. Regional lymphadenopathy is occasionally present but
malaise and fever are not regularly found. Furunculosis should be
differentiated from hidradenitis suppurativa and inflamed epidermoid
cysts (see below).

    The diagnosis is usually made on a clinical basis; pus from
fluctuant lesions may be aspirated or drained for culture.

COURSE AND PROGNOSIS

Furuncles left untreated resolve spontaneously in 10 to 20 days. During this time fluctuant lesions may rupture and drain. The pus from such lesions often causes bacterial contamination of adjacent skin leading to the development of multiple new lesions. In debilitated or immunocompromised patients furunculosis sometimes progresses to more serious, systemic staphylococcal infection.

PATHOGENESIS

Furunculosis is a bacterial infection due to <u>Staphylococcus aureus</u>. The infection develops around the hair follicle and is similar to, but much deeper than, that found in folliculitis. Events favoring the development of furunculosis include tissue trauma and the presence of heat and moisture. Persons with recurrent furunculosis are often chronic staphylococcal nose and throat carriers. Diabetes mellitus is said to be more common in patients with recurrent furunculosis but such a relationship, if it exists, is rarely of clinical importance.

THERAPY

Patients with furunculosis should be treated with systemically administered antibiotics. The use of phenoxymethyl penicillin may be sufficient but generally those penicillins resistant to penicillanase degradation (see Chapter 4) are preferred. Erythromycin is also appropriate and is the drug of choice for those allergic to penicillin.

Traditionally, warm soaks have been used as adjunctive therapy but data demonstrating their usefulness are lacking. Incision and drainage are appropriate only for those lesions where fluctuance is present. The placement of drains or gauze packing following incision and drainage is occasionally necessary in the largest lesions.

INFLAMED EPIDERMOID CYSTS

DIAGNOSTIC HALLMARKS

1. Distribution: Random but some predilection for the back
2. History of a preceding noninflammatory cyst or nodule
3. Characteristic fragments of white keratin on incision and drainage

CLINICAL PRESENTATION

Asymptomatic, skin colored epidermoid cysts (see Chapter 9) occasionally become red and tender. When this occurs differentiation from a furuncle may become difficult. However, the history of a preceding noninflammatory nodule, the absence of a pustule on the summit, and somewhat lesser pain suggest a cystic process. Inflamed cysts can occur almost anywhere but most are encountered on the trunk with special predilection for the back.

COURSE AND PROGNOSIS

Inflamed cysts generally are accompanied by sufficient pain to bring the patient to medical attention quickly. If left untreated most resolve spontaneously over 2 to 4 weeks. However, a few will spontaneously rupture to the surface with subsequent chronic drainage. Treated lesions are likely to recur unless the entire cyst wall has been successfully removed.

PATHOGENESIS

The inflammatory changes are rarely the result of true bacterial infection. They occur instead because of the extrusion of keratinous material (and possibly nonpathogenic follicular bacteria) through a ruptured cyst wall. Sometimes the rupture of the wall occurs as a result of trauma but often it appears to occur spontaneously.

THERAPY

Small lesions can be excised but most lesions will first require incision and drainage. When this procedure is carried out there is usually a larger than expected amount of purulent, foul smelling material that can be expressed. Generally some pieces of solid, yellow-white keratin are mixed in with the fluid material. This contrasts with the situation in fluctuant furunculosis wherein only a small amount of pure pus is present. A significant cavity is left when large lesions are incised and drained. Such "dead space" should be filled with gauze packing, the tail of which is left to extend through the incision site. Cultures can be taken from the expressed material but they are rarely productive of pathogenic bacteria. Systemically adminstered antibiotics are used routinely by some clinicians but they are seldom medically necessary. Attempts to remove all of the cyst wall through the incision site are not often successful. I prefer to let the process heal completely over a 2-month period and then consider elliptical excision of the small papule which remains.

CELLULITIS (ERYSIPELAS)

DIAGNOSTIC HALLMARKS

1. Distribution: no characteristic pattern
2. Sudden onset
3. Pain and tenderness
4. Response to therapy

CLINICAL PRESENTATION

Cellulitis occurs as a tender, edematous, bright red plaque 5 to 20 cm in diameter. Generally only a single lesion is present. A thin red line progressing proximally from the lesion (lymphangitis) is seen in about 20% of patients. The initial lesion of cellulitis appears suddenly. Centrifugal growth of the lesion is rapid during the first 24 hours but thereafter it occurs more slowly. Cellulitis is less painful than furunculosis and areas of fluctuance never develop. Fever, malaise, and regional lymphadenopathy may or may not be present. Differentiation of cellulitis from an acute urticarial plaque such as occurs following bee stings is sometimes difficult but generally the course of events over the succeeding 24 hours allows for appropriate identification.

The diagnosis of cellulitis is made on a clinical basis. It is theoretically possible to culture the lesion by way of injection and subsequent aspiration of sterile saline but most clinicians do not find this helpful or necessary. If this test is carried out one should be careful not to use saline from multiple dose vials since such preparations usually contain antibacterial agents for the maintenance of vial sterility.

COURSE AND PROGNOSIS

Most instances of cellulitis resolve spontaneously over 10 to 20 days. However, in debilitated or otherwise immunocompromised individuals, progressive spread and systemic infection may develop. The process is particularly troublesome when it occurs in patients taking systemic steroids, since not only is resistance reduced but the signs and symptoms of the infection may be greatly masked by the anti-inflammatory action of the steroids.

Special attention should be given to cellulitis of the central face since, left untreated, there is a significant risk of extension to the cavernous sinus.

Cellulitis is not usually recurrent. However, in patients with chronic lymphedema there is a tendency both for the simultaneous presence of multiple lesions and for the development of repeated episodes. The presence of hypalgesia, anesthesia, or blister formation over an area of cellulitis, especially if the fluid is yellow or blood tinged, should warn the clinician of possible underlying necrotizing fasciitis.

PATHOGENESIS

Cellulitis is a nonfollicular, connective tissue infection due to <u>Staphylococcus aureus</u> or <u>Streptococcus pyogenes</u>. Clinical signs indicating which of the two organisms is responsible are unreliable, but lymphangitis is more commonly found in staphylococcal infection. Fever, on the other hand, is more often seen in streptococcal infection. Trauma to the skin predisposes to the development of cellulitis but such a history is not regularly present. Patients with chronic lymphedema seem particularly susceptible to the development of cellulitis.

THERAPY

Systemic antibiotics, as described for the treatment of furunculosis (see also Chapter 4), should be administered to all patients with cellulitis. It is not necessary to decide whether the problem is staphylococcal or streptococcal before initiating therapy and, in fact, culture is not usually possible even with saline injection and aspiration (see above). Incision and drainage are never carried out. Hot packs or hot soaks are often recommended but there is little evidence that this approach speeds resolution.

SELECTED READING

Binnick AN, Klein RB, Banghaman RD: Recurrent erysipelas caused by Group B streptococcus organisms. <u>Arch Dermatol 116</u>:798, 1980.
Hook EW III, Hooton TM, Horton CA, <u>et al</u>: Microbiologic evaluation of cutaneous cellulitis in adults. <u>Arch Intern Med 146</u>:295, 1986

HIDRADENITIS SUPPURATIVA

DIAGNOSTIC HALLMARKS

1.   Distribution: axillae and groin
2.   Nonresponsiveness to antibiotic therapy
3.   Recurrence in the same sites

CLINICAL PRESENTATION

The individual lesions of hidradenitis suppurativa arise as firm, tender, dome shaped papules and nodules 1 to 3 cm in size. The larger lesions often develop an area of fluctuance and drain spontaneously. Pustule formation is sometimes present. Lesions are most commonly found in the groin and in the axilla; the buttocks and breasts are occasionally involved. Individual lesions are easily

confused with the lesions of furunculosis. However, the distinctive
location, multiple recurrences at the same site, the recovery of a
panoply of organisms on culture, and the failure to respond promptly
to antibiotic therapy are helpful clues to the diagnosis of
hidradenitis suppurativa. The disease is considerably more common
in women than in men; blacks are affected more often than are
Caucasians. Those who are obese are at greater risk than are those
who are thin.

COURSE AND PROGNOSIS

Hidradenitis first develops during late puberty and then
continues sporadically throughout the next 10 to 20 years. Disease
activity often seems to be directly related to the degree of
obesity. There is considerable variation in severity from patient
to patient. Some individuals develop only two or three small
papules each year whereas in others new lesions appear and drain as
rapidly as old ones resolve.
Individual lesions, whether they drain spontaneously or not,
heal slowly over a period of 10 to 30 days. Healing is almost
always accompanied by some scarring. In a few patients recurrent
scarring results in the development of lymphedema and contracture
formation. On the other hand, scarring may also contribute to the
apparent "burning out" of the disease over a period of many years.

PATHOGENESIS

Hidradenitis suppurativa appears to be an acne-like process of
those pilosebaceous units to which apocrine sweat glands are
attached. Such units generally occur only in the axilla and groin.
Apocrine glands do not become active until hormonal stimulation
begins during puberty. If at that time the outlet of one or more
glands is blocked the pilosebaceous follicle becomes distended. The
distention is then followed by rupture and extrusion of apocrine
sweat and follicular bacteria into the surrounding tissue. This in
turn results in a massive inflammatory response and the formation of
a painful nodule. The reasons for blockage of the apocrine follicle
are not known but some possibilities include embryologic
malformation of the apocrine duct, compression of the duct due to
sweat retention (miliaria), and bacterial infection of the ostium.
However, in my opinion, pathogenic bacteria (as opposed to normal,
follicular bacteria) recovered on culture are usually secondary
invaders rather than a primary cause of the disease.

THERAPY

Hidradenitis suppurativa is an extremely difficult disease to
control. The first step in therapy is to improve those

environmental factors which might cause follicular blockage.
Attempts should be made to minimize the amount of heat and
sweating. Constrictive clothing should be avoided and as much
weight as possible should be lost. Second, if patients are having
continuous problems, 2 months or more of tetracycline or
erythromycin therapy should be administered. Third, if long term
antibiotic therapy is insufficient, the administration of birth
control pills (see under acne, Chapter 8) should be considered.
Fourth, individual lesions can be treated locally. Tender lesions,
regardless of whether or not fluctuance is present, can be injected
intralesionally with depot-type steroids such as triamcinolone (see
Chapter 4). Fluctuant lesions should be incised and drained prior
to injection. If, in spite of all this, activity of the disease
continues consideration should be given to excisional surgery. A
strip of apocrine gland bearing skin, several centimeters wide, is
removed and the defect is sutured closed. The presence of draining
lesions is not a contraindication to the performance of surgery
since the pus which is present is primarily due to noninfectious
inflammation. Finally, one can consider the oral administration of
retinoids. About 50% of patients receiving 4 months of
13-cis-retinoic acid in doses similar to those used for acne obtain
appreciable improvement but relapse quickly occurs after the
medication is discontinued.

SELECTED READING

Dicken CH, Powell ST, Spear KL: Evaluation of isotretinoin
    treatment of hidradenitis suppurativa. J Am Acad Dermatol
    11:500, 1984.
Mortimer PS, Gales MA, Moore RA, Dawber RPR: Hidradenitis
    suppurativa -- An androgen-dependent condition. Br J Dermatol
    113:27, 1985.
Fitzsimmons JS, Guilbert PR, Fitzsimmons EM: Evidence of genetic
    factors in hidradenitis suppurativa. Br J Dermatol 113:1, 1985.

MISCELLANEOUS ERYTHEMATOUS NODULES

Patients with severe acne frequently develop tender inflamed
cystic lesions. These are dome shaped or slope shouldered nodules 1
to 3 cm in diameter. The distribution of lesions on the face and
upper trunk is characteristic. Pustules and comedones always occur
in association with acne cysts. Topical therapy is of no help and
may even be counterproductive in these individuals. Systemically
administered antibiotics are administered and adjunctive therapy
such as intralesionally injected steroids may be necessary as well
(see acne, Chapter 8).

Erythema nodosum (see Chapter 14) sometimes presents as
inflammatory nodules instead of inflammatory plaques. For this
reason it is listed both here and in Group 8.

Nodular hemangiomas of either the strawberry or cavernous type may be present at birth or may develop during the first few months of life. These red, cool, nontender lesions are easily recognized. Small lesions are best left untreated. Large lesions and those occurring around the nose, eyes, and mouth may be troublesome enough to require therapy. In particular one should be aware of the possibility of disseminated intravascular coagulation (DIC) due to platelet consumption within the lesion (Kasabach-Merritt syndrome) and to the risk of surface necrosis with subsequent infection. Systemically or intralesionally administered corticosteroids are sometimes used in treatment as are cryotherapy and laser surgery.

SELECTED READING

Nelson LB, Melick JE, Harley RD: Intralesional corticosteroid
    injections for infantile hemangiomas of the eyelid. Am J
    Ophthalmol 93:496, 1982.
Esterly NB: Kasabach-Merritt syndrome in infants. J Am Acad
    Dermatol 8:504, 1983.

Chapter 14

Group 8:
Vascular Reactions

GROUP IDENTIFICATION

The vascular reactions are characterized by the presence of smooth surfaced, nonscaling erythematous papules and plaques. Since these characteristics are shared by the diseases of Group 7 (the erythematous papules and nodules) some rules of thumb are necessary to separate the two groups. The first rule regards the profiles, or cross-sectional appearance of lesions. Lesions belonging to Group 7 generally are dome shaped or hemispherical whereas lesions of Group 8 are generally flattopped. Second, solitary lesions are almost always assigned to Group 7. Third, purpuric lesions are always assigned to Group 8. Fourth, confluence of lesions, when present, favors assignment to Group 8.

In spite of these general rules one cannot always be certain to which of the two groups a nonscaling erythematous eruption belongs. For this reason it may sometimes be necessary to assemble one's list of differential diagnoses from among the diseases in both groups.

THE VASCULAR REACTIONS AS A SPECTRUM

The diseases of the vascular reaction group are not as precisely separable as are the diseases in the other groups. Thus, the lesions of secondary syphilis and those of pityriasis rosea may look remarkably similar, but there is no doubt that, no matter how much alike they look, they are completely different diseases. The vascular reactions, on the other hand, exist on a spectrum in which overlap occurs in clinical features, etiology, and pathophysiology.

This spectrum is displayed in Table 14-1. Examination of the table demonstrates that as one travels along the spectrum there is an ever increasing severity of vascular pathology which finally results in the absence of vascular flow and the necrosis of tissue.

SELECTED READING

Russell Jones R, Bhogal B, Dash A, et al: Urticaria and vasculitis: A continuum of histologic and immunopathologic changes. Br J Dermatol 108:695, 1983.

TABLE 14-1
SPECTRUM OF THE VASCULAR REACTIONS

CLINICAL CONDITION	PATHOPHYSIOLOGY
1. Flushing syndromes	Vessel dilation only; no structural damage
2. Urticarias	Vessels dilate; leak plasma; no structural damage
3. Persistent erythemas	Vessels dilate, leak plasma and lymphocytes; minimal structural damage
4. Vasculitic purpuras	Vessel walls partially destroyed by neutrophils; red blood cells escape
5. Vascular ulcers	Vessel walls completely destroyed; no nutritional flow

The first (flushing syndromes) and final (vascular ulcers) positions on this spectrum are too rarely encountered to warrant discussion in this book. The remaining three conditions will be discussed individually, but since they share, to a remarkable degree, a common pathogenesis, this feature will be covered only once at the end of the chapter.

URTICARIA AND ANGIOEDEMA

DIAGNOSTIC HALLMARKS

1.   Distribution: no characteristic distribution but some
     tendency for lesions to appear at sites of pressure or
     trauma
2.   Lesions evolve and resolve in minutes to hours
3.   Pigskin type dimpling on surface of lesion

CLINICAL PRESENTATION

The primary lesion in urticaria is an edematous papule called a
wheal. Wheals are sharply marginated and predominantly flattopped.
Their color varies from light pink to dark red depending on the
amount of fluid present between the skin surface and the underlying
dilated vascular bed. Wheals frequently have a dimpled surface
because of the anchoring effect of hair follicles as fluid fills the
papillary dermis surrounding them.
Wheals often undergo very rapid centrifugal growth to form
large, flat plaques. The coalescence of adjacent lesions lends a
notable gyrate (serpiginous) configuration to these large plaques.
Annular patterns are also seen as a result of the central clearing
which sometimes occurs within the plaques.
Urticaria can involve any areas of the body including the scalp,
lips, palms, and soles. Itching, severe at times, is usually
present but excoriations are rarely seen.
Angioedema, which is the development of skin colored soft
swelling, often accompanies urticaria. The eyelids and lips are the
area most typically affected. Laryngeal edema (see below) does not
usually occur.

COURSE AND PROGNOSIS

Perhaps the most characteristic feature of urticaria is the
transient nature of the individual papules and plaques. Lesions
appear, change shape, resolve, and reappear in a matter of minutes
to hours. This rapid metamorphosis occurs with no other skin
disease. It can be dramatically demonstrated by viewing, at hourly
intervals, a patient whose lesions have been previously outlined
with a marking pencil. As lesions evolve the spontaneous resolution
which occurs is often most notable in the center of lesions. As a
result of this process many annular lesions with serpiginous
outlines are formed.
It is usually not possible to predict the total course of the
disease at the time the patient is first seen. Obviously, if a
medication reaction or acute viral infection is believed to be the
cause, a short course is likely. Unfortunately, such instances

account for a minority of the cases. Many cases of urticaria go on
for months and a few even last for years.

Systemic symptoms and signs accompany urticaria only in
hypocomplementemic vasculitis, anaphylactic reactions, and
hereditary angioedema. In the latter two conditions death from
laryngeal edema is a distinct possibility. Laryngeal edema does not
otherwise occur in patients with chronic urticaria.

PATHOGENESIS

The etiology and pathophysiology is discussed in a separate
section at the end of this chapter.

THERAPY

If hypotension, facial swelling, or any indication of laryngeal
edema accompanies an episode of urticaria, subcutaneously or even
intramuscularly injected epinephrine should be administered.
Generally 0.3 to 0.5 cc of a 1/1000 solution of aqueous epinephrine
is used. This can be repeated in 15 to 30 minutes if necessary.
Venous access for the administration of fluids is established and,
depending on the degree of bronchoconstriction, consideration can be
given to the intravenous adminstration of aminophylline. Oxygen is
used as necessary. Diphenhydramine (Benadryl) 50 to 75 mg, or
similar antihistamine, is usually administered intramuscularly at
the same time as epinephrine is given. Orally administered
antihistamines are then continued at 6-hour intervals as needed.

Urticaria that has been present for hours or days does not
require the use of injected medications. Antihistamines are given
orally starting in conventional dosage (see Chapter 4). If, after
48 hours, there is no improvement the dosage is gradually increased
until side effects interfere or until relief is obtained. It
probably matters very little which antihistamine is chosen.
Dermatologists and allergists generally prefer the use of
hydroxyzine (Atarax) but it is rather expensive and does cause a
good deal of drowsiness. Terfenadine (Seldane) is a particularly
good choice if sedation is to be avoided. It is possible that an
additional beneficial effect can be obtained when H2 antagonists
such as cimetidine are used concomitantly with conventional
antihistamines but proof of this hypothesis is lacking.

If patients do not respond satisfactorily to antihistamines,
orally administered ephedrine or terbutaline can be added.
Unfortunately, unacceptable jitteriness often accompanies their
use. Systemically administered corticosteroids are quite effective
but the need for long term adminstration with resultant drug
toxicity markedly detracts from their usefulness. Psychotropic
agents will be helpful in some cases and should be tried in all
resistant cases. Tricyclic agents, because of their excellent

antihistaminic effects, are widely recommended, but in my experience benzodiazepines are also often helpful. Topically applied steroids are totally noneffective. Considerable work is now going into the development of orally absorbed cromolyn-like compounds but as yet no products are commercially available.

SELECTED READING

Monroe EW, Cohen SH, Kalbfleisch J, Schulz CI: Combined H1 and
    H2 antihistamine therapy in chronic urticaria. Arch Dermatol
    117:404, 1981.
Monroe EW: Urticaria. Int J Dermatol 20:32, 1981.
Juhlin L: Recurrent urticaria: Clinical investigation of 330
    patients. Br J Dermatol 104:369, 1981.
Jorizzo JL, Smith EB: The physical urticarias. An update and
    review. Arch Dermatol 118:194, 1982.
Champion RH, Highet AS: Investigation and management of chronic
    urticaria and angio-oedema. Special Symposium on Dermatological
    Therapy: VI. Dermatitis in urticaria. Clin Exp Dermatol
    7:291, 1982.
Singh G: H2 blockers in chronic urticaria. Int J Dermatol
    23:627, 1984.
Warin RP: The effect of large doses of H1 antagonists in
    urticaria. Br J Dermatol 111:121, 1984.
Cerio R, Lessof MH: Treatment of chronic idiopathic urticaria with
    terfenadine. Clin Allergy 14:139, 1984.
Monroe EW: Treatment of urticaria. Dermatol Clinics 3:51, 1985.
Guin J: The evaluation of patients with urticaria. Dermatol
    Clinics 3:29, 1985.
Farham J, Grant JA: Angioedema. Dermatol Clinics 3:85, 1985.

MISCELLANEOUS URTICARIAS AND OTHER TRANSIENT ERYTHEMAS

Anaphylaxis is a medical emergency characterized by the sudden onset of urticaria, angioedema, dyspnea, and hypotension. It is most commonly encountered after the administration of penicillin or the ingestion of shellfish or nuts in individuals who have specific IgE antibodies attached to their mast cells as a result of previous sensitization. The therapy of anaphylaxis is given in the section above.

The physical urticarias include cholinergic urticaria and urticarial reactions due to heat, ultraviolet light, cold, and pressure. In a simplistic way dermographism, which is the appearance of urticaria at sites of stroking, can be considered as a variant of pressure urticaria.

Hereditary angioedema is a rare familial disease in which affected individuals lack the Cl esterase inhibitor for complement. In these individuals many nonspecific events trigger an unregulated development of the complement cascade with the consequent onset of

sudden and severe angioedema. A few patches of reticulate erythema
may also appear but urticarial wheals are essentially absent. Long
term administration of androgenic hormones such as danazol is quite
effective in preventing recurrent episodes.

Urticarial vasculitis is somewhat of a misnomer. The disease is
characterized by the appearance of flattopped erythematous papules
but these lesions remain in place for days at a time rather than
possessing the transient nature of true urticarial wheals. Biopsy
reveals a neutrophilic vasculitis. These patients are often
hypocomplementemic and they may have symptoms and signs suggestive
of a lupus-like syndrome.

SELECTED READING

Sanchez NP, Winkelmann RK, Schroeter AL, Dicken CH: The clinical
    and histopathologic spectrums of urticarial vasculitis: Study
    of forty cases. J Am Acad Dermatol 7:599, 1982.
Lucke WC, Thomas H Jr: Anaphylaxis: Pathophysiology, clinical
    presentations and treatment. J Emerg Med 1:83, 1983.
Brickman CM, Hosea SW: Hereditary angioedema. Int J Dermatol
    22:141, 1983.
Greenberger PA: Life-threatening idiopathic anaphylaxis associated
    with hyperimmunoglobulinemia E. Am J Med 76:553, 1984.
Sheffer AL: Anaphylaxis. J Allergy Clin Immunol 75:227, 1985.
Gammon WR: Urticarial vasculitis. Dermatol Clinics 3:97, 1985.
Sibbald RG: Physical urticaria. Dermatol Clinics 3:57, 1985.

ERYTHEMA MULTIFORME

DIAGNOSTIC HALLMARKS

1. Distribution: trunk, but palm and sole involvement is
    often present
2. Target lesions
3. Less transient than urticaria

CLINICAL PRESENTATION

Erythema multiforme is characterized by the presence of
flattopped, sharply marginated papules 1 to 2 cm in diameter. The
color is generally duskier than the bright red color of urticarial
lesions. Typically, at least a few of the larger papules will be of
the "target" type in which three concentric rings are found: an
outermost red ring, a lighter colored intermediate ring, and a
central, dark colored bulls-eye. Bullous changes, when they are
present (see Chapter 7), develop from the center of such lesions.
The lesions of erythema multiforme seem to exist on a spectrum with
those of urticaria. They differ from urticarial papules by being
considerably less transient (they change in days rather than hours),

by being a duskier red in color (less edema to "dilute" the
redness), and by showing less tendency for coalescence or plaque
formation.

The lesions of erythema multiforme may occur anywhere on the
body but the presence of palm and sole involvement is quite
characteristic. The amount of pruritus which accompanies erythema
multiforme varies from minimal to moderate; it is usually less
troublesome than that which occurs in urticaria.

The diagnosis of erythema multiforme is made on the basis of
clinical examination. Biopsies can be used to support a clinical
diagnosis.

Atypical Clinical Presentations. Many patients present with a
condition which exists between urticaria and erythema multiforme in
clinical appearance. The flattopped papules are bright red and show
some tendency for coalescence. However, unlike the lesions of
urticaria, once present they remain unchanged for days. On the
other hand, target lesions are not present and mucous membranes are
not involved. Such a picture is hardly "multiform." The term
erythema multiforme simplex has been used for this condition but I
prefer the term erythema monoforme.

Erythema multiforme occurring with bullous changes, mucous
membrane involvement, and fever is known as the Stevens-Johnson
syndrome (see Chapter 7). The etiologies and pathogenesis are the
same as for conventional erythema multiforme but morbidity is
considerably greater.

Toxic epidermal necrolysis of the Lyell type is a variant of
erythema multiforme in which blister formation is tremendously
extensive; sheets of skin lift off as might occur in a severe
thermal burn. The clinical presentation is somewhat similar in
appearance to that of the staphylococcal scalded skin syndrome
(toxic epidermal necrolysis of the Ritter type) but the histologic
site of blister formation is different and there is considerably
greater morbidity with the erythema multiforme variant.

COURSE AND PROGNOSIS

Most cases of erythema multiforme continue at an active level
for 10 to 15 days at which point slow, spontaneous resolution
occurs. Postinflammatory pigmentation may be left at the site of
some lesions. Recurrent episodes are not common except when the
process is triggered by herpes simplex infections. Controversy
exists as to whether or not a chronic, persistent form of erythema
multiforme exists, but in most instances, immunofluorescent studies
suggest that "chronic" erythema multiforme is actually pemphigoid or
dermatitis herpetiformis.

Morbidity in erythema multiforme varies considerably. Few
systemic symptoms and signs occur in most cases but patients with

Stevens-Johnson syndrome and toxic epidermal necrolysis are quite
ill and death can occur.

PATHOGENESIS

The etiology and pathophysiology of erythema multiforme is
discussed in a separate section at the end of this chapter.

THERAPY

The lesions of erythema multiforme respond poorly to therapy.
Patients with the more severe forms of the disease are usually
treated with systemically administered steroids, but proof of
efficacy and for that matter, proof of safety, is lacking. Milder
cases do not require steroid therapy. Orally administered
antihistamines may be helpful when itching is a problem but they
will have little or no effect on the lesions themselves. Topical
applications, including topically applied steroids, are not
effective.

SELECTED READING

Tonnesen MG, Harrist TJ, Wintroub BU, et al: Erythema multiforme:
    Microvascular damage and infiltration of lymphocytes and
    basophils. J Invest Dermatol 80:282, 1983.
Huff JC, Weston WL, Tonnesen MG: Erythema multiforme: A critical
    review of characteristics, diagnostic criteria, and causes. J
    Am Acad Dermatol 8:763, 1983.
Westly ED, Wechsler HL: Toxic epidermal necrolysis. Granulocytic
    leukopenia as a prognostic indicator. Arch Dermatol 120:721,
    1984.
Ting HC: Erythema multiforme -- Response to corticosteroid.
    Dermatologica 169:175, 1984.
Howland WW, Golitz LE, Weston WL, Huff JC: Erythema multiforme:
    Clinical, histopathologic, and immunologic study. J Am Acad
    Dermatol 10:438, 1984.
Huff JC: Erythema multiforme. Dermatol Clinics 3:141, 1985.

ERYTHEMA NODOSUM

DIAGNOSTIC HALLMARKS

    1.   Distribution: anterior lower legs
    2.   Pain and tenderness

CLINICAL PRESENTATION

Erythema nodosum is characterized by the presence of large (4-
to 10-cm) nonscaling, red, painful lesions on the anterior surface

of the lower legs. The smaller lesions appear as slope shouldered
nodules whereas the larger lesions appear as flattopped plaques.
Because of this bimorphic appearance, erythema nodosum is listed
with the erythematous papules and nodules (Group 7) as well as with
the vascular reactions. Ulceration is never seen. On palpation the
lesions are slightly warm and very tender. The distribution may be
unilateral at first but later in the course of the disease both legs
become involved. Generally no more than six lesions are present at
any one time. The lesions usually occur on the anterior shins or
around the ankles. Occasional lesions develop above the knee, on
the thigh, or posteriorly on the calf. Ankle and knee swelling with
redness and tenderness in and around the joint is rather commonly
found. Erythema nodosum occurs considerably more often in women
than in men.

The rapidity of onset, together with tenderness and warmth on
palpation, often suggests the presence of cellulitis. However, the
presence of more than a single lesion, a duration of more than
several days, and the failure to respond to antibiotics usually
allow for differentiation. Superficial thrombophlebitis also
occasionally mimics erythema nodosum but it is rarely if ever
bilateral. Biopsy can be used to confirm a clinical diagnosis of
erythema nodosum.

COURSE AND PROGNOSIS

Individual lesions resolve over a period of 15 to 20 days but
even as the first lesions disappear one or more new ones begin to
develop. Because of this sequential development, the entire course
of the disease may last for months. Recurrent episodes, following
long periods of inactivity, occur in about 5% of patients. Healing
is accompanied by postinflammatory hyperpigmentation but no
permanent scarring develops.

PATHOGENESIS

The etiology and pathophysiology of erythema nodosum is
discussed in a separate section at the end of this chapter.

THERAPY

The discomfort of erythema nodosum is due to tissue distention
which is in turn caused by the presence of inflammation. Treatment
revolves around the use of nonsteroidal anti-inflammatory agents,
leg elevation, and bed rest. For patients who wish to be up and
around, the use of elastic wraps or support stockings may be very
helpful. In rare instances systemically administered steroids may
be necessary. Hot soaks and topically applied medications are not
useful.

SELECTED READING

Ubogy Z, Persellin RH: Suppression of erythema nodosum by
    indomethacin. _Acta Derm Venereol_ _62_:265, 1982.
White JW Jr: Erythema nodosum. _Dermatol Clinics_ _3_:119, 1985.

MISCELLANEOUS PERSISTENT ERYTHEMAS

Fixed drug eruptions present as one (but sometimes two or more)
flat patches of sharply marginated, nonscaling erythema rather than
as a blistering disease. Lesions may occur anywhere but the hands
and penis are the most commonly involved sites. The lesions fade in
7 to 10 days but are often followed by intense postinflammatory
hyperpigmentation. Readministration of the responsible drug causes
recurrent lesions to develop in exactly the same location. Thus it
is the location rather than the duration that accounts for the term
"fixed." Many drugs are listed as possible causes, but the most
common among these are the various tetracyclines, phenolphthalein-
containing laxatives, and some antipyretic medications.

Bacterial cellulitis may present as inflammatory nodules or as
flat plaques of sharply marginated erythema. Thus it is listed in
both Group 8 (the vascular reactions) and in Group 7 (the
inflammatory papules and nodules). The lesions of cellulitis may be
confused with those of erythema nodosum when they occur on the lower
legs (see above). Cellulitis is discussed in greater detail in
Chapter 13.

The annular and gyrate erythemas are flat or slightly elevated
plaques of erythema in which central resolution is so marked that
only the advancing, peripheral border is visible. Scale is usually
absent and, when present, is never prominent. Postinflammatory
hyperpigmentation is sometimes seen in the central areas of the
lesions as the border advances. Understandably, these lesions are
regularly mistaken for tinea corporis ("ringworm"), but of course,
the KOH and cultures will be negative. Four varieties of this
condition exist.

Erythema annulare centrifugum is the most common of the four
types. These lesions occur in mid or late adult life and usually
begin on the lower portion of the trunk. The peripheral extension
changes visibly over a matter of days. Individual lesions resolve
while others appear and grow. Occasionally a second ring develops
in the center of the larger first ring. Systemic malignancy or
fungal infection of the feet have been historically listed as
possible causes.

Erythema chronicum migrans, which is a tick-borne spirochetal
infection, generally presents as a single, slowly expanding ring. A
solitary red papule is sometimes present in the middle of the
expanding circle. This papule occurs at the site of a tick bite.
Lesions are most commonly found on exposed surfaces, particularly

the lower legs. In this country the lesion is usually seen as a component of the Lyme arthritis syndrome.

Erythema marginatum consists of very thin, fast moving red lines. The size of the circle is often so large the lines appear wavy or straight; a circular component may not be recognized. Movement of the lines takes place over a matter of hours. Entire lesions may disappear overnight only to reappear the next day. No scale is present and postinflammatory hyperpigmentation is not seen. This condition is particularly likely to be seen with rheumatic fever or, less often, juvenile rheumatoid arthritis (Still's disease).

Erythema gyratum repens consists of waves of erythematous lines occurring in association with systemic malignancy. It is rarely encountered.

Mucocutaneous lymph node syndrome (Kawasaki's disease) and toxic shock syndrome may have as one of their components the presence of persistent erythema. In the toxic shock syndrome multiple areas of flat erythema accompany the sudden onset of fever, hypotension, and gastrointestinal disturbance. Postinflammatory desquamation of the palms and soles is a late finding. In Kawasaki's disease flat redness in a scarlatiniform pattern is found in association with marked redness of the hands, feet, lips, tongue, and conjunctivae. There is a history of preceding fever and enlarged cervical lymph nodes can be palpated. Here, too, postinflammatory desquamation of the palms and soles is frequently encountered.

SELECTED READING

Everett ED: Acute febrile mucocutaneous lymph node syndrome -- Kawasaki syndrome. Int J Dermatol 21:506, 1982.
Korkij W, Soltani K: Fixed drug eruption. A brief review. Arch Dermatol 120:520, 1984.
Shrestha M, Grodzicki RL, Steere AC: Diagnosing early Lyme disease. Am J Med 78:235, 1985.
White JW Jr: Gyrate erythema. Dermatol Clinics 3:129, 1985.
Kauppinen K, Stubb S: Fixed eruptions: Causative drugs and challenge tests. Br J Dermatol 112:575, 1985.
Koren G, Rose V, Lavi S, Rowe R: Probable efficacy of high-dose salicylates in reducing coronary involvement in Kawasaki disease. J Am Acad Dermatol 254:767, 1985.

LEUKOCYTOCLASTIC VASCULITIS

DIAGNOSTIC HALLMARKS

1.   Distribution: especially marked on the lower legs
2.   Nonblanchable petechiae
3.   The petechiae are slightly palpable

CLINICAL PRESENTATION

Purpura is the general name for the escape of red blood cells into the skin. Purpura occurs in two forms: petechiae and ecchymoses. Petechiae are small lesions: macules and papules. Ecchymoses are large lesions: patches and plaques. The purpuric lesions of neutrophilic vasculitis consist entirely of petechiae; ecchymoses are not found. Moreover, since the petechiae form in association with the presence of a perivascular inflammatory infiltrate, the petechiae are usually palpable. This accounts for one of the synonyms for this disease: palpable purpura. Other synonyms include hypersensitivity angiitis, allergic vasculitis, and necrotizing vasculitis.

The smallest lesions of neutrophilic vasculitis occur as pinpoint dots which, early in the course of the disease, are bright red in color. As the lesions age they become increasingly violaceous or even blue-black in color. The smallest lesions may not be palpable, but they are usually accompanied by at least a few larger, palpable papules. These larger lesions are sharply marginated violaceous papules 2 to 10 mm in diameter. They are characterized by the presence of a minute centrally located blue-black infarct or tiny hemorrhagic vesicle. Both the small and the large lesions of neutrophilic vasculitis fail to blanch when they are compressed by a glass microscope slide. The lesions are asymptomatic.

The lesions of vasculitic purpura first develop on the lower legs but in the more severe cases there may be spread to the rest of the body. Some clustering of lesions, particularly over joints, is often notable.

The lesions of vasculitic purpura are easily recognizable on a clinical basis. A coagulation survey is usually carried out to eliminate nonvasculitic diseases such as thrombocytopenic purpura.

Atypical Presentations. Anaphylactoid purpura (Henoch-Schonlein purpura) is a neutrophilic vasculitic disease occurring primarily in children. The skin lesions are quite similar to those described above, though they are usually accompanied by scattered, intermingled dusky red flattopped papules 1 to 2 cm in diameter. These, too, fail to blanch on diascopy. Renal and gastrointestinal involvement are regularly present.

COURSE AND PROGNOSIS

The prognosis of vasculitic purpura depends largely on whether or not internal organs are involved. When internal involvement is not present there is little morbidity and the disease runs an uneventful course over 2 or 3 weeks. On the other hand, involvement of the nervous system, kidneys, or lungs results in considerable morbidity and even the possibility of death. Intermediate syndromes

with only skin, joint, and gastrointestinal involvement are less
troublesome.

PATHOGENESIS

The etiology and pathogenesis of leukocytoclastic vasculitis is
discussed in a separate section at the end of this chapter.

THERAPY

Milder cases of vasculitic purpura require no therapy at all.
Systemically administered steroids will be required in most
instances where internal organ involvement is recognized. The
response to such therapy is good but relapse often follows cessation
of steroid usage. There have recently been anecdotal reports
suggesting that nonsteroidal anti-inflammatory agents such as
colchicine, indomethacin, and dapsone are helpful. Antihistamines,
while often administered, do not seem to be particularly effective.

SELECTED READING

Mackel SE, Jordon RE: Leukocytoclastic vasculitis. A cutaneous
expression of immune complex disease. Arch Dermatol 118:296,
1982.
Saulsbury FT: Henoch-Schonlein purpura. Pediatr Dermatol 1:195,
1984.
Ekenstam E, Callen JP: Cutaneous leukocytoclastic vasculitis.
Clinical and laboratory features of 82 patients seen in private
practice. Arch Dermatol 120:484, 1984.
Sanchez NP, Van Hale HM, Su WPD: Clinical and histopathologic
spectrum of necrotizing vasculitis. Report of findings in 101
cases. Arch Dermatol 121:220, 1985.
Callen JP: Colchicine is effective in controlling chronic cutaneous
leukocytoclastic vasculitis. J Am Acad Dermatol 13:193, 1985.

MISCELLANEOUS PURPURAS

Purpura which occurs without inflammatory change (i.e.,
nonvasculitic purpura) can be divided into two groups: 1) an
intravascular type characterized by disorders of coagulation and 2)
an extravascular type characterized by faulty mechanical support for
blood vessel walls. Both of these types of purpura are
characterized by the presence of ecchymoses as well as petechiae.

The intravascular purpuras include conditions such as
thrombocytopenia, hemophilia, and platelet aggregation disorders.
Clinically these intravascular disorders are accompanied by the
presence of nonpalpable petechia, cutaneous ecchymoses, and evidence
of internal bleeding in the form of nosebleeds and gingival oozing.

The extravascular purpuras include conditions such as steroid induced purpura and actinic (senile) purpura. Clinically these extravascular disorders are accompanied by the presence of nonpalpable petechiae and cutaneous ecchymoses but they lack evidence of systemic bleeding. That is, nosebleeds and gingival oozing do not occur. Actinic purpura occurs only on sun damaged skin, primarily the lateral arms, whereas steroid purpura occurs anywhere on the body.

PATHOGENESIS OF THE VASCULAR REACTIONS

ETIOLOGY

A specific etiology (one that, when removed or treated, is followed by clearing of the vasculitis) is found in only about 10% of cases. These causes can be placed in six major groups: medications, infections, immune diseases, dysproteinemias, malignancies, and food, food dyes, and food preservatives. Specific items within these groups are listed in Table 14-2. These possibilities must be considered for any patient presenting with urticaria, erythema multiforme, erythema nodosum, or leukocytoclastic vasculitis. Of course, some causes are more often associated with one of these conditions than with the others. Thus penicillin reactions often occur as urticaria but rarely occur as vasculitis; on the other hand, sulfa reactions are more commonly associated with vasculitis than they are with urticaria. In order to simplify the identification of these many etiologies I have listed the most frequent causes for each of the clinical syndromes in the paragraphs below.

Urticaria. The most frequently identified causes of urticaria include penicillin, the sulfa related medications (antibiotics, thiazide diuretics, sulfonylureas, phenothiazines, and procainamide), streptococcal infection, acute viral syndromes, hepatitis B, coccidioidomycosis, lupus erythematosus, chronic inflammatory bowel disease, cryoglobulinemias, leukemia, and, in infants, all of the items listed under foods.

Erythema Multiforme. The most frequently identified causes of erythema multiforme include sulfa related medications as noted under urticaria, streptococcal infection, herpesvirus infection, mycoplasma pneumonia, coccidioidomycosis, histoplasmosis, lupus erythematosus, and chronic inflammatory bowel disease.

Erythema Nodosum. The most commonly identified causes of erythema nodosum include sulfa derived medications, yersinial enterocolitis, tuberculosis, coccidioidomycosis, histoplasmosis, inflammatory bowel disease, and sarcoidosis.

Leukocytoclastic Vasculitis. The most commonly identified causes of leukocytoclastic vasculitis include sulfa related medications, allopurinol, streptococcal infection, hepatitis B,

TABLE 14-2
COMMON CAUSES FOR URTICARIA, ERYTHEMA MULTIFORME, ERYTHEMA NODOSUM,
AND LEUKOCYTOCLASTIC VASCULITIS

Medications
    Antibiotics: penicillin, sulfas, cephalosporins
    Cardiovascular: thiazides, quinidine, procainamide
    Anticonvulsants: phenytoin, phenobarbital
    Miscellaneous: sulfonylureas, phenothiazines, allopurinol,
        some nonsteroidal anti-inflammatory agents (NSAIA)

Infections
    Bacterial: staphylococcal, streptococcal, yersinial, and
        mycobacterial infections
    Viral: many acute viral infections; chronic viral infections due
        to Epstein-Barr virus, hepatitis B virus, cytomegalovirus,
        and herpesvirus hominis
    Fungal: coccidioidomycosis and histoplasmosis
    Miscellaneous: mycoplasma, spirochetal, and rickettsial
        infection

Immune (autoimmune) disease
    Lupus erythematosus
    Dermatomyositis
    Polyarteritis nodosa
    Rheumatoid arthritis
    Juvenile rheumatoid arthritis
    Subacute bacterial endocarditis (see also bacterial infections)
    Sjogren's syndrome
    Chronic inflammatory bowel disease (all types)
    Sarcoidosis

Dysproteinemias
    Cryoglobulinemia
    Monoclonal and polyclonal gammopathies

Malignancies
    Leukemia (several types)
    Lymphoma (several types)
    Myeloma

Foods, food dyes, and food preservatives
    Foods: milk, eggs, nuts, shellfish, berries, chocolate, pork
    Food dyes: tartrazine; other azo dyes
    Food preservatives: monosodium glutamate

---

lupus erythematosus, rheumatoid arthritis, chronic inflammatory
bowel disease, cryoglobulinemia, polyclonal gammopathies, leukemia,
and myeloma.

There are, in addition to the causes discussed in the paragraphs
above, many precipitating factors which seem to enhance the
development of vascular reactions. Many of these act by way of
vasodilation (exercise, bathing, alcohol, spicy foods, hot foods,
and beverages); other precipitating factors include psychologic
stress, depression, pregnancy, chronic renal failure, and ingestion
of aspirin.

Finally, one must recognize that since a cause will only be
found for 10% of the patients, extensive laboratory testing in the
absence of clinical clues is not likely to be helpful. In most
cases a careful history and a thorough physical examination will
represent the most efficacious and cost saving approach.

PATHOPHYSIOLOGY

Most often urticaria, erythema multiforme, erythema nodosum, and
leukocytoclastic vasculitis develop as a result of immunologic
reactions to antigens listed in Table 14-2. For example when
erythema multiforme occurs as a result of herpes simplex infection,
the eruption is due to the antigenic rather than infective
properties of the virus. Thus the herpes simplex virus can cause
vesicles of the lip due to direct infection and can also cause a
bullous erythema multiforme through immunologic mechanisms.
Specific aspects of the immunologic reactions for each of the
vascular reactions are discussed in the paragraphs below.

Urticaria. The prototypic explanation for the development of
urticaria invokes a type 1, IgE mediated, hypersensitivity
response. During the process of sensitization IgE antibody is
synthesized and is attached to the cytoplasmic membrane of mast
cells. The next exposure to the sensitizing agent results in the
attachment of antigen to two adjacent antibody molecules on the mast
cell. This "bridging" attachment then results in mast cell
degranulation and release of a number of inflammatory mediators.
However, reactions of this type have only been documented in the
anaphylactic type of urticarias such as are sometimes seen with
penicillin allergy.

Urticarias can also be caused through complement mediated events
(e.g., cryoglobulin induced urticaria) and through nonimmunologic
mechanisms such as direct pharmacologic stimulation of mast cells
and induction of the lipoxygenase pathway of arachidonic acid
metabolism.

Erythema Multiforme. The specific immunologic mechanism
responsible for the development of erythema multiforme is unknown.
Circulating immune complexes are frequently present and, at least in
those instances due to herpes simplex infection, they may be

deposited at the site of the lesions. However, this immune complex
disease differs from that which occurs in leukocytoclastic
vasculitis in that immunoglobulins are not usually deposited in
lesional sites and only rarely does there appear to be deposition of
complement. The marked histologic presence of lymphocytes in the
lesions have caused some to suggest that cell mediated (type IV)
mechanisms are important. Mediator release as a result of mast cell
degranulation probably occurs but the mechanism through which this
occurs is unknown.

Erythema Nodosum. Essentially nothing is known about the
pathway(s) through which the lesions of erythema nodosum arise.
Histologically the process is a mixed lymphocytic and histiocytic
mediated panniculitis; some minor degree of lymphocytic vasculitis
is often present as well. The presence of lymphocytes suggests the
possibility of a cell mediated (type IV) reaction, perhaps existing
in the special granulomatous subset of these reactions. No
immunoreactants are deposited within the lesions suggesting that a
standard type III immune complex mechanism is not an important
component of the reaction.

Leukocytoclastic Vasculitis. Studies suggest that all, or
nearly all, examples of leukocytoclastic vasculitis develop as a
result of immune complex (type III) mechanism. In this process
circulating immune complexes are deposited on the basement membrane
of venules. This deposition requires some disturbance of the
endothelial cells (possibly occurring as a result of mediator
release from mast cells) in order to gain direct exposure of the
underlying basement membrane. Once complexes are deposited,
complement is activated. As part of the complement cascade
chemoattractant molecules are released which draw neutrophils into
the area. These neutrophils attempt to phagocytize the deposited
immune complexes and in so doing release destructive proteolytic
lysosomal enzymes. The vascular wall damage done by these enzymes
allows for the characteristic extravasation of erythrocytes. This
whole process requires only 24 to 72 hours, at which time the
neutrophils are slowly replaced by mononuclear cells as part of the
reparative phase of the reaction.

SELECTED READING

Orton PW, Huff JC, Tonnesen MG, Weston WL: Detection of a herpes
    simplex viral antigen in skin lesions of erythema multiforme.
    Ann Intern Med 101:48, 1984.
Yancey KB, Lawley TJ: Circulating immune complexes: Their
    immunochemistry, biology, and detection in selected dermatologic
    and systemic diseases. J Am Acad Dermatol 10:711, 1984.
Keahey TM: The pathogenesis of urticaria. Dermatol Clinics
    3:13, 1985.

Group 9: The Papulosquamous Diseases

GROUP IDENTIFICATION

Groups 9 and 10 are characterized by the presence of scaling erythematous papules and plaques. The scaling, which differentiates these two groups from Groups 7 and 8, may or may not be readily appreciable. Psoriatic-type scale (large white or gray flakes) can be easily seen but pityriasis-type scale is fine and powdery. One needs to loosen it with the edge of scalpel blade before the fine white powder becomes visible. Lichen-type scale is tightly compacted on the surface of the lesion. Its flatness and tight attachment gives it a shiny, translucent appearance. These three types of scale are discussed in greater detail in Chapter 3. Sometimes, however, lesions which are by nature scaly have been modified by the patient in such a way that no evidence of scale can be found. Thus if the patient has vigorously bathed shortly before the examination, if the patient has applied any hand cream or lubricant, or if the patient's disease is partially treated, no scale may be discernible.

Differentiation between the lesions of Group 9 (the papulosquamous diseases) and Group 10 (the eczematous diseases) depends on the sharpness of margination and on the presence or absence of epithelial disruption. Thus the papulosquamous diseases are characterized by the presence of sharp margination and the absence of epithelial disruption. The clinical features of epithelial disruption are discussed in Chapter 3 and again, under group identification, in Chapter 16.

PSORIASIS

DIAGNOSTIC HALLMARKS

    1.   Distribution: scalp, elbows, knees, gluteal fold
    2.   Koebner phenomenon
    3.   Nail pitting

CLINICAL PRESENTATION

    Psoriasis is characterized by the presence of sharply marginated
red plaques which are covered by copious amounts of white or silver
scale. The scale is made up of fairly large flakes, some of which
are large enough to grasp and strip off. Doing so may reveal
underlying pinpoint spots of bleeding (Auspitz sign). Newly
developed lesions are small (1- to 3-mm) papules but centrifugal
growth with coalescence of adjacent lesions results in the formation
of large plaques. The coalescence results in the formation of some
plaques which have a gyrate or serpiginous configuration. Linear
lesions are also often present. This linearity is a reflection of
the Koebner phenomenon, wherein lesions preferentially arise at the
site of cutaneous trauma. The Koebner phenomenon is highly
distinctive and it is found in only one other commonly encountered
disease, lichen planus.
    Lesions of psoriasis can occur anywhere on the body, but they
are most commonly located on the scalp, elbows, and knees. The
extensor surfaces of the arms and legs are also often involved.
Involvement of the gluteal fold and umbilicus is less commonly seen
but is a very distinctive sign of psoriasis when present.
    Nail changes are present in many patients. Early changes
include nail plate pitting and onycholysis. Later changes include
marked nail plate dystrophy and marked buildup of subungual, soft
yellow keratin. The latter changes are very similar to those which
occur in fungal infections of the nail; differentiation depends on
KOH examination and fungal culture. Nail changes are said to be
more common in those patients who have associated psoriatic
arthritis of the hands.
    In most instances the lesions of psoriasis are not pruritic but
those plaques which occur in the scalp and intertriginous folds are
sometimes associated with considerable itching. A few patients,
presumably those who are genetically atopic, will complain of
generalized itching.
    Atypical Clinical Presentations. Very rarely the lesions in
psoriatics become extensive enough to involve the entire body
surface. In such instances itching is often severe and there is
evidence of eczematization with weeping and crusting. Distinction
from other forms of exfoliative erythrodermatitis (see Chapter 16)

is assisted by the presence of typical nail changes, seronegative arthritis, and a past history of more typical lesions.

Children and young adults sometimes develop guttate psoriasis. This form of psoriasis is recognized by the sudden outbreak of hundreds of small, red, nonconfluent papules. Scale formation on these papules is often scanty. Plaque formation is usually minimal but a careful search will usually reveal one or more slightly linear lesions due to the Koebner phenomenon. The appearance of guttate psoriasis is sometimes triggered by a preceding streptococcal infection. Children with guttate psoriasis that has resolved sometimes experience long periods of complete remission.

Pustular psoriasis (see also Chapter 8) occurs in two forms: that which involves primarily the palms and soles and is accompanied by nonpustular lesions of psoriasis elsewhere (Barber type) and that which is completely generalized (Von Zumbusch type). The latter often evolves into an exfoliative erythrodermatitis and is often accompanied by fever, anemia, leukocytosis, and general debilitation.

COURSE AND PROGNOSIS

Psoriasis is a lifelong, chronic disease characterized by exacerbations and remissions. Individual lesions tend to be in a constant state of flux. Plaques are continually growing, resolving, and changing in shape. The overall course of the disease is highly unpredictable. The patient's initial lesions offer no clue as to the future course. Months of mild involvement may be followed by a period of severe flaring but then again sometimes the reverse occurs.

Little disability occurs as a result of the skin lesions but about 10% of psoriatics develop arthritic changes. Many of these individuals will experience considerable pain and joint deformity. This is particularly true for those few patients who develop spondylitis and sacroiliitis.

PATHOGENESIS

The cause of psoriasis is unknown but genetic factors play a role in the development of the disease. About 30% of psoriatic patients have a positive family history. Moreover, psoriatics have a significantly increased incidence of several HLA antigens. Immunologic factors may also be important but no consistent explanation of specific immunologic abnormalities has as yet been elucidated.

Psoriatic lesions examined histologically reveal the presence of inflammatory cells, an increase in the number of epidermal cells (acanthosis), and increased keratin production. The influx of inflammatory cells (especially the neutrophils) is probably due to the presence of one or more leukotrienes with potent chemotactic properties within the stratum corneum. The increased keratin production is most likely due to changes in epidermal cell kinetics. Specifically, the keratinocyte cell cycle is greatly shortened and there is extraordinarily fast movement of cells from the basal layer to the stratum corneum. This increased proliferative activity is accompanied by elevated epidermal cell levels of cyclic guanosine monophosphate (cGMP), prostaglandins (notably PGE_2), and polyamines. It is not known whether these biochemical changes account for, or result from, the proliferative activity.

THERAPY

Sunlight is beneficial to many patients with psoriasis. Some individuals can control their own disease solely with sunbathing. Most patients, however, require additional therapy, such as intermittent use of the mid and high potency topically applied steroids. Where necessary, penetration of these topically applied steroids can be enhanced by the use of occlusive dressings or, alternately, individual lesions may be intralesionally injected with triamcinolone acetonide.

Topically applied tar products are also useful but, because of odor and appearance, are often not acceptable to patients. Most tar therapy is administered during hospitalization as part of the modified Goeckerman program. In this regimen crude coal tar ointment is applied each day after UVB ultraviolet light has been administered. The tar is reapplied several times during the day, but prior to the next day's light treatment, a bath is taken and the tar products are washed off. This cycle is carried out for about 3 weeks, during which time most patients will have achieved a satisfactory remission. Such remissions can often be maintained for 4 to 8 months. This approach is expensive in time and money but the results are good and the safety factor is high. The Goeckerman program can also be carried out in day care centers when these are available in the community.

Anthralin, a tar-like product, is gaining acceptance for home therapy. In this setting 0.1 to 1.0% concentrations are applied for 15 to 60 minutes; the anthralin is then completely washed off. This "short application" program avoids much of the staining and odor problem associated with tars.

Alternatively, PUVA therapy can be used. This therapy (see Chapter 4) is remarkably effective in the treatment of psoriasis, but this efficacy is balanced by high cost, need for continued maintenance treatment, and some uncertainty about possible later development of cutaneous malignancy and cataract formation. Approximately 95% of patients can obtain complete clearing when PUVA treatments are given two or three times a week over a 2-month period.   Thereafter the frequency of treatments can be gradually reduced.

Psoriasis unresponsive to the approaches described above may require cytotoxic drugs. Methotrexate, the most widely used agent, is generally given orally in a weekly 25-mg dose (see Chapter 4). Usually ten tablets (2.5 mg each) are taken in a single dose but split schedule dosages may also be used. Improvement is noted within 4 weeks and appreciable clearing can be expected by the end of the second month. The dose is then tapered to whatever maintenance level keeps the psoriasis under acceptable good control. Short term toxicity is not a major problem but long term hepatotoxicity is. For this reason periodic liver biopsies are required. Methotrexate is discontinued if and when fibrosis is found. Fortunately psoriatics receiving long term methotrexate have shown no propensity for the development of nosocomial infection or drug induced malignancies.

The role for retinoids in the treatment of psoriasis is not yet settled. There is little doubt that they are extremely effective, but concern remains about long term toxicity, especially as regards hyperlipidemia and calcification of the spine. Short term administration of 13-cis-retinoic acid, isotretinoin, is very useful in treating the acute phase of pustular psoriasis, whereas long term administration of etretinate in doses of 0.5 to 1.0 mg per kg results in nearly complete clearing of patients with more classical plaque-type psoriasis.

The presence of scalp and nail disease presents special problems in the treatment of psoriasis. Scalp lesions sometimes respond to the use of a tar shampoo alone but often steroid lotions must be applied as well. Penetration of the steroid solution can be enhanced by using shower cap occlusion at night. The presence of thick scale sometimes prevents adequate topical application. In such instances softening solutions such as Baker's P & S or T-Derm solution can be applied along with the steroid lotion. Both are left on overnight. The softened scale is then appreciably easier to remove during the morning shampoo.

Local treatment of nail dystrophy is difficult. High potency topical steroids are applied to the nail matrix and a finger cot is used for occlusion. This must be continued for 3 months due to the slow growth of nails. Unfortunately the onset of cutaneous atrophy often occurs before normal nails have regrown. Alternately, the nail matrix can be injected with triamcinolone acetonide but this approach is severely limited by patient discomfort. Methotrexate, retinoid, or PUVA therapy may be necessary to obtain satisfactory clearing and often concerns about toxicity limit the applicability of these approaches.

The arthritis of psoriasis often improves when skin lesions are successfully treated. To the degree that this does not occur, consideration should be given to the use of methotrexate, retinoids

or even intramuscularly administered gold. Symptomatic treatment
with nonsteroidal anti-inflammatory agents (NSAIA) is, of course,
also carried out. However, there is at least theoretical concern
that some of the agents, by way of blocking the cyclo-oxygenase
pathway of arachidonic acid metabolism, may increase production of
leukotrienes and actually worsen psoriasis.

SELECTED READING

Cram DL: Psoriasis: Current advances in etiology and treatment. J
    Am Acad Dermatol 4:1, 1981.
Weiss VC, van den Broek H, Barrett S, West DP: Immunopathology of
    psoriasis: A comparison with other parakeratotic lesions. J
    Invest Dermatol 78:256, 1982.
Miller RAW: The Koebner phenomenon. Int J Dermatol 21:192, 1982.
Maibach H: Topical treatment of psoriasis with corticosteroids.
    Efficacy screening in relationship to clinical psoriasis. Acta
    Derm Venereol Suppl 112:17, 1983.
Muller SA: Topical treatment of psoriasis with tar. Acta Derm
    Venereol Suppl 112:7, 1983.
Farber EM, Abel EA, Charuworn A: Recent advances in the treatment
    of psoriasis. J Am Acad Dermatol 8:311, 1983.
Kouskoukis CE, Scher RK, Lebovits PE: Psoriasis of the nails.
    Cutis 31:169, 1983.
Greaves MW: Neutrophil polymorphonuclears, mediators and the
    pathogenesis of psoriasis. Br J Dermatol 109:115, 1983.
Boer J, Hermans J, Schothorst AA, Suurmond D: Comparison of
    phototherapy (UV-B) and photochemotherapy (PUVA) for clearing
    and maintenance therapy of psoriasis. Arch Dermatol 120:52,
    1984.
Zachariae H: Cytostatic treatment of psoriasis -- present status.
    Acta Derm Venereol Suppl 113:127, 1984.
Edells LD, Wolff JM, Garloff J, Eaglstein WH: Comparison of
    suberythemogenic and maximally aggressive ultraviolet B therapy
    for psoriasis. J Am Acad Dermatol 11:105, 1984.
Armstrong RB, Leach EE, Fleiss JL, Harber LC: Modified Goeckerman
    therapy for psoriasis. Arch Dermatol 120:313, 1984.
Baker BS, Swain AF, Valdimarsson H, Fry L: T-cell subpopulations in
    the blood and skin of patients with psoriasis. Br J Dermatol
    110:37, 1984.
Oriente CB, Scarpa R, Pucino A, et al: Prevalence of psoriatic
    arthritis in psoriatic patients. Acta Derm Venereol Suppl
    113:109, 1984.
Krueger GG, Bergstresser PR, Lowe NJ, et al: Psoriasis. J Am Acad
    Dermatol 11;937, 1984.
Grabbe J, Czarnetzki BM, Rosenbach T, Mardin M: Identification of
    chemotactic lipoxygenase products of arachidonate metabolism in
    psoriatic skin. J Invest Dermatol 82:477, 1984.

Weinstein GD, McCullough JL, Ross PA: Cell kinetic basis for
    pathophysiology of psoriasis. J Invest Dermatol 85:579, 1985.
Braverman IM, Sibley J: The response of psoriatic epidermis and
    microvessels to treatment with topical steroids and oral
    methotrexate. J Invest Dermatol 85:584, 1985.
Schwarz T, Gschnait F: Anthralin minute entire skin treatment.
    Arch Dermatol 121:1512, 1985.
Moy RL, Kingston TP, Lowe NJ: Isotretinoin vs. etretinate therapy
    in generalized pustular and chronic psoriasis. Arch Dermatol
    121:1297, 1985.
Dubertret L, Chastang C, Beylot C, et al: Maintenance treatment of
    psoriasis by Tigason: A double-blind randomized clinical
    trial. Br J Dermatol 113:323, 1905.

TINEA PEDIS, TINEA CRURIS, TINEA CORPORIS, AND TINEA CAPITIS

DIAGNOSTIC HALLMARKS

    1.   Distribution: feet, groin, face, hands, and arms
    2.   KOH preparations and fungal cultures

CLINICAL PRESENTATION

    The clinical appearance of these diseases depends to a very
large extent on the location of the disease. Each of these three
conditions is discussed separately below.
    Tinea pedis usually begins with the development of a fissure in
the web space betwen the fourth and fifth toes. Keratin buildup
occurs on the edges of the fissures and, because of maceration, the
keratin usually appears white and soggy. From there the infection
can spread to the toenails and to the bottom of the feet. Fungal
infection on the plantar aspect of the foot occurs as a red scaling
plaque which curves a short way up the sides of the foot. However,
extension onto the dorsal surface of the foot does not occur.
Vesiculation occasionally develops on the instep of the foot (see
Chapter 7). Tinea pedis is found in teenagers and adults; for
practical purposes it does not develop in children. Patients with
mild disease are usually asymptomatic but in some instances heat and
sweating cause considerable itching. Resultant scratching converts
the original papulosquamous process to that of an eczematous disease
(see Chapters 16 and 17). When that occurs the dorsal surface of
the feet often becomes eczematized. A suspected clinical diagnosis
must be confirmed by KOH preparation or culture.
    Tinea cruris is characterized by the development of sharply
marginated, red plaques on the upper inner thighs. Lesions first
appear close to the inguinal-scrotal crease and slowly advance down
the inner sides of the thighs. As advancement occurs, healing of
previously involved skin is sometimes seen. This results in the

appearance of an advancing, thin, semicircular line ("ringworm") on the inner thighs. A small amount of scale formation is present at the active border but it is often obscured because of the moisture retained in the groin. The penis and scrotum are not involved but extension onto the buttocks may be seen. Tinea cruris does not develop prior to puberty. Men are much more commonly infected than are women. The lesions are usually asymptomatic but retention of heat and sweating sometimes cause considerable itching. Resultant scratching converts the papulosquamous appearance to that of an eczematous process (see Chapters 16 and 17). KOH preparations or cultures should be used to confirm a clinical diagnosis.

Tinea corporis occurs in two forms: zoophilic infections acquired from animals and anthropophilic infections acquired from personal contact or fomites. Zoophilic infections appear as circular, bright red, sharply marginated, scaling plaques. Often only a single plaque is present but occasionally three or four may be seen. Each plaque is usually less than 5 cm in diameter. The plaques are often solid but annular forms are also seen. Those infections which are acquired from pets or farm animals occur in both children and adults. Anthropophilic infections, on the other hand, are found only in adults. They occur as larger, annular lesions with gyrate or serpiginous borders. Anthropophilic lesions are annular rather than solid. However, incomplete forms may be present such that only fragments of the circles are recognized. The erythematous, thin border of the lesions is a dull red and the amount of scale present is highly variable. Lesions are most commonly found on the buttocks and around the waist but involvement of the face or dorsal surface of the hands also occurs. Most lesions of tinea corporis are asymptomatic, but excoriations may be present, especially in areas where sweat is retained. In both types of tinea corporis a clinical diagnosis must be confirmed by KOH preparations or culture.

Tinea capitis, or "ringworm" of the scalp, presents as one or more sharply marginated plaques of partial alopecia. Inflammation and scale are present but often these two changes are quite minimal. The recognition of broken hairs in the form of stubble and black dots at the follicular orifices is the best clue to correct diagnosis. Nearly all cases occur in children but the diagnosis should be considered in any adult presenting with evidence of localized alopecia (see Chapter 18). Kerion formation is a complication which occurs in about 10% of cases. This represents a sensitization phenomenon where the fungi present induce a remarkably brisk inflammatory reaction in the infected plaques with pustulation, crusting, and edema formation. Wood's lamp examination is negative and KOH preparations are difficult for the inexperienced to interpret. For this reason any suspected diagnosis requires the removal of infected hairs for fungal culture.

COURSE AND PROGNOSIS

Tinea capitis and zoophilic tinea corporis usually resolve
spontaneously after 6 to 12 months of activity. Tinea pedis, tinea
cruris, and anthropophilic tinea corporis continue indefinitely.
There are, however, periods of relative quiescence and
exacerbation. All of these fungal diseases respond well to
treatment, but with the exception of tinea capitis and zoophilic
tinea corporis infections, recurrence following treatment is rather
likely.

PATHOGENESIS

Tinea pedis, tinea cruris, and anthropophilic tinea corporis are
most commonly caused by Trichophyton rubrum. Trichophyton
interdigitale and Epidermophyton floccosum infections also are
seen. Generally one cannot predict the causative organism on the
basis of clinical appearance. Zoophilic tinea corporis can be
caused by Microsporum canis, Trichophyton mentagrophytes, and
Trichophyton verrucosum. Tinea capitis is caused by Trichophyton
tonsurans in 90% of cases.
The likelihood of inoculation with any of these fungi is
enhanced if cuts and scratches are present on the skin. Infection
following inoculation is encouraged by the presence of warmth and
moisture, such as occurs in the groin and under footwear.
Depression of cell mediated immune responsiveness, such as is found
in atopic individuals, is a major predisposing factor for the
development of T. rubrum infection.

THERAPY

Tinea cruris and tinea pedis which involves only the web spaces
can be treated with any of the topical antifungal agents discussed
in Chapter 4. Other forms of tinea pedis usually require the use of
griseofulvin. Mild cases of tinea corporis also respond well to
topical agents. Extensive disease and those with a component of
follicular pustulation are best treated with griseofulvin. Tinea
capitis requires the use of griseofulvin. Orally administered
ketoconazole therapy is rarely appropriate for either tinea corporis
or capitis. Kerion formation, if present, can be treated with
intralesional steroid injections or with a short burst of
systemically administered steroids.

SELECTED READING
Hay RJ, Shennan G: Chronic dermatophyte infections II. Antibody
    and cell-mediated immune responses. Br J Dermatol 106:191, 1982.
Solomon LM: Tinea capitis: Current concepts. Pediatr Dermatol
    2:224, 1985.

Rudolph AH: The diagnosis and treatment of tinea capitis due to trichophyton tonsurans. Int J Dermatol 24:426, 1985.

LUPUS ERYTHEMATOSUS

DIAGNOSTIC HALLMARKS

1. Distribution: face, neck, and sun exposed areas of the upper trunk and arms
2. Sunlight sensitivity

CLINICAL PRESENTATION

Lupus erythematosus (LE) is a disease which has a very broad spectrum of clinical symptoms and signs (Fig. 15-1). The spectrum is seamless but it is convenient to consider four points on the spectrum as if they were four separate conditions. The cutaneous aspects of the four conditions are described in the paragraphs below; the polar aspects of the various skin lesions are summarized in Table 15-1. Discussion regarding the systemic aspects of the disease can be found in reference textbooks.

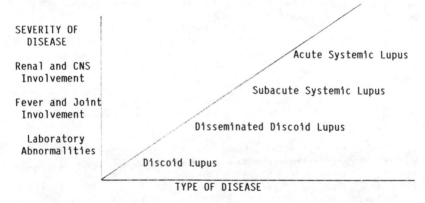

Figure 15-1. The spectrum of lupus erythematosus extends from the purely cutaneous forms to severe, systemic disease. There is no sharp cutoff between the various categories and one type of the disease may, with the passage of time, merge with the next. There is, however, no inexorable progression from mild to severe disease. Patients who begin with the purely cutaneous forms are unlikely ever to develop significant systemic disease.

As is apparent from the discussion below, only the discoid type skin lesions possess all of the characteristics of papulosquamous disease. The skin lesions which occur in patients with systemic disease lack one or more papulosquamous characteristics and thus overlap with disease of the vascular reaction and eczematous disease groups.

The lesions in all types of LE are, in a general sort of way, correlated with sunlight exposure. They are primarily found on the sun exposed portions of the body and in many cases the patient will have noted the development of new lesions (or the worsening of old lesions) following one or more episodes of sunlight exposure. Nevertheless, a specific history of photosensitivity is lacking in some patients.

The patches and plaques of LE are generally asymptomatic but a sensation of swelling and burning is sometimes described by patients with the lesions of systemic LE.

The diagnosis of LE involving the skin can usually be made on the basis of clinical examination. However, confirmation should be obtained through biopsy. Immunofluorescent biopsies of skin lesions (the lupus band test) are particularly helpful since they regularly reveal the deposition of complement and immunoglobulin at the dermal-epidermal junction. Similar deposits can also be present in the nonlesional skin of those patients who have systemic disease. Discussion of serologic tests useful in the diagnosis of LE is beyond the scope of this chapter.

Discoid Lupus Erythematosus. The skin lesions of discoid LE consist of sharply marginated, erythematous plaques 1 to 4 cm in diameter. The larger of these lesions are often annular. In such lesions a thin erythematous scaling border surrounds a white, scarred center. Smaller lesions are solid, flattopped papules and plaques diffusely covered with scale. The lesions of discoid LE occur anywhere on the face but are most often found on the lateral cheeks, particularly at the jawline. The distribution, although usually bilateral, is often not symmetrical. Lesions in the scalp occur as sharply localized patches of hair loss (see Chapter 18). Gray-white plaques are sometimes found on the lips and oral mucous membranes (see Chapter 21). Discoid lupus erythematosus occurs with approximately equal frequency in men and women. The disease develops at any point from childhood to late adult life (see also Table 15-1).

Disseminated Discoid Lupus Erythematosus. In disseminated discoid LE the skin lesions are similar to those described above. There is, however, less tendency for central clearing and for scarring. Moreover, the distribution pattern is widened; lesions are found on the sun exposed surfaces of the arms and hands as well as on the face. Scarring alopecia is not often present.

Subacute Lupus Erythematosus. Two types of subacute LE exist. The first consists of lesions which are predominantly distributed on

TABLE 15-1
POLAR ASPECTS OF SKIN LESIONS IN LUPUS ERYTHEMATOSUS

| MORPHOLOGY | TYPE OF LUPUS ERYTHEMATOSUS | |
	DISCOID	SYSTEMIC
Distribution	Face, scalp	Face, trunk, arms, hands
Symmetry of distribution	Asymmetrical	Symmetrical
Scarring	Present	Absent
Margination	Sharp	Diffuse
Scaling	Present	Minimal
Hair loss	Localized	Diffuse

the chest and shoulders. These lesions are usually annular plaques 2 to 10 cm in diameter. The outer red ring is 3 to 5 mm wide and has little or no scale. The central portion appears as normal skin. Coalescence of these lesions to form larger plaques with a gyrate configuration sometimes occurs. More rarely psoriasiform lesions may be found in the same distribution. The second type of subacute LE occurs on the face, trunk, and arms in the form of erythematous, psoriatic-type plaques which are intermediate in morphology between those of discoid and those of systemic LE. Thus symmetry is usually present but scale and central atrophy are less prominent. Margination is sharp in some areas but diffuse in others.

  Acute Systemic Lupus Erythematosus. The cutaneous hallmark of acute systemic LE is the presence of a symmetrical, poorly marginated, erythematous plaque which extends over the bridge of the nose and onto the upper malar prominences. Scale formation in this so-called butterfly eruption is minimal and the plaque is usually somewhat edematous. When lesions occur other than on the face, there is a marked tendency for coalescence, as opposed to the smaller discrete lesions of discoid LE. Hair loss when present is diffuse rather than localized. Mucous membrane lesions occur in about 25% of patients; they are identical with those seen in discoid LE (see Chapter 21). Both sides of the hands are regularly involved. Small patches of erythema are located on the dorsal surface of the phalanges but the area over the knuckles is spared. Reddening and telangiectasia are frequently present in a narrow band

at the posterior nail folds. The palmar surfaces of the hands are
often a dusky, violaceous color. This is particularly notable over
the tips of the fingers and on the thenar and hypothenar eminences.
Small, bright red, blanching macules or violaceous vasculitic
lesions may be superimposed against these duskier color changes.
Acute LE develops most often during the second, third, and fourth
decades. Women outnumber men by a considerable margin (see also
Table 15-1).

COURSE AND PROGNOSIS

The course and prognosis of LE correlate rather well with
various types of cutaneous lesions (see Fig 15-1). Patients with
discoid lesions confined to the face may have a few minor laboratory
abnormalities but rarely, if ever, have symptoms and signs of
systemic disease. Moreover, 95% of such patients will have a normal
life span with nothing more than cutaneous morbidity as a
manifestation of their disease.
Patients with disseminated discoid skin lesions usually have a
number of minor laboratory abnormalities, but they, too, rarely
develop significant systemic disease.
Patients with lesions of subacute LE often have fever and
arthralgia, but cardiac, central nervous system, and renal
involvement are usually mild or absent. Patients with lesions of
acute LE are highly likely to have serious systemic symptoms and
signs.
The lesions of discoid LE heal with scarring and sometimes "burn
out" altogether after 10 to 20 years of activity. The lesions of
subacute and acute LE heal without scarring. These latter lesions
tend to mirror the activity of the underlying systemic disease.
That is, they fade during periods of remission and reappear during
exacerbations.

PATHOGENESIS

The cause of skin lesions in lupus erythematosus is not known.
In most instances, sunlight seems to play an important precipitating
role. Exposure to wavelengths of 280- to 320-nm UVL (the UVB or
sunburn spectrum) presumably leads to damage of epithelial cell
DNA. It is hypothesized that this modified DNA then acts as a new
antigen which stimulates the production of "autoimmune" antibodies.
The production of these antibodies by B cells is enhanced by the
reduction in suppressor T cells usually found in LE patients.
Antibodies, once formed, are deposited along with complement in the
skin and other organs. Genetic factors, as manifest by the
frequency of familial cases and the presence of certain HLA
patterns, are undoubtedly important. Since the more serious forms
of LE occur primarily in women it is suspected that the presence of
estrogens (or absence of androgens) may play a role.

THERAPY

All patients should be protected from ultraviolet light
irradiation in the UVB (sunburn) spectrum. This can be accomplished
rather well by regular application of sunscreens with high SPF
factors (see Chapter 4). In addition, protective clothing is
recommended and a change in lifestyle which moves outdoor activities
to the beginning and end of the day is suggested.

The cutaneous lesions of LE resolve with steroid treatment.
Discoid lesions respond poorly to topical steroids but do improve
with intralesional injections of triamcinolone. The lesions of
subacute and acute LE clear when associated systemic disease is
treated with systemic steroids. The oral administration of
hydroxychloroquine (Plaquenil) in a daily dose of 200 to 400 mg is
very helpful in the treatment of both types of skin lesions.

SELECTED READING

Callen JP: Chronic cutaneous lupus erythematosus. Clinical,
    laboratory, therapeutic, and prognostic examination of 62
    patients. Arch Dermatol 118:412, 1982.
Sontheimer RD, Maddison PJ, Reichlin M, et al: Serologic and HLA
    associations in subacute cutaneous lupus erythematosus, a
    clinical subset of lupus erythematosus. Ann Intern Med 97:664,
    1982.
Sontheimer RD, Deng J-S, Gilliam JN: Antinuclear and
    anticytoplasmic antibodies. Concepts and misconceptions. J Am
    Acad Dermatol 9:335, 1983.
Zamansky GB: Sunlight-induced pathogenesis in systemic lupus
    erythematosus. J Invest Dermatol 85:179, 1985.
Callen JP, Fowler JF, Kulick KB: Serologic and clinical features of
    patients with discoid lupus erythematosus: Relationship of
    antibodies to single-stranded deoxyribonucleic acid and of other
    antinuclear antibody subsets to clinical manifestations. J Am
    Acad Dermatol 13:748, 1985.
Callen JP: Systemic lupus erythematosus in patients with chronic
    cutaneous (discoid) lupus erythematosus. J Am Acad Dermatol
    12:278, 1985.
Christian CL, Elkon KB: Autoantibodies to intracellular proteins.
    Clinical and biologic significance. Am J Med 80:53, 1986.

PARAPSORIASIS AND MYCOSIS FUNGOIDES

DIAGNOSTIC HALLMARKS

    1. Distribution: trunk, buttocks, and thighs
    2. Stability of plaque shape and size

Parapsoriasis is not itself a very important disease. It is rarely seen, is not contagious, and cannot be cured. Its importance lies in its relationship to the cutaneous T cell lymphoma mycosis fungoides. These two diseases exist on a spectrum such that over a number of years the lesions have some predilection towards evolution into those of mycosis fungoides. Recognition of these evolving lesions at earliest possible time is important from a therapeutic standpoint.

CLINICAL PRESENTATION

Several varieties of parapsoriasis exist, but only the most common one, parapsoriasis en plaque, is discussed here. The lesions of parapsoriasis en plaque consist of sharply marginated, scaling, red plaques. As the name suggests, the appearance of these plaques is somewhat similar to that of psoriasis plaques. However, in parapsoriasis the color is brown-red rather than bright red; the scale is fine and powdery (pityriasis type) rather than flaky; and evidence of the Koebner phenomenon is not found. Finally, the plaques of parapsoriasis are extraordinarily stable in shape and size whereas those of psoriasis are constantly changing over a period of weeks to months. The lesions of tinea corporis are also somewhat similar in appearance to those of parapsoriasis. KOH preparations and cultures will allow for differentiation.

The lesions of parapsoriasis can occur anywhere on the trunk and proximal extremities but are most commonly seen on the abdomen, buttocks, and thighs. In women the breasts are often involved. Parapsoriasis does not appear until the mid or late adult years. The lesions are asymptomatic.

The evolution of parapsoriatic plaques into those of mycosis fungoides is marked by a gradual thickening. Scale becomes less apparent and the brown-red color gradually develops dusky, violaceous hues. The round or oval outline of the plaques gradually takes on a more irregular shape. Indented (kidney shaped) and polycyclic forms are seen. Biopsies show more atypicality in the lymphocytes which crowd the upper dermis and clusters of these atypical cells begin to appear within the epidermis. These clinical and histologic changes characterize the second, or plaque, stage of mycosis fungoides. The final stage of mycosis fungoides is identified by the formation of large nodular tumors many of which develop deep ulcerations. Patients with advanced cutaneous disease are likely to have systemic involvement as well.

Atypical Clinical Presentations. Mycosis fungoides may also begin as an exfoliative erythrodermatitis. This generalized eczematous process may be indistinguishable from that due to other causes (see Chapter 16), but in some instances there is associated alopecia, palmar and plantar hyperkeratosis, and cutaneous hyperpigmentation. This constellation of findings is known as

Sezary's syndrome. Patients with Sezary's syndrome usually have evidence of systemic involvement as noted by lymphadenopathy and the presence of mycosis (Sezary) cells on examination of the peripheral white blood cell smear.

Rarely, the first manifestation of mycosis fungoides is the sudden onset of multiple tumors. The patches and plaques of earlier stages are entirely lacking. This condition is known as d'emblee-type mycosis fungoides.

COURSE AND PROGNOSIS

Parapsoriasis is an extraordinarily stable and slow moving disease. Gradual centrifugal enlargement of individual plaques does occur but years go by before light microscopic and clinical evidence of malignancy is seen. Patients frequently develop other health problems and die long before mycosis fungoides becomes a problem.

The course of mycosis fungoides, once present, is extremely variable. A few individuals will develop evidence of systemic disease in as little as several years but most will go for 5 to 10 years before internal involvement is recognized. However, once the latter develops, the pace of the disease picks up appreciably. At that point one can predict death from the disease within 2 to 5 years. In spite of this slow and highly variable course, one thing is clear. Mycosis fungoides is inevitably fatal. One escapes death from mycosis fungoides only by dying from some other process.

PATHOGENESIS

The cause of parapsoriasis and mycosis fungoides is unknown. However, a current, attractive hypothesis suggests that mycosis fungoides develops as an uncontrolled immunologic reaction to a persistent antigen which is deposited on, or is developed in, the skin. This hypothesis, which is based on the large number of Langerhans cells present in the early inflammatory infiltrate, suggests that Langerhans cells process and convey an unknown antigen to helper T cell lymphocytes. These T cells in turn activate a clone of T cells which, perhaps because of persistent stimulation, eventually develops malignant characteristics. Once formed, these malignant T cells (known as mycosis cells, Lutzner cells, or Sezary cells) increase in number and collect in the skin and eventually in the lymph nodes and other internal organs. In the early lesions of mycosis fungoides the proportion of malignant to benign inflammatory cells is low. In the tumor stage a much higher proportion of malignant cells is found.

Discovery of the HTLV-I virus has added another dimension to our understanding of cutaneous T cell lymphomas. Infection of T helper lymphocytes with this virus results in eventual proliferation of infected cells. It seems likely that at first this is a latent infection which only subsequently (perhaps due to antigenic stimulation) leads to transformation and proliferation. It is not presently known why HTLV infection leads to a proliferative response, whereas infection with the related HTLV-III virus (the agent responsible for acquired immunodeficiency syndrome [AIDS]) leads to the death of T helper cells. However, it should be noted that most patients in the United States with cutaneous T cell lymphoma do not seem to have evidence of this virus infection and for this reason it alone cannot be used to explain the etiology of mycosis fungoides.

THERAPY

Patients with parapsoriasis are often first treated with topically applied steroids. Unfortunately, the degree of response is usually unsatisfactory and at that point a decision must be made regarding the use of more vigorous therapies. The more conventional approach revolves around the use of topically applied nitrogen mustard or the administration of PUVA therapy. Both types of therapy are discussed in Chapter 4. With either modality 70 to 80% of patients can obtain a complete cutaneous remission. These remissions must be maintained by continuous treatment; once treatment is stopped relapse is certain. Those who fail to respond and those who break through during treatment can be treated with electron beam radiation.

The more radical approach involves the initial use of total body electron beam irradiation. Complete remissions are obtained in 90% of the patients treated and, more importantly, about 20% of these patients maintain their remissions indefinitely without further therapy. Thus a small but significant proportion of the patients appear to be cured. Unfortunately, this approach exposes patients to a considerable amount of radiation (about 3000 rads), is time consuming and expensive, and can only be carried out in a limited number of institutions.

Patients with evidence of systemic disease are usually given multiple drug chemotherapy in addition to total body electron beam therapy. Unfortunately, no matter how aggressive an approach to therapy is taken, cure is not possible in those with evidence of systemic disease. Death inevitably occurs within a matter of 2 to 5 years. Because of this terribly poor prognosis there is currently considerable interest in the experimental use of agents such as retinoids, various interferons, photophoresis of lymphocytes, and nodal irradiation.

SELECTED READING

Lambert WC, Everett MA: The nosology of parapsoriasis. J Am Acad Dermatol 5:373, 1981.

Abel EA: Clinical features of cutaneous T cell lymphoma. <u>Dermatol</u>
    <u>Clinics</u> <u>3</u>:647, 1983.
McFadden NC: Mycosis fungoides. Unsolved problems of diagnosis and
    choice of therapy. <u>Int</u> <u>J</u> <u>Dermatol</u> <u>23</u>:523, 1984.
Van Vloten WA, De Vroome H, Noordijk EM: Total skin electron beam
    irradiation for cutaneous T-cell lymphoma (mycosis fungoides).
    <u>Br</u> <u>J</u> <u>Dermatol</u> <u>112</u>:697, 1985.
Zachariae H, Thestrup-Pedersen K, Sogaard H: Topical nitrogen
    mustard in early mycosis fungoides. A 12-year experience. <u>Acta</u>
    <u>Derm</u> <u>Venereol</u> <u>65</u>:53, 1985.
Rosenbaum MM, Roenigk HH Jr, Caro WA, Esker A: Photochemotherapy in
    cutaneous T cell lymphoma and parapsoriasis en plaques. <u>J</u> <u>Am</u>
    <u>Acad</u> <u>Dermatol</u> <u>13</u>:613, 1985.
Ralfkiaer E, Wantzin GL, Mason DY, <u>et</u> <u>al</u>: Phenotypic
    characterization of lymphocyte subsets in mycosis fungoides. <u>Am</u>
    <u>J</u> <u>Clin</u> <u>Pathol</u> <u>84</u>:610, 1985.
Vonderheid EC, Micaily B: Treatment of cutaneous T-cell lymphoma.
    <u>Dermatol</u> <u>Clinics</u> <u>3</u>:673, 1985.
McMillan EM: Monoclonal antibodies and cutaneous T cell lymphoma.
    <u>J</u> <u>Am</u> <u>Acad</u> <u>Dermatol</u> <u>12</u>:102, 1985.
Solomon AR: Retroviruses and lymphoproliferative disease. <u>Dermatol</u>
    <u>Clinics</u> <u>3</u>:615, 1985.
Toback AC, Edelson RL: Pathogenesis of cutaneous T cell lymphoma.
    <u>Dermatol</u> <u>Clinics</u> <u>3</u>:605, 1985.

MISCELLANEOUS PAPULOSQUAMOUS DISEASES WITH PLAQUE FORMATION

<u>Pityriasis</u> <u>rubra</u> <u>pilaris</u> (PRP) is a disease which looks very
much like psoriasis. However, in PRP the scalp is diffusely
involved; the palms and soles are markedly thickened; and small
follicular papules are noted on the dorsal surface of the hands and
fingers. The plaques of PRP are huge and often the entire trunk is
covered with disease. The treatment is similar to that given in
psoriasis.

<u>Reiter's</u> <u>syndrome</u> consists of a migratory pauciarticular
arthritis of the large joints, inflammatory disease of the eyes,
urethritis, balanitis, and psoriatic-like lesions on the palms and
soles. The degree of overlap with psoriasis is considerable and at
times a distinction between the two diseases cannot be made. The
course of the disease is chronic but is characterized by
exacerbation and remissions. Methotrexate therapy is indicated in
the more severe cases.

<u>Bowen's</u> <u>disease</u> and <u>superficial</u> <u>basal</u> <u>cell</u> <u>carcinoma</u> (both
representing malignancy confined entirely to the epidermis) present
as sharply marginated, slightly scaling, erythematous plaques.
These lesions range from 2 to 6 cm in diameter. Such lesions are
usually singular but on occasion several may be present. Any
solitary papulosquamous plaque, claimed by the patient to have been

present and unchanged for years, should be biopsied with the possibility of carcinoma in situ in mind.

Darier's disease is a familial condition characterized by the presence of large, red-brown, scaling plaques with peripheral, satellite papules. The lesions occur primarily in a seborrheic distribution. Biopsy is diagnostic.

SELECTED READING

Callen JP, Headington J: Bowen's and Non-Bowen's squamous intraepidermal neoplasia of the skin. Arch Dermatol 116:422, 1980.

Soppi A-M, Soppi E, Eskola J, Jansen CT: Cell-mediated immunity in Darier's disease: Effect of systemic retinoid therapy. Br J Dermatol 106:141, 1982.

Thomas JR III, Cooke JP, Winkelmann RK: High-dose vitamin A therapy for Darier's disease. Arch Dermatol 118:891, 1982.

Keat A: Reiter's syndrome and reactive arthritis in perspective. N Engl J Med 309:1606, 1983.

Fox BJ, Odom RB: Papulosquamous diseases: A review. J Am Acad Dermatol 12:597, 1985.

PITYRIASIS ROSEA

DIAGNOSTIC HALLMARKS

1. Distribution: trunk and proximal extremities
2. Oval shaped lesions
3. The oval lesions run parallel to the rib lines
4. Herald patch

CLINICAL PRESENTATION

Pityriasis rosea usually has an easily recognized, highly distinctive appearance. The full blown eruption consists of 30 to 100 isolated, nonconfluent papules 1 to 2 cm in diameter. Many of these papules will have a characteristic oval or football shape. Moreover, the long axes of these ovals lie parallel to each other and correspond roughly to the rib lines of the patient. These lesions are distributed over the central trunk, the neck, and the inner aspects of the arms and thighs. The face is always spared.

Approximately half of the patients will have one considerably larger plaque which historically will have preceded the appearance of the smaller lesions. This so called "herald" patch is often round rather than oval and frequently has an annular configuration. Because of the annularity, this lesion may be mistaken for tinea corporis. A KOH preparation allows one to distinguish between the two.

The amount of scale present on the lesions of pityriasis rosea is highly variable. The herald patch, if present, usually has visible scale, but the other lesions may have little or none. Itching also varies considerably. Most patients are asymptomatic but pruritus is a major complaint for a few. Pityriasis rosea is almost exclusively seen between the ages of 10 and 30.

Diagnosis is made on the basis of the clinical appearance. Diagnostic certainty is very high in the presence of a herald patch and oval lesions. On the other hand, in instances where a herald patch is lacking and where only a few oval lesions are present, one can easily confuse the eruption with that of secondary syphilis or guttate psoriasis. The lack of associated symptoms and signs, together with a negative serologic test for syphilis, help to confirm an uncertain diagnosis. Biopsy in pityriasis rosea is not generally helpful.

COURSE AND PROGNOSIS

The herald patch (if it occurs at all) precedes the remainder of the eruption by 7 to 10 days. Once the major portion of the eruption has begun to appear it evolves rather quickly. New lesions continue to develop only during the first 2 weeks and thereafter the number of lesions and their size are stable.

Pityriasis rosea is a self-limited disease. All cases resolve spontaneously within 10 weeks and most have started their resolution phase in the fourth to the sixth week. Recurrence of the eruption is very unlikely; only 5% of the patients will have a second episode. The disease is not contagious and epidemiologic clusters do not seem to occur.

PATHOGENESIS

The cause of pityriasis rosea is unknown. The predilection for young people, the lack of recurrences, and the occasional presence of a preceding pharyngeal or upper respiratory infection suggests the possibility of a viral etiology. However, the lack of antibody development and the failure to identify viruses microscopically or on culture would seem to negate this hypothesis. An attractive alternative possibility suggests that the eruption occurs as part of a postviral, immunologic reaction.

THERAPY

Most patients will require no therapy. Itching, if present, can be treated with topical or systemic antipruritic preparations (see Chapter 4). A rare patient might require a short burst of systemic steroids to reduce the itching. Steroids, however, have only a minimal effect on the eruption itself. Some clinicians believe that

UVB ultraviolet light exposure decreases the severity and duration of the lesions.

SELECTED READING

Chuang T-Y, Ilstrup DM, Perry HO, Kurland LT: Pityriasis rosea in Rochester, Minnesota, 1969 to 1978. J Am Acad Dermatol 7:80, 1982.

Chuang T-Y, Perry HO, Ilstrup DM, Kurland LT: Recent upper respiratory tract infection and pityriasis rosea: A case-control study of 249 matched pairs. Br J Dermatol 108:587, 1983.

Arndt KA, Paul BS, Stern RS, Parrish JA: Treatment of pityriasis rosea with UV radiation. Arch Dermatol 119:381, 1983.

Aiba S, Tagami H: Immunohistologic studies in pityriasis rosea. Evidence for cellular immune reaction in the lesional epidermis. Arch Dermatol 121:761, 1985.

LICHEN PLANUS

DIAGNOSTIC HALLMARKS

1. Distribution: trunk and extremities; special predilection for the wrists and penis
2. Violaceous color
3. Shiny, flattopped papules
4. Koebner phenomenon
5. White patches in mouth

CLINICAL PRESENTATION

The primary lesion of lichen planus is a violaceous, flattopped papule 2 to 4 mm in diameter. Scale is not visible in the form of flakes, but the shiny, mirror-like surface indicates that the papule is in fact covered with compacted, lichen-type scale. These papules of lichen planus generally occur in clusters (sometimes taking on an annular configuration) and they frequently coalesce to form small plaques 1 to 2 cm in diameter. Plaques larger than this are not often seen. Papules may also be arranged in a linear configuration as a result of the Koebner phenomenon (see psoriasis). Rarely, a fine network pattern of gray-white lines (Wickham's striae) can be noted on the surface of the papules.

The lesions of lichen planus can occur anywhere on the body, but the volar surface of the wrists and forearms, the anterior surface of the lower legs, and the shaft and glans of the penis are particularly likely to be involved. Striking postinflammatory hyperpigmentation sometimes develops at sites where lesions have resolved. Gray-white, lacy plaques may be present on oral mucous membranes (see Chapter 21).

Lichen planus is by far the most pruritic of the papulosquamous diseases. This itching, however, is not commonly accompanied by scratching to the point of visible excoriations. Lichen planus occurs at any age but it is particularly common in mid adult life.

COURSE AND PROGNOSIS

Lichen planus is a chronic disease in which new lesions appear as old lesions resolve. Thus, like psoriasis, lichen planus is a disease of constantly changing patterns. A few fortunate individuals have attacks which last only a matter of months but most patients experience many years of intermittent activity. Lichen planus seems to occur more commonly than would be expected in patients with biliary cirrhosis, especially when penicillamine is used in therapy.

PATHOGENESIS

Lichen planus is a disease of unknown etiology. A role for immunologic factors has been postulated based on globular deposits of IgM and fibrin in the papillary dermis. Moreover, lesions similar to those of lichen planus often occur in the immunologic graft versus host reaction.

Clinical experience suggests that stress is a common and important precipitating factor but it is not identifiable in all instances. Some cases of lichen planus occur as the result of medication reactions. This pattern is most likely to occur with chlorthiazides, quinidine, benzodiazepines, and quinacrine.

THERAPY

Lichen planus is a difficult disease to treat. Topically applied steroids should be tried, but even with occlusion, such therapy is often disappointing. Orally administered steroids can be used to bring an acute flare-up under control but recrudescence is very likely when the steroids are stopped. The usefulness of orally administered retinoids is currently under study. In some circumstances psychologic counseling, the administration of tranquilizers, or the use of behavior modification for stress reduction may be beneficial. Pruritus can be treated symptomatically with topically applied or systemically administered antipruritic agents.

SELECTED READING
Gonzalez E, Momtaz-T, K, Freedman S: Bilateral comparison of
    generalized lichen planus treated with psoralens and ultraviolet
    A. J Am Acad Dermatol 10:958, 1984.

Korkij W, Chuang T-Y, Soltani K: Liver abnormalities in patients
    with lichen planus. J Am Acad Dermatol 11:609, 1984.
Fox BJ, Odom RB: Papulosquamous diseases: A review. J Am Acad
    Dermatol 12:597, 1985.

SECONDARY SYPHILIS (SECONDARY LUES)

DIAGNOSTIC HALLMARKS

1.   Distribution: trunk and extremities; special predilection
      for the palms, soles, and face
2.   White plaques on mucous membranes
3.   Patchy alopecia
4.   Lymphadenopathy
5.   Positive serologic tests for syphilis

CLINICAL PRESENTATION

The eruption of secondary syphilis is characterized by the
presence of numerous nonconfluent, dome shaped, red papules 1 to 4
mm in diameter. The amount of scale present is variable. Smaller
lesions tend to have little visible scale whereas larger lesions may
be quite scaly. The papules sometimes form a small annular lesion
but coalescence with resultant plaque formation is not otherwise
seen. Annular lesions are particularly likely to be found on the
face and genitalia.

The papules of secondary syphilis are randomly distributed on
the trunk and extremities. In addition, they are regularly found on
the face, palms, and soles. Those papules which occur on the palms
and soles are often larger, firmer, and more brown-red in color than
are those found elsewhere. Itching, when present at all, is not
usually troublesome.

Other distinctive lesions of secondary syphilis include white
plaques on the mucous membranes and flattopped, red or white, moist
papules (condyloma lata) in intertriginous sites. Patchy alopecia
of the scalp and loss of the lateral eyebrows occurs in some
patients. Lymphadenopathy, fever, and malaise may also be present.
A history of an ulcerating primary lesion (chancre) may or may not
be obtainable.

A clinical diagnosis of secondary syphilis must be confirmed
either by identification of typical treponemes on dark field
examination or through serologic testing (see Chapter 5). The
histologic pattern on biopsy is also quite distinctive and from time
to time cases are first identified during examination of a biopsy
specimen taken from an otherwise unrecognized papulosquamous
eruption.

COURSE AND PROGNOSIS

The ulcerative lesion of primary syphilis (the chancre) appears 2 to 3 weeks after exposure to an infected person (see Chapter 20). It reaches its maximum size of 1 to 2 cm quickly and then remains stable until it undergoes spontaneous resolution 3 to 4 weeks later. The eruption of secondary syphilis begins at about this time, that is, 6 weeks after original contact. Occasionally there is a short period of overlap during which both primary and secondary lesions are present. Of course, if the primary lesion occurs in a hidden site, the first apparent evidence of infection will be the secondary eruption. The lesions of secondary syphilis contain motile treponemes and thus contagion, particularly from moist lesions, is entirely possible.

Left untreated, the lesions of secondary syphilis remain in place for about 2 months and then gradually undergo spontaneous resolution. Over the next 6 to 12 months recurrent crops of secondary lesions may redevelop. Secondary syphilis is not simply a cutaneous infection; systemic involvement in the form of lymphadenopathy, uveitis, hepatitis, or glomerulonephritis is frequently present.

About one-third of the patients who remain untreated through the secondary stage develop tertiary disease. Another one-third remain free of clinical disease but continue to have serologic evidence of activity (latent syphilis). The final one-third experience complete, spontaneous, clinical and serologic cure.

Treatment of patients with primary or secondary syphilis effectively halts all clinical progress of the disease. The serologic tests in these patients gradually become negative over a 12- to 36-month period. Unfortunately, little or no immunity is conferred as a result of primary or secondary infection and thus reinfection is quite possible.

PATHOGENESIS

Syphilis is caused by the spirochete Treponema pallidum. This organism is passed from person to person during close skin-to-skin contact such as occurs during sexual activity. Spirochetemia results in the subsequent presence of infectious organisms in the mucocutaneous lesions of secondary syphilis. Antibody reaction to infections with T. pallidum is brisk but their reappearance does not result in resolution of the disease. Moreover, reinfection is possible even in the face of antibody formation. The formation of these antibodies, together with the continued presence of treponemal antigen, results in the development of circulating immune complexes. These in turn appear to be responsible for some of the systemic symptoms and signs which occur during the secondary stage of the disease.

THERAPY

Penicillin is the treatment of choice for syphilis. Penicillin
is only effective during the process of microbial replication and,
since T. pallidum   replicates rather slowly, serum levels must be
maintained for 10 to 20 days. This is most conveniently
accomplished through the use of intramuscularly administered
benzathine penicillin. The product Bicillin L-A should be specified
since Bicillin C-R contains a 50% mixture of short acting procaine
penicillin. Current recommendations for the treatment of primary
and secondary syphilis suggest that 2.4 million units be given in a
single injection. Most clinicians, however, administer an
additional 2.4 million units 1 week later. Erythromycin 2.0 grams
per day for 15 days can be used for patients allergic to
penicillin. Following treatment, serologic tests for syphilis
should be monitored at 3-month intervals until the titer of antibody
has returned to zero. A rising titer following treatment suggests
reinfection and the need for retreatment.

SELECTED READING
Chapel TA: Physician recognition of the signs and symptoms of
    secondary syphilis. J Am Acad Dermatol 246:250, 1981.
Felman YM, Nikitas JA: Sexually transmitted diseases. Secondary
    syphilis. Cutis 29:322, 1982.
Alessi E, Innocenti M, Ragusa G: Secondary syphilis. Clinical
    morphology and histopathology. Am J Dermatopathol 5:11, 1983.
Chapel TA: Primary and secondary syphilis. Cutis 33:47, 1984.
Fiumara NJ: Treatment of primary and secondary syphilis: Serologic
    response. J Am Acad Dermatol 14:487, 1986.

MISCELLANEOUS PAPULOSQUAMOUS DISEASES WITHOUT PLAQUE FORMATION

Psoriasis is usually associated with plaque formation. However,
some individuals (mostly children and young adults) explosively
develop 50 to 100 small, nonconfluent papules over the trunk and
proximal extremities. This phenomenon, known as guttate psoriasis,
is particularly likely to be precipitated by a preceding
streptococcal infection or by an episode of severe emotional
stress. The Koebner phenomenon and nail pitting are often absent.
    The eruption of rubella (German measles) occurs after several
days of mild upper respiratory symptoms. It consists of light red
macules or very slightly elevated papules which first appear on the
face and neck but quickly spread to the trunk and extremities.
Cervical, postauricular, and suboccipital lymphadenopathy is usually
present. Strictly speaking, the lesions of rubella are not scaling,
but at the time the patient is first examined postinflammatory
desquamation has usually started, resulting in the appearance of a
fine, pityriasis-like scale over the earliest lesions. Facial

lesions often become confluent but those elsewhere usually remain discrete.

The eruption <u>rubeola</u> (measles) occurs in association with marked fever, coryza, conjunctivitis, and cough. It consists of macules and barely palpable papules which first appear on the forehead and behind the ears. Spread rapidly occurs to the face, trunk, and limbs. Koplik spots (white dots with surrounding red rings) are usually present on the buccal surfaces opposite the molars. Here, too, postinflammatory desquamation leads to a minor amount of scale formation. Coalescence of lesions occurs on the face but limb lesions remain discrete.

Group 10:
The Eczematous Diseases

GROUP IDENTIFICATION

Both the papulosquamous diseases (Group 9) and the eczematous diseases (Group 10) are characterized by the presence of erythematous scaling papules and plaques. Separation of these two groups is based on the predilection of the eczematous lesions to demonstrate evidence of epithelial disruption and nonsharp margination.

Epithelial Disruption. The most easily recognized evidence for epithelial disruption is the presence of linear or angular erosions (excoriations) secondary to scratching, but as can be seen above, such lesions will not always be present. Thus careful examination for weeping, crusts, yellow scale, and minute fissures should be carried out whenever red scaling plaques are present. Weeping is easily recognized by a sense of wetness on palpation. This wetness is due to the presence of serum on the surface of the skin and can only be found when the barrier layer of the epithelium has been broached. Crusting occurs when water from the serum on the surface

of the skin evaporates, leaving behind solid serum proteins. The
physical appearance of crusts is described in Chapter 3. Yellow
scale occurs when the amount of serum exuded is very slight. In
this situation there is insufficient protein to form crusts and the
serum instead lightly coats the scale which is present. The
presence of small fissures is the most subtle sign of epithelial
disruption and is all too often overlooked. These fissures are too
narrow to be easily recognized as erosions and instead appear as
thin red lines which wend their way in and around small islands of
scale. They represent small cracks in the outer portion of the
epidermis which are not deep enough or wide enough to allow for the
visible escape of serum.

Nonsharp Margination. In the papulosquamous diseases the
transition from normal to abnormal skin occurs so abruptly it is
possible to place a pencil point at the exact point where the lesion
ends and normal skin begins. This is not so in the eczematous
diseases; the zone of transition generally occurs over a space of 2
or more mm. However, it must be recognized that the entire 360° of
the circumference of any lesion must be taken into consideration as,
in many eczematous diseases, some portion of any one lesion may well
be sharply marginated. The key feature is that nonsharp ("diffuse")
margination will be present in some significant portion of
eczematous lesions whereas the sharp margination will occur around
the entire lesion in papulosquamous disease.

The separation of the eczematous diseases from the
papulosquamous diseases is probably the single most difficult task
in dermatologic diagnosis. Because of this, in uncertain cases, it
is both expedient and desirable to form one's list of differential
diagnoses from diseases in both groups.

Finally, a word on terminology may be useful. For the purpose
of this book the words "eczema" and "dermatitis" can be considered
as synonyms. Thus the eczematous group could just as easily have
been called "the dermatitic diseases" and individual diseases can be
identified either way, such that atopic dermatitis is synonymous
with atopic eczema.

ATOPIC DERMATITIS (NEURODERMATITIS,
LICHEN SIMPLEX CHRONICUS, INFANTILE ECZEMA)

DIAGNOSTIC HALLMARKS

1. Distribution: cheeks and groin (infants); feet,
    antecubital and popliteal fossae (children, adolescents);
    hands, feet, ankles, and groin (adults)
2. Presence of the itch-scratch cycle
3. Evidence of atopy

CLINICAL PRESENTATION

The distribution pattern, as noted above, appears to be determined by irritant factors which lead to cutaneous nerve stimulation. Sweat retention is the most important of these and probably accounts for development of lesions on the genitalia, in the groin, on the dorsal surface of the feet, around the ankles, and in the antecubital and popliteal fossae. Drooling during sleep and urine soaked diapers greatly influence the localization of disease in infants whereas xerosis secondary to soap and water exposure accounts for dorsal hand involvement in adults. Other less common sites such as the occipital region of the scalp and extensor surfaces of the arms and legs are probably also influenced by these same factors.

The most highly characteristic feature of atopic dermatitis is the presence of uncontrolled scratching in a pattern termed the itch-scratch cycle. In this pattern, stimulation of cutaneous nerve endings leads to the central nervous system recognition of itching which in turn is followed by vigorous rubbing and scratching. This response leads to greater peripheral nerve stimulation, heightened appreciation of itching, and ever more vigorous scratching. The cycle then continues until the pain of nail-induced skin damage supplants the sensation of itching.

Clinical recognition of the itch-scratch cycle is usually not difficult. Most patients acknowledge its presence and will voluntarily discuss the role it plays in their disease. Sometimes, however, the scratching occurs almost entirely at the subconscious level. In such instances identification of the cycle depends on a family member's description of habitual scratching, particularly at night. The importance of nighttime scratching can hardly be over-emphasized. Many patients can control, at least to some degree, the amount of scratching that occurs during the day but then virtually destroy their skin as a result of accompanying sleep. Frustration over the inability to control this scratching and fatigue which occurs as a result of scratching induced sleep disturbance lead to daytime irritability and a continued worsening of the problem. In my view the importance of nighttime scratching is such that identification of its presence (and the ruling out of scabies and dermatitis herpetiformis) is usually sufficient to warrant a diagnosis of atopic dermatitis even in the absence of the other characteristic features listed as diagnostic hallmarks.

The presence of numerous excoriations can in itself be a clue to the existence of the itch-scratch cycle. Most other pruritic diseases (urticaria and lichen planus, for example) are not accompanied by prominent excoriations even though patients complain vigorously about the severity of itching. From this observation one can conclude that the itching in atopic dermatitis is qualitatively different than that which exists in most other pruritic processes.

As noted above, however, there are at least two diseases, scabies and dermatitis herpetiformis, wherein all patients, regardless of whether or not they are atopic, scratch to the point of prominent excoriation.

Lichenification (see definition in Chapter 3) is to rubbing as excoriation is to scratching. Not surprisingly then, lichenification can also be used as a clue to the existence of the itch-scratch (or itch-rub?) cycle and, in fact, is probably an even more reliable indicator of atopic dermatitis since it is not often encountered in scabies and dermatitis herpetiformis.

The reason why the itch-scratch cycle is so closely related to atopic dermatitis is not known but it probably depends at least in part on the marked sensation of pleasure noted by atopics when they scratch or rub. This sensation of pleasure probably acts in a Pavlovian way to reinforce the habituation of scratching. Adults can be asked directly about the degree of pleasure associated with scratching but the same process is observable in infants: they are quiet while scratching but cry vigorously when their hands are even gently restrained.

The third and, to my mind, the least useful hallmark of atopic dermatitis is the identification of the patient as possessing the atopic diathesis. The features which are said to identify atopy include: 1) drier than normal skin (xerosis); 2) keratosis pilaris (see Chapter 10); 3) pityriasis alba (see Chapter 10); 4) a second wrinkle, the Dennie-Morgan fold, on the lower eyelid; 5) abnormal cutaneous vascular reactions to mechanical and pharmacologic stimuli; 6) a personal history of hay fever or asthma; 7) idiopathic peripheral eosinophilia; and 8) elevated levels of IgE antibodies. The problem with the use of these features is the variability with which they are present and the fact that, even if present, they only identify the patient as being atopic without identifying the disease in question as being atopic dermatitis. For example, since about 20% of the population is atopic, approximately one-fifth of all psoriatics will possess some or all of these characteristics.

The diagnosis of atopic dermatitis is made on a clinical basis; biopsy is not particularly helpful.

COURSE AND PROGNOSIS

Atopic dermatitis is a chronic disease characterized by exacerbations and remissions. A few patients have a single episode and then remain clear indefinitely, but for most individuals, once the initial episode has occurred future problems may be anticipated.

Individual episodes of atopic dermatitis left untreated generally continue chronically. Treatment, on the other hand, is usually quite successful and may lead to prolonged periods of remission. Most initial episodes of atopic dermatitis occur during childhood and 90% of patients will have had their first episode by age 35.

Patients with atopic dermatitis are at considerable risk of developing the noncutaneous atopic diseases of hay fever and asthma. There is also some evidence to suggest that these patients are more likely to develop alopecia areata, vitiligo, otitis media, urticaria, and dyshidrosis, but proof of these associations is lacking.

Patients with atopic dermatitis, as a reflection of the mild depression of cell mediated immune responsiveness which accompanies the disease, are also more likely to develop cutaneous fungal and viral infections. Moreover, these infections when present may be unusually severe. For instance, atopics are at considerable risk for the development of disseminated cutaneous herpetic or vaccinia infection in the syndrome known variously as Kaposi's varicelliform eruption or eczema herpeticum.

Staphylococcal organisms regularly colonize the lesions of atopic dermatitis. However, in spite of the large number of organisms which are present, clinical signs of true infection are not often present.

PATHOGENESIS

The potential for development of atopic dermatitis is known as the atopic diathesis. This diathesis appears to be a genetic trait which is inherited in an autosomal dominant manner. It occurs in about 20% of the population. The expression of this trait in the form of atopic dermatitis is seen in only about one-fourth of the individuals who have inherited the diathesis.

Several factors seem to be important in determining just who will develop atopic dermatitis and at what point in their lives it will appear. These can be viewed as precipitating factors. They include adverse environmental conditions such as sweat retention, maceration due to other fluids, and excess dryness, all of which result in stimulation of cutaneous nerve endings. This stimulation might lead to irritation or mild discomfort in nonatopics but is perceived as pruritus in those who are atopic. This in turn results in scratching and initiation of the itch-scratch cycle.

Psychological factors are also very important. Most atopic individuals experience considerable itching during times of stress and fatigue. The mechanism through which this occurs is unknown. Some believe that atopic individuals have distinctive personalities characterized by restlessness, high productivity, obsessive-compulsive behavior, and suppressed hostility toward parents and authority figures. This may well be so, but even if true, it offers no explanation as to why it should be expressed in the form of a pruritic eruption. Atopic disease does seem to be expressed more commonly in those of higher socioeconomic standing but it is not

clear whether this is a result of that position or is simply a
reflection of greater access to medical attention.

In any event, the presence of one or more of these precipitating
factors in atopic individuals frequently results in scratching of
what appears to be normal skin. This sequence of events had led to
the tongue-in-cheek definition of atopic dermatitis as the itch that
rashes. However, it seems likely to me that this clinically normal
skin has undergone some subclinical histologic or molecular changes
and that these changes are responsible for the itching. Certainly
once scratching has occurred, various inflammatory mediators such as
histamine are released; these in turn no doubt intensify the
pruritus.

Immunologic changes in both the humoral and cell mediated
systems are regularly present but their role in the pathogenesis of
atopic dermatitis is not known. The mild but consistent depression
of T cell responsiveness does lead to more frequent cutaneous viral
and fungal infections but no direct relationship can be shown
between this propensity and the appearance of atopic dermatitis.
Serum levels of IgE are frequently elevated in individuals who have
severe atopic dermatitis. It would be tempting to relate this
immunoglobulin elevation to the presence of a causative (inhaled,
injested, or contacted) antigen, particularly since antigenic
stimulation seems to play such an important role in the associated
atopic diseases of hay fever and asthma. Unfortunately, with the
exception of some evidence incriminating food antigens in infancy,
few hard data support this view. Interest in an immunologic
explanation as the cause of atopic dermatitis is further stimulated
by the observation that an eruption indistinguishable from atopic
dermatitis occurs in infants with certain congenital
immunodeficiency diseases, but here, too, no clear-cut mechanisms
are recognized.

THERAPY

One absolute rule exists regarding therapy of atopic
dermatitis: scratching must be stopped. Therapy which fails to
interrupt the itch-scratch cycle will not lead to consistent,
prolonged clinical improvement.

Soaks (see Chapter 4) are indicated in the treatment of acute
episodes accompanied by weeping and crusting. Such soaks serve two
purposes. First, they restore a more physiologic environment to the
sensory nerve endings. Presumably this reduces nerve stimulation
and thus decreases the transfer of itch sensations to the brain.
Second, by removing crust, maceration is reduced and bacterial
overgrowth is minimized.

Topically applied steroids are almost indispensable in the
treatment of atopic dermatitis. Infants and adults with involvement
of the face and groin should be treated with low potency products

such as 1% hydrocortisone whenever possible. In other areas of the
body higher potency products will be required. Cream vehicles are
generally used because of easy spreading and cosmetic
acceptability. However, if stinging on application is a problem,
ointments can be substituted. If ointments are used, they should be
applied sparingly and should be spread as thinly as possible in
order to minimize sweat retention and the development of
maceration. A more detailed discussion of topical steroid usage can
be found in Chapter 4.

Patients with severe or extensive disease may initially require
a burst of prednisone (see Chapter 4). Clinical response is
extraordinarily good but rapid exacerbation can be expected unless a
good topical program is also being conscientiously carried out.
Failure to recognize this point defeats the rationale for the short
term use of systemic steroids.

Systemically administered antihistamines are often necessary to
help control pruritus. Part of their effectiveness is no doubt
related to inhibition of inflammatory mediators, but an additional,
important component of efficacy is undoubtedly obtained through
central, sedative mechanisms. In fact, I believe that tranquilizers
and other sedatives reduce pruritus about as well as
antihistamines. Because of the sedation, all of these agents are
generally best administered in the evening and the dosage should be
adjusted to the point where, because of deeper sleep, nighttime
scratching is stopped. The best possible daytime therapeutic
program will be completely undone if the patient scratches during
the nighttime hours. In addition, a good night's sleep decreases
the fatigue that is usually present. The patient starts the day
well rested and is then better able to handle the stresses of
everyday life.

Long term lifestyle adjustments to reduce stress and increase
relaxation are necessary in some cases and are particularly helpful
in tense patients who cannot relax easily. Some of these
adjustments occur as the patient develops insight, but often the use
of counseling or behavior modification techniques such as vigorous
athletics, transcendental meditation, yoga, hypnosis, and
biofeedback is necessary.

Modifications in routine skin care are necessary. Lubricants
retard moisture loss from superficial epidermal cells, reducing the
nerve stimulation which occurs through dry, chapped skin. Hands
should be lubricated four to six times a day; full body lubrication
should be carried out twice daily. Fingernails should be trimmed
and filed such that no sharp edges remain. Hot water bathing and
the use of soap ought to be decreased as much as possible since both
remove lipids necessary to keep the skin from becoming xerotic. The
use of cotton clothing minimizes the deleterious effect of sweat
retention. Wool clothing should be specifically avoided since the
prickly wool fibers tend to have an irritating effect on atopic

242 DERMATOLOGY FOR THE HOUSE OFFICER

skin. Finally, patients should, where possible, set room
temperatures at a level which prevents heat buildup and sweat
production.

The therapeutic program described above is representative of the
way most clinicians care for patients with atopic dermatitis. Three
additional approaches strongly favored by some dermatologists ought
to be mentioned. The first of these is the modified Scholz regimen,
which avoids all use of soaps and lipids. Cleaning is carried out
with the nonlipid preparation Cetaphil. Cetaphil lotion is also
used as the vehicle for all medications. The second approach
substitutes coal tar products for topical steroids wherever
possible. This avoids the potential side effects of steroids and is
also quite inexpensive. Unfortunately, improvement occurs rather
slowly and patient compliance is poor because of the staining and
odor associated with tar products. The third approach suggests the
routine use of systemically administered antibiotics when weeping or
crusting is present on the surface of the skin. Advocates of this
approach believe that the bacteria which grow readily on eczematous
skin play a role in the pathogenesis of the disease. The use of
antibiotics does sometimes speed up healing but, of course, also
raises the potential problem of eventual bacterial resistance.

Marsh DG, Meyers DA, Bias WB: The epidemiology and genetics of
    atopic allergy. N Engl J Med 305:1551, 1981.
Hanifin JM: Atopic dermatitis: J Am Acad Dermatol 6:1, 1982.
Beer DJ, Osband ME, McCaffrey RP, et al: Abnormal histamine-induced
    suppressor-cell function in atopic subjects. N Engl J Med
    306:454, 1982.
Soppi E, Viander M, Soppi AM, Jansen CT: Cell-mediated immunity in
    untreated and PUVA treated atopic dermatitis. J Invest Dermatol
    79:213, 1982.
Cooper KD, Kazmierowski JA, Wuepper KD, Hanifin JM: Immuno-
    regulation in atopic dermatitis: Functional analysis of T-B
    cell interactions and the enumeration of Fc receptor-bearing T
    cells. J Invest Dermatol 80:139, 1983.
Chandra RK, Baker M: Numerical and functional deficiency of
    suppressor T cells precedes development of atopic eczema.
    Lancet 2:1393, 1983.
Larsen FS, Jorgensen AS, Grunnet N: Natural killer cell function in
    atopic dermatitis. Clin Exp Dermatol 10:104, 1985.
Friedman SJ, Schroeter AL, Homburger HA: IgE antibodies to
    Staphylococcus aureus. Arch Dermatol 121:869, 1985.
Esterly NB: Significance of food hypersensitivity in children with
    atopic dermatitis. Pediatr Dermatol 3:161, 1986.

DYSHIDROTIC ECZEMA

DIAGNOSTIC HALLMARKS

1. Distribution: sides and tips of the digits; palms and soles
2. History of preceding noninflammatory vesicles (i.e., dyshidrosis)

CLINICAL PRESENTATION

Dyshidrosis, a disease of noninflammatory vesiculation, is discussed with the vesicular diseases in Chapter 7. Eczematization of dyshidrosis develops under two conditions. The first occurs when itching leads to uncontrolled scratching. This superimposition of the itch-scratch cycle leads to vesicle roof disruption and causes excoriations in surrounding, previously normal, skin. Weeping and crusting are present because of the broken epithelium. The second condition occurs when closely set vesicles appear fast enough to form fragile multilocular bullae. These break easily, leading to profuse weeping and crusting. New vesicles develop before re-epithelialization has occurred and the process continues indefinitely even without superimposition of the itch-scratch cycle.

In either event additional eczematization occurs through the process of autosensitization and spreads onto the previously uninvolved dorsal surface of the fingers and hands. Moreover, the eczematization obscures the noninflammatory nature of the original underlying vesicles. Because of the these two changes, the clinician may miss the correct diagnosis unless the patient is asked about the possible presence of noninflammatory vesicles which might have existed prior to the onset of eczematization. The differential diagnoses of hand and foot eczema are considered in greater detail in Chapter 17.

The diagnosis of dyshidrotic eczema is made on a clinical basis; biopsy is not usually helpful.

COURSE AND PROGNOSIS

The superimposition of the itch-scratch cycle on dyshidrosis converts an intermittently active process into one that is chronically troublesome. New crops of vesicles continue to appear on the skin that is already eczematized; this triggers new bouts of scratching and further skin damage. Moreover, mild irritation due to soap and water exposure, which might have been insufficient to harm normal skin, tends to aggravate the condition further.

PATHOGENESIS

The development of dyshidrotic eczema occurs in only about 10% of patients with dyshidrosis. In some instances dyshidrotic eczema is simply an extension in severity of dyshidrosis. New vesicles appear more rapidly than old ones heal. But in most instances the eczematous appearance occurs as a result of the superimposition of the itch-scratch cycle (atopic dermatitis) directly over the noninflammatory vesiculation of dyshidrosis. Not surprisingly, dyshidrotic eczema (as opposed to dyshidrosis itself) preferentially occurs in those who are genetically atopic. The pathogenesis of dyshidrosis is discussed in Chapter 7.

THERAPY

Soaks, sedatives, and application of mid to high potency topical steroids may be sufficient for mild cases of dyshidrotic eczema. Patients with more severe disease will require a "burst" of systemic steroids (see Chapter 4). Because of the importance of psychologic factors in both dyshidrosis and dyshidrotic eczema, it is sometimes necessary to consider counseling, behavior modification, and the use of psychotropic medication. In general, the approach to treatment is similar to that for dyshidrosis (see Chapter 7) and atopic dermatitis (see above).

SELECTED READING

Shelley WB, Shelley ED: Chronic hand eczema strategies. Cutis 29:569, 1982.
Forsbeck M, Skog E, Asbrink E: Atopic hand dermatitis: A comparison with atopic dermatitis without hand involvement, especially with respect to influence of work and development of contact sensitization. Acta Derm Venereol 63:9, 1983.
Stocker WW: Hand dermatitis and psychosomatic factors. J Am Acad Dermatol 11:523, 1984.
Epstein E: Hand dermatitis: Practical management and current concepts. J Am Acad Dermatol 10:395, 1984.
Thelin I, Agrup G: Pompholyx -- a one year series. Acta Derm Venereol 65:214, 1985.

STASIS DERMATITIS

DIAGNOSTIC HALLMARKS

1. Distribution: ankle
2. History of preceding noninflammatory swelling (stasis)
3. Presence of varicosities

CLINICAL PRESENTATION

The term stasis refers to the presence of chronic, noninflammatory edema of the lower leg. Stasis dermatitis occurs when the itching which often accompanies stasis leads to scratching, excoriations, weeping, crusting, and inflammation. The color of the inflammation in stasis dermatitis is violaceous rather than bright red because of pooling and deoxygenation of venous blood. In long standing cases of stasis dermatitis postinflammatory hyper-pigmentation adds a distinctive brown hue to the underlying violaceous color. The initial changes of stasis dermatitis are almost invariably found at the ankles but extension onto the foot and remainder of the lower leg is commonly seen.

Many types of eczematous disease occur around the foot and ankle (see Chapter 17). Correct identification of stasis dermatitis depends on evidence that noninflammatory edema preceded the appearance of the eruption. Other eczematous conditions which occur in this area include atopic dermatitis and contact dermatitis, which is usually the result of sensitization to topical agents used in the treatment of already existing stasis dermatitis. Stasis ulcers frequently accompany stasis dermatitis.

COURSE AND PROGNOSIS

Stasis dermatitis generally runs a chronic course with intermittent exacerbations and remissions. Postinflammatory hyperpigmentation remains present for months after each exacerbation.

The presence of trauma (cuts, bruises, and excoriation) to the weakened skin in stasis dermatitis sometimes leads to the development of stasis ulcers. Healing of these ulcers causes the development of tightly constricted, thickened skin around the ankle. Residual edema may be found above and below the constricted area. Squamous cell carcinoma occasionally develops in the edges of long standing stasis ulcers.

PATHOGENESIS

The chronicity of stasis dermatitis depends on the continuous presence of edema. For this reason stasis dermatitis is commonly seen when the edema is due to venous valve incompetency (varicose veins) but occurs only infrequently with the intermittent lower leg swelling of congestive heart failure.

Only a small proportion of patients with stasis develop stasis dermatitis. This situation is analogous to the infrequency with which dyshidrosis evolves into dyshidrotic eczema. In both diseases the eczematization occurs primarily because of the superimposition of the itch-scratch cycle, thus suggesting that atopic individuals are at particular risk.

Most stasis ulcers begin as a result of trauma to edematous, eczematized skin. This ulcerated skin, both because of anatomically poor arterial blood supply to the lower leg and the further compromise in blood flow due to edema, heals very slowly. When healing finally occurs it is accompanied by scarring. This in turn further compromises blood flow, allowing even minor episodes of trauma to initiate a whole new cycle. Bacterial infection in the ulcers or in the surrounding eczematized skin sometimes further complicates the process.

THERAPY

Neither stasis dermatitis nor stasis ulcers will heal unless the edema which is invariably present can be reduced. Leg elevation (heels higher than knees) is worth trying but is rarely successful. Likewise, compression stockings of either the individually fitted (Jobst) or nonfitted type are excellent in theory but less useful in practice. Generally, compression stockings can only be used for the most compliant of patients and in the presence of the least severe disease. I favor the use of elastic wraps such as Ace bandages since the tension can be adjusted frequently through rewrapping. Unna boots are also helpful since they require no attention from the patient but they can only be used where the lesions are fairly dry. The Unna boot is formed by the wrapping of moist zinc oxide bandages (Gelocast) in overlapping strips from the toes to the knee. These bandages dry to a semisolid consistency which restricts further edema formation and prevents scratching. Each week the bandages are cut off, the skin is cleansed and lubricated, and the boot is reapplied.

Patients with appreciable weeping and crusting will require bed rest, soaks, and intermittently wrapped elastic bandages. Soaks may be applied as either intermittent or constant wet wraps (see Chapter 4). After each soak topical steroids are applied. Lubricants can be applied over the topical steroids if weeping and crusting are not too prominent. Fine mesh gauze or nonstick bandages such as Telfa pads are placed over the eczematized areas and any ulcers which are present are filled with Gelfoam or dextranomer (Debrisan) particles. Large ulcers can be covered with oxygen permeable dressings such as Duoderm. The leg is then wrapped with gauze strips and, finally, an elastic bandage (Ace bandage) is snugly applied.

There is no consensus regarding the use of antibiotics in the treatment of stasis dermatitis and stasis ulcers. Bacterial organisms are regularly recovered but it is difficult to determine if their presence represents anything more than colonization. Nevertheless, some clinicians believe that healing occurs more quickly if antibiotics are used. Antibiotics, whether topically applied or systemically administered, should be chosen on the basis of culture reports. Neomycin and bacitracin containing products should be used with care since prolonged application is sometimes followed by the development of allergic sensitization.

Once the skin has healed every effort must be made to avoid recurrence of the edema. Compression stockings, here used for prophylaxis rather than for treatment, are quite helpful in this regard. Lubricants ought to be used twice daily to prevent xerosis and fissuring, either of which might trigger a new itch-scratch cycle.

SELECTED READING

Mertz PM, Marshall DA, Eaglstein WH: Occlusive wound dressings to prevent bacterial invasion and wound infection. J Am Acad Dermatol 12:662, 1985.
Hendricks WM, Swallow RT: Management of stasis leg ulcers with Unna's boots versus elastic support stockings. J Am Acad Dermatol 12:90, 1985.
Eriksson G: Comparison of two occlusive bandages in the treatment of venous leg ulcers. Br J Dermatol 114:227, 1986.
Falanga V, Eaglstein WH: A therapeutic approach to venous ulcers. J Am Acad Dermatol 14:777, 1986.

SCABIES (SCABETIC ECZEMA)

DIAGNOSTIC HALLMARKS

1. Distribution: finger webs, elbows, axillary folds, buttocks, breasts, penis
2. History of contagion (family members or sexual partners with evidence of similar disease)
3. Identification of the mites, feces, or ova in scrapings from lesions
4. Response to therapy

CLINICAL PRESENTATION

Scabies is basically a vesicular disease (see also Chapter 7) but the intensity of itching leads to such vigorous scratching that vesicles are destroyed as quickly as they are formed. This results in a presentation which is predominantly eczematous in morphology. Careful examination, however, in a suspected case will usually reveal an occasional intact oval or linear vesicle (burrow). The width of these burrows is about 1 mm and the length is generally 1.5 to 3.0 mm. Inflammation is prominent in excoriated lesions but is variable around intact burrows.

The distribution of lesions is quite characteristic. Burrows and excoriated papules are most commonly found in the web spaces of the fingers, around the elbows, on the anterior axillary folds, and

over the buttocks. The breasts in women and the shaft and glans of
the penis in men are also frequently affected. In patients with
chronic infestation widespread involvement of the trunk and
extremities may also be noted. The face, except occasionally in
infants, is normally spared.

Early on burrows and eczematous papules are isolated and widely
separated. The resulting absence of both confluence and large
plaque formation is a valuable diagnostic clue during the first few
weeks of infestation but this feature is lost in well established
cases of many months' duration.

A history of contagion is an important diagnostic feature. For
this reason a query should probably be made about the presence of
pruritic eruptions in family members, friends, and sexual partners
to any patient who presents with eczematous disease.

In instances where clinical suspicion is high it is permissible
to attempt confirmation of one's diagnosis through a therapeutic
trial (see below) of antiscabetic medication. Rapid response, as
measured by abrupt cessation of itching, is tantamount to proof of
diagnosis.

Identification of the mite in scrapings from lesions is
theoretically desirable but is not always possible. In fact,
scrapings carried out from any lesion other than an intact burrow
are so rarely positive they are not worth the effort. When an
intact burrow is present the roof can be lifted off with a thin
scalpel shave technique. This roof, together with material
subsequently scraped from the base of the burrow, is then
transferred to a microscope slide. A drop of immersion oil is
placed over the scrapings and a cover slip is applied. Examination
under low power is carried out in an attempt to identify mites, ova,
or feces. Unfortunately, it requires considerable practice and
skill before positive scrapings can routinely be obtained.

Atypical Manifestations. In a small number of patients a
residuum of long lasting, dome shaped, erythematous, pruritic
nodules remains after treatment has been completed. They are most
commonly seen in young men, particularly around the waist and in the
groin. These nodules do not contain live mites but instead
apparently form as a tissue reaction to scabetic antigenic material
which remains after treatment. The lesions do eventually disappear
but their resolution can be hastened by the intralesional injection
of triamcinolone.

Under some circumstances (very poor hygiene or in
institutionalized individuals) scabetic infestation can become
overwhelming to the point where the entire body is involved in an
exfoliative erythrodermatitis. Such widespread infestation has in
the past been known as Norwegian scabies.

COURSE AND PROGNOSIS

Pruritus disappears quickly after treatment in most individuals. No new lesions develop and all evidence of infestation ordinarily disappears within 7 to 14 days. However, approximately 20% of patients are apparent treatment failures. In about half of these patients new lesions continue to appear and one must assume that either therapy has been inadequately carried out or that reinfection has occurred. Such individuals and all of their contacts should be retreated. In the other half, no new lesions develop, but itching and scratching persist at the site of old lesions. These individuals, most of whom are genetically atopic, have developed an itch-scratch cycle and they will continue to scratch indefinitely unless topical steroids and antihistamines are used to break up the cycle.

Scabies, if left untreated, persists for years. During this time there is a gradual resolution of old lesions and subsequent development of new lesions. This prolonged course accounts for the colloquial name of the disease: "the seven year itch."

PATHOGENESIS

Scabies is due to an infestation with the human variety of the mite Sarcoptes scabiei. The female of the species burrows within the stratum corneum, depositing eggs which over a 3-week period mature into adult mites. The adult mite is just at the threshold of visibility and can sometimes be recognized as a tiny red or brown-red dot at the end of an intact burrow.

Transmission of the disease ordinarily depends on direct person-to-person contact. However, in a small percentage of cases, the contagion occurs through the use of shared clothing or bed linen. Infestation occurs in individuals at all ages and from all socioeconomic groups but for unknown reasons it rarely develops in blacks. Once present, the disease spreads by scratching; mites and eggs are transferred from one location to another by way of fingernail contamination.

Early in the course of infestation there is little in the way of host inflammatory reaction but with the passage of several weeks allergic sensitization with accompanying pruritus and inflammation takes place. The role of immunologic response in the resolution of scabies has not been adequately studied but the occurrence of epidemics at 20- to 30-year intervals suggests that the development and waning of herd immunity may be important from an epidemiologic standpoint.

THERAPY

For many years lindane (gamma benzene), sold under the trade names of Kwell and Scabene, has been the treatment of choice for scabetic infestations. Problems with chemical resistance have not developed. Patients and all of their close contacts are instructed to bathe and then apply a thin layer of lindane over the entire body. The medication is left in place for 8 to 12 hours, at which time the patient bathes a second time. Clothing or bed linen used prior to or during therapy is washed with soap and water in a normal fashion. No special attention is needed for furniture and other inanimate objects. A single treatment carried out in this manner will result in clearing of 80% of patients. As mentioned above, an additional 10% will require retreatment because of problems with therapeutic compliance or reinfection. The remaining 10% will require the additional use of steroids and antihistamines in order to break up the itch-scratch cycle.

Unfortunately, lindane is well absorbed from the surface of the skin. This absorption, particularly in youngsters, has the potential for the induction of neurotoxicity. As a result most clinicians recommend that infants under the age of 1 be treated with crotamiton (Eurax) cream instead. The method of application is similar to that used for lindane. Unfortunately, the failure rate for patients treated with crotamiton is fairly high and retreatment with lindane, in spite of its potential dangers, is sometimes necessary.

SELECTED READING

Burkhart CG: Scabies: An epidemiologic reassessment. Ann Intern Med 98:498, 1983.
Davies JE, Dedhia HV, Morgade C, et al: Lindane poisonings. Arch Dermatol 119:142, 1983.
Taplin D, Rivera A, Walker JG, et al: A comparative trial of three treatment schedules for the eradication of scabies. J Am Acad Dermatol 9:550, 1983.
Orkin M, Maibach HI: Current views of scabies and pediculosis pubis. Cutis 33:85, 1984.

MISCELLANEOUS EXCORIATED ECZEMATOUS DISEASES

Almost any skin disease can become secondarily eczematized. The three major factors which determine the circumstances under which this is likely to happen include the following. First, those patients who are genetically atopic (20% of the population) are particularly likely to initiate the itch-scratch cycle in the presence of almost any dermatologic condition. Second, those lesions which occur in areas of sweat retention (groin, feet, scalp) and those which occur on skin likely to be xerotic (hands, lower

legs) are much more likely to be scratched than those which occur
elsewhere. Third, those diseases which are inherently pruritic are
more likely to engender scratching than those which are
nonpruritic. One can see that, based on these factors, diseases
from Groups 1 through 9 will from time to time take on an
excoriated, eczematous appearance. To the degree that this obscures
the true nature of the underlying disease one can simply (and
temporarily) assign the condition to the eczematous disease group
and can then procede to treat the itch-scratch cycle. Once this
cycle has been interrupted (and the scratching has stopped) the true
nature of the underlying condition can be recognized and it can be
more correctly reassigned.
     This secondary eczematization is particularly likely to occur
with psoriasis, dermatophyte fungal disease, and candidiasis. In
situations such as these one can see that the process involved is
very much analogous to the development of stasis dermatitis in
patients with stasis and dyshidrotic eczema in patients with
dyshidrosis.
     Dermatitis herpetiformis, like scabies, represents a special
case. Both of these conditions, though basically vesicular in
nature, are so severely pruritic that they are virtually always
excoriated and eczematized. Thus, though both scabies and
dermatitis herpetiformis are listed in both the vesiculobullous
group and in the eczematous group, they will present as eczematous
diseases about 95% of the time. Nevertheless, dermatitis
herpetiformis is discussed primarily in Chapter 7 because of its
pathogenetic relationship to the other immunobullous diseases.

SEBORRHEIC DERMATITIS

DIAGNOSTIC HALLMARKS

1. Distribution: scalp and other hairy areas; nasal folds,
    glabella, retroauricular folds, external os of the ear, and
    mid sternum

CLINICAL PRESENTATION

     Seborrheic dermatitis is particularly likely to occur in areas
where moisture is easily trapped. Thus as a general rule it is
likely to affect hairy regions and intertriginous folds. The most
common of these areas are listed above under diagnostic hallmarks.
     In hairy areas seborrheic dermatitis is characterized by the
presence of diffuse, poorly marginated plaques of scaling erythema.
The scale is often compacted against the underlying skin by the
anchoring effect of the hair shafts. In such instances the
scaliness will not be appreciated until the involved area is scraped
with a fingernail. In very young infants scale buildup may be

extensive enough to deserve the colloquial term "cradle cap." When the scalp is involved, oiliness (seborrhea) of the scale may be noticeable, but in the other locations this is not a prominent finding. In men seborrheic dermatitis sometimes occurs in the beard, mustache, and hairy area of the mid sternum.

Evidence of epithelial disruption is usually not prominent. Pruritus is present but few excoriations are found. Often the only clue to the presence of epithelial disruption is the yellow color of the overlying scale. This yellow color occurs because of small amounts of serum which have exuded onto the surface of the scale. Frank crusting, with less prominent scale formation, occurs in patients with more severe disease.

Seborrheic dermatitis of the scalp must be distinguished from tinea capitis and psoriasis. In these two latter diseases sharply marginated individual plaques rather than diffuse involvement are found. Notable hair loss occurs with tinea capitis but this is not seen with psoriasis or seborrheic dermatitis. In both psoriasis and seborrheic dermatitis, extension onto the nonhairy, marginal skin surrounding the scalp is occasionally seen.

Seborrheic dermatitis also occurs on nonhairy (glabrous) skin. It is particularly likely to be found in the retroauricular folds, the external os of the ears, the nasal fold, and the glabella. Less commonly, intertriginous areas such as the inframammary and inguinal folds may be involved. In a general sort of way seborrheic dermatitis in these areas can be considered as an eczematous variant of intertrigo.

The plaques of seborrheic dermatitis occurring on glabrous skin are often rather sharply marginated and for this reason are easily mistaken for papulosquamous lesions. Confusion with psoriasis is particularly likely and the term "seboriasis" is sometimes used when differentiation is not possible.

Pruritus is usually present but it rarely provokes scratching to the point of excoriation.

The diagnosis of seborrheic dermatitis is made on a clinical basis; biopsies are not helpful.

COURSE AND PROGNOSIS

Seborrheic dermatitis is a chronic disease characterized by exacerbations and remissions. It can occur at any age. In infancy it is frequently seen as "cradle cap" and as one form of diaper dermatitis (see Chapter 17). Seborrheic dermatitis is not very prominent during the childhood years but it frequently develops in the early teens as a manifestation of puberty. Thereafter it occurs at any time throughout adult life. The acute onset of what appears to be severe seborrheic dermatitis of the face can occur as one of the manifestations of acquired immunodeficiency syndrome (AIDS).

PATHOGENESIS

The cause of seborrheic dermatitis is unknown. Its name is derived from the fact that it was first recognized in the scalp, where the flow of sebum (seborrhea) is prominent. Since seborrheic dermatitis occurs in many other areas unassociated with sebum production, this relationship is probably more coincidental than causal. Likewise, the relationship between simple dandruff and seborrheic dermatitis is not completely clear. It is true that all patients with seborrheic dermatitis of the scalp have dandruff in the sense that scale is present, but a large portion of the population has dandruff, sometimes rather severely, without ever developing the inflammatory component of seborrheic dermatitis. Possibly the retention of sweat, with or without subsequent overgrowth of normally present yeast organisms, is an initiating factor for the conversion of dandruff to seborrheic dermatitis.

Hygiene and environmental factors seem important. Seborrheic dermatitis of the scalp generally first appears or worsens when shampooing is not carried out on a regular basis. The converse is also true. Frequent, vigorous shampooing (regardless of the type of soap used) is remarkably effective in keeping the disease under control. As mentioned above, perhaps the simple accumulation of scale, anchored in place by hair shafts, causes maceration and inflammation by way of sweat retention. Support for this hypothesis is offered by the observation that when a man with no skin disease on the face grows a beard he may then suddenly develop seborrheic dermatitis in that area.

Climate may also play a role. Seborrheic dermatitis regularly worsens in the fall and winter and improves considerably in the spring and summer. Additionally the disease does seem to be more troublesome in tropical areas than it is in equally warm but dry desert areas.

Factors relating to the central nervous system are of considerable interest. Clinicians have long recognized that seborrheic dermatitis sometimes accompanies Parkinson's disease. Moreover, seborrheic dermatitis seems to occur far more frequently in those patients bedridden with cerebral vascular accidents than it does in patients equally debilitated by non-neural illnesses such as myocardial infarction. Psychologic factors also seem important since nearly all patients agree that their seborrheic dermatitis worsens appreciably during times of stress and fatigue.

Finally, as mentioned above, recent evidence suggests that at least some forms of seborrheic dermatitis may be caused by overgrowth of the common yeast organisms which inhabit normal skin.

THERAPY

The mainstay of therapy for seborrheic dermatitis of the scalp is frequent, vigorous shampooing. The type of shampoo used seems much less important than the aggressiveness and frequency with which it is applied. Shampooing ought to be done initially on a daily basis; thereafter, the intervals can be lengthened as tolerated. The fingernails should be used to mechanically loosen scale and scrubbing ought to be carried out for at least 5 minutes. For mild to moderate seborrheic dermatitis shampoos such as Sebulex, Head and Shoulders, and Selsun Blue can be used. For more severe involvement, tar shampoos (Sebutone, Zetar, T-Gel) or prescription strength (2.5%) selenium sulfide (Exsel, Selsun) will be required. In these more severe cases topical steroid lotions applied after shampooing may be required in order to bring itching and inflammation under control.

Perhaps surprisingly, attention to the scalp is equally important in the treatment of seborrheic dermatitis occurring elsewhere. However, topical steroids, such as 1% hydrocortisone cream applied twice daily, are usually also necessary.

Recent reports suggest that antiyeast therapy such as oral administration of ketoconazole or topical administration of various imidazoles may represent a very useful adjunct in the treatment of some forms of seborrheic dermatitis.

SELECTED READING

Sheth RA, Desai SC: Dandruff: Assessment and management. Int J Dermatol 22:511, 1983.

Shuster S: The aetiology of dandruff and the mode of action of therapeutic agents. Br J Dermatol 111:235, 1984.

Ford GP, Farr PM, Ive FA, Shuster S: The response of seborrheic dermatitis to ketoconazole. Br J Dermatol 111:603, 1984.

Skinner RB Jr, Noah PW, Taylor RM, et al: Double-blind treatment of seborrheic dermatitis with 2% ketoconazole cream. J Am Acad Dermatol 12:852, 1985.

Marks R, Pearse AD, Walker AP: The effects of a shampoo containing zinc pyrithione on the control of dandruff. Br J Dermatol 112:415, 1985.

Soeprono FF, Schinella RA, Cockerell CJ, Comite SL: Seborrheic-like dermatitis of acquired immunodeficiency syndrome. J Am Acad Dermatol 14:242, 1986.

IRRITANT CONTACT DERMATITIS

DIAGNOSTIC HALLMARKS

1. Distribution: areas of expected solvent exposure or maceration (weak irritant); areas conforming to patient history of specific contact (strong irritant)
2. Discontinuation of exposure leads to improvement

CLINICAL PRESENTATION

The relatively common problem of irritant contact dermatitis occurs because of important environmental changes in the outer layers of the epidermis. Two types are recognized: that due to strong irritants and that due to weak irritants.

Strong irritant contact dermatitis occurs after a single exposure and a short latent period. Because of the direct connection between the exposure and the reaction, patients can usually identify the cause with little difficulty. Examples of strong irritants include chemicals which markedly change pH (acid and alkali "burns") or temperature (thermal burns and frostbite). Sunburn can also be conceptualized as a strong irritant contact dermatitis. The reactions caused by strong irritants are characterized by inflammation, pain, and epithelial disruption. The latter often occurs in the form of skin necrosis. The relative lack of pruritus and scale formation often results in an appearance that only marginally meets the morphologic requirements of the eczematous group.

Weak irritant contact dermatitis requires multiple exposures and, consequently, a long latent period. The connection between the exposures and the reaction is often not apparent to the patient. Fortunately, only one environmental modification, that of a change in moisture content of the skin, is very frequently responsible for the development of a weak irritant contact dermatitis. This change in moisture content results in skin that is too dry (xerosis) or too wet (maceration). Thus on the one hand solvents (of which detergents and hot water exposure are the most common) dry the skin by removing the lipid layer on the outer surface of the epidermis. Without a normal lipid layer the superficial epidermal cells lose moisture to the environment and the cells shrink in size. This shrinkage leads to cell separation with resultant cracking and fissuring. When the fissures are very shallow and are noninflammatory the process is known as chapping or xerosis. When the fissures are deeper and are accompanied by inflammation, it is appropriate to use the term irritant contact dermatitis or xerotic eczema (see below). Some scale formation occurs and the skin feels dry on palpation. Weeping, crusting, and excoriation are usually not prominent. Irritant contact dermatitis due to solvent exposure

occurs mostly on the hands. A history of excess solvent exposure
can usually be elicited.

Alternatively, in the process known as maceration, the constant
entrapment of too much fluid (water, sweat, urine, etc.) against the
skin results in overhydration, swelling, and eventually epidermal
cell death. Irritant contact dermatitis due to maceration is
suggested by localization of the eczematous process to the feet or
to intertriginous areas. When maceration is mild and is
unaccompanied by evidence of epithelial disruption the process is
known as intertrigo. When the inflammation of intertrigo is
accompanied by epithelial disruption in the form of a small amount
of weeping or yellow scale, the term irritant contact dermatitis can
be used. When maceration occurs intermittently rather than
constantly, the picture becomes more like that seen with excess
solvent exposure. The shiny, dry, cracked appearance of the toes in
"tennis shoe foot" and the fingers in those with hyperhidrosis
represent good examples of this phenomenon.

The diagnosis of either type of irritant contact dermatitis is
made clinically; proof of the correct diagnosis requires the
demonstration of improvement following modification of the suspected
environmental factors.

COURSE AND PROGNOSIS

Removal of the offending environmental irritant is usually all
that is needed to end the episode of dermatitis. In most cases this
is easy to do but in other instances (notably hand eczema due to
solvent exposure and diaper dermatitis due to urine retention) it
may be quite difficult. In such situations the addition of
topically applied steroids will also be necessary. Finally, in some
cases the itch-scratch cycle will become superimposed on the
irritant contact dermatitis. Failure to end the scratching (see
therapy section under atopic dermatitis) results in continuation of
eczematous disease even though the environmental factors are
suitably modified.

PATHOPHYSIOLOGY

In most cases of strong irritant contact dermatitis, damage is
caused because of a direct destructive effect on the exposed
epithelial cells. In weak irritant contact dermatitis the damage is
done more indirectly. Epithelial cells, like cells elsewhere in the
body, require a certain moisture content for health and function.
Loss of moisture (solvent action) or the presence of excess moisture
(maceration) eventually results in cell death. In all instances of
irritant contact dermatitis, epithelial cell death leads to exposure
of cutaneous nerve endings and the conveyance of burning, tingling,
or itching to the central nervous system. If the itching sensation

is translated into scratching (such as often happens in atopic individuals) prolongation and worsening of the epithelial damage can be expected.

Weak irritant contact dermatitis, as mentioned above, is most often caused from excess exposure to the solvent action of soap and water. Our hands will generally tolerate about five soap and water exposures per day. Five to ten exposures result in mild chapping which can be controlled by lubrication. More than ten exposures per day (a level frequently reached by housewives and mothers) result in more severe damage, with superimposition of inflammatory changes against a background of cracking and fissuring. The skin over the rest of our body is not as resistant. Bathing twice a day leads to mild xerosis; more frequent bathing frequently results in the development of inflammatory changes as well.

The deleterious effect of maceration is harder to quantitate. Skin of the groin and feet tolerates entrapment of moisture for several hours quite well but exposures longer than this (chronically wet diapers and chronic hyperhidrosis of the feet) result in the appearance of eczematous disease.

Less often, weak irritant contact dermatitis develops as a result of direct, repetitive mild trauma. Thus the constant handling of rough materials, such as stone or brick, or repeated wiping of the hands because of wet work will eventually cause the hands to become eczematized. This trauma causes direct damage to epithelial cells but it also causes removal of the protective lipid layer, as occurs in solvent exposure.

THERAPY

The first step in the treatment of contact dermatitis is the removal of the offending contactant. Of course to do this, the correct contactant must be identified. In instances of irritant contact dermatitis this is generally not too difficult since one can usually obtain a reasonably accurate history regarding solvent exposure, moisture entrapment, and mechanical trauma. In an industrial setting this may be somewhat more difficult but even here the number of possible solvents can usually be narrowed down to a few prime suspects. In all instances the use of solvents such as soap and detergents should be minimized. Bath oils or Cetaphil can be used instead of soap for washing, and the skin can be patted, rather than rubbed, dry. The temperature of wash water can be decreased. In situations of maceration, wet clothing (stockings, diapers, etc.) can be changed frequently and nonporous items of clothing made of nylon, plastic, or rubber can be avoided.

Once the environment has been modified the second step is to restore a protective lipid layer. This is carried out through the application of lubricants as described in Chapter 4. In general one cannot overemphasize the frequency with which these emollients need

to be applied but some care should be taken in treating
intertriginous areas such that excess sweat is not trapped.
      Topically applied steroids may or may not be necessary.
Generally if itching is present or if more than a minimal degree of
inflammation is present their use is desirable.

SELECTED READING

Steck WD: Juvenile plantar dermatosis: the "wet and dry foot
      syndrome." _Cleve Clin Q_ _50_:145, 1983.
Rietschel RL: Irritant contact dermatitis. _Dermatol Clinics_ _2_:545,
      1984.
Early SH, Simpson RL: Caustic burns from contact with wet cement.
      JAMA 254:528, 1985.

ALLERGIC CONTACT DERMATITIS

DIAGNOSTIC HALLMARKS

   1.   Distribution: location of the lesions suggests a
        specific contactant to the clinician; unilateral or
        asymmetrical distribution, if present, suggests external
        causation
   2.   Shape of the lesions suggests a specific contactant to the
        clinician
   3.   Removal of the suspected contactant leads to resolution of
        the dermatitis
   4.   Positive patch test

CLINICAL PRESENTATION

      The lesions of allergic contact dermatitis are quite different
in appearance than those of irritant contact dermatitis. Erythema
and edema are prominent and pruritus is often troublesome. In the
more acute cases weeping and crusting will be present while in
chronic cases scale and fissuring are the dominant findings. In
either instance some minor degree of excoriation may be found.
Blistering is seen only in those cases due to contact with plants of
the poison ivy type. This bullous variant of allergic contact
dermatitis is discussed in Chapter 7.
      The distribution and shape of individual lesions often provide
clues to the diagnosis of allergic contact dermatitis.
Asymmetrically or unilaterally located lesions of any type suggest
that the eruption was externally caused. If the morphology of the
lesions is eczematous the likelihood is great that they are due to
externally contacted antigens. The presence of lesions with a
nonround (especially linear or angular) configuration is likewise a
clue to possible external causation. In many instances the location

and shape of the lesions suggests to the examiner, unaided by patient history, a single, specific contactant.

COURSE AND PROGNOSIS

Removal of the responsible contactant results in spontaneous resolution of lesions over a 7- to 10-day period. Immunologic sensitivity to these contactants remains intact for many years and for this reason re-exposure, even to very small concentrations, is rapidly followed by exacerbation of the eczematous changes. Occasionally the itch-scratch cycle becomes superimposed on allergic contact dermatitis. In such instances removal of the contactant alone is insufficient to obtain resolution; attention directed towards disruption of the itch scratch cycle is also necessary.

PATHOPHYSIOLOGY

Allergic contact dermatitis is an immunologic event. The external factor (the antigen) does not itself cause any direct damage. The eczematous change occurs instead as a result of the inflammatory response which the antigen provokes. Moreover, development of allergic contact dermatitis requires the presence of a suitably sensitized host. Thus one's first exposure is never accompanied by a significant cutaneous reaction and instead simply initiates the process of sensitization. During sensitization the antigen on the skin is intercepted by epidermal dendritic macrophages known as Langerhans cells. Once processed by the Langerhans cells the antigen is presented to helper T cell lymphocytes. These cells in turn (probably through the release of interleukin 2) activate a clone of responder T cells. This process begins in the epidermis but is concluded in the regional lymph nodes which drain the contact site. At this point the host is primed to react to subsequent antigen re-exposure. When contact with the antigen next occurs these sensitized lymphocytes migrate to the skin where they attack the offending antigen through the creation of a vigorous cell mediated immune response.

Our understanding of why some substances stimulate this sensitization reaction and others do not is limited. Nevertheless, it is fortunate that of the thousands of substances we contact daily only a miniscule number have any significant antigenic potential. Molecules which seem to be the most potent antigens are characterized by the presence of one or more chemically active sites which can form stable, covalent bonds with other substances. Small molecules (generally those under 5000 daltons in molecular mass) may not in themselves be troublesome, but by binding to a carrier protein present in the host these haptens can become antigenic. Larger molecules do not require carrier proteins and can instead bind directly to macrophage cell membranes.

The stratum corneum plays an important role in sensitization. Thickly keratinized surfaces such as the palms and soles resist sensitization whereas skin with a disrupted stratum corneum is rather easily sensitized. Moreover, chemicals which are soluble in the lipid layer of the stratum corneum may possess stronger antigenic potential than do those which are not soluble.

The substances most likely to cause contact dermatitis and the circumstances under which they are most likely to be contacted include the following. The most commonly recognized antigenic contactant is probably that of the pentadecylcatechol responsible for poison-ivy-type contact dermatitis. The second most frequent offender is undoubtedly nickel. Nickel is found in most metals used in snaps, buckles, and jewelry. Thus nickel contact dermatitis can be found in association with rings, bracelets, watch bands, earrings, and metal closures used in various types of clothing. Other common causes of allergic contact dermatitis include reactions to formaldehyde used in the preparation of permanent press clothing; reactions to neomycin, benzocaine, parabens, and ethylenediamine used in many topically applied medications; reactions to chromates used in cements and cutting oils; uncured epoxy resins used in many industries; several chemicals used in sunscreens; fragrances used in perfumes; and permanent wave solutions used by beauty operators. The antigens on this list account for more than 90% of all instances of allergic contact dermatitis. Note that soaps, detergents, and most types of clothing are not on this list. These latter items are only rarely responsible for allergic reactions and should not be incriminated simply because there is a history of their use.

THERAPY

The first step in therapy is the identification of suspected contactants. As indicated above this identification is often possible simply because the location or shape of the lesions suggests a specific contactant. In more subtle cases one has to work with statistical probability based on the knowledge of which contactants are among the most frequent offenders. Rarely there may even be justification for the application of a series of screening patch tests in hopes that one or more positive responses will provide at least an initial clue.

Once identified, exposure to the contactant needs to be discontinued. In most cases this is not difficult but in some instances the offending chemical may be found in several unsuspected alternative sources or the chemical may cross-react with other substances. Textbooks on contact dermatitis offer considerable information about these problems but in many instances the complexities involved warrant referral of patients with allergic contact dermatitis to a dermatologist.

Treatment of the dermatitis itself depends on the use of

steroids. In most instances topically applied steroids of mid or
high potency will suffice. In instances of greater severity
systemically administered steroids may be desirable.

SELECTED READING

Adams RM: Patch testing -- A recapitulation. J Am Acad Dermatol
    5:629, 1981.
Keil JE, Shmunes E: The epidemiology of work-related skin disease
    in South Carolina. Arch Dermatol 119:650, 1983.
Bergstresser PR: Immunologic mechanisms of contact
    hypersensitivity. Dermatol Clinics 2:523, 1984.
Burrows D: The dichromate problem. Int J Dermatol 23:215,
    1984.
Storrs FJ: Permanent wave contact dermatitis: Contact allergy to
    glyceryl monothioglycolate. J Am Acad Dermatol 11:74, 1984.
Nishioka K: Allergic contact dermatitis. Int J Dermatol 24:1, 1985.
Adams RM, Maibach HI: A five-year study of cosmetic reactions. J
    Am Acad Dermatol 13:1062, 1985.
Larsen WG: Perfume dermatitis: J Am Acad Dermatol 12:1, 1985.
Adams RM, Fisher AA: Contact allergen alternatives: 1986. J Am
    Acad Dermatol 14:951, 1986.
Bajaj AK, Gupta SC: Contact hypersensitivity to topical
    antibacterial agents. Int J Dermatol 25:103, 1986.

XEROTIC ECZEMA (ASTEATOTIC ECZEMA, WINTER ITCH)

DIAGNOSTIC HALLMARKS

    1.   Distribution: legs, hands
    2.   Minute, thin fissures
    3.   Minimal inflammation

CLINICAL PRESENTATION

    Xerotic eczema is closely related both in appearance and cause
to solvent-type weak irritant contact dermatitis. The difference
lies in the fact that the patient with xerotic eczema is
constitutionally unable to provide an adequate lipid layer, whereas
in weak irritant contact dermatitis the lipid layer is removed by
contactants. The end result, too little epidermal lipid, is the
same for both conditions. The patches and barely elevated plaques
of xerotic eczema are nummular in appearance. They are 2 to 5 cm in
diameter and are usually very sharply marginated. Mild inflammation
may be present within the plaques but redness is most pronounced
within the cracks and fissures which encircle and criss-cross the
surface of the plaque. These cracks do not usually penetrate the
full thickness of the epidermis and for this reason there is little
weeping and crusting. Scale, particularly lying along the edges of

the fissures, is usually present but is usually not very prominent.
Excoriations are seldom numerous. The plaques of xerotic eczema can
occur anywhere on the body but they are found most commonly on the
legs. Burning and stinging usually accompany the moderately severe
pruritus which is present.

The diagnosis of xerotic eczema is made on a clinical basis.
Biopsy is not helpful.

COURSE AND PROGNOSIS

Xerotic eczema, once present, tends to persist simply because
the damaged skin tolerates the normal trauma of everyday life very
poorly. In fact, patients often unintentionally worsen the process
by increasing the frequency and intensity of bathing in a misguided
attempt to treat their rash through better cleanliness. Healing of
xerotic skin requires that excess water loss through the epidermis
be stopped long enough for regrowth of epithelial cells to bridge
the cracks. Once healed the skin may remain normal for considerable
periods of time.

PATHOGENESIS

Xerotic eczema is the inflammatory end stage of xerosis or
chapping. This process begins when, because of insufficient lipid
on the surface of the skin, epidermal water loss as a result of
evaporation exceeds replenishment from below. In this setting
epithelial cells shrink to the point where islands of cells begin to
separate in a process similar to that seen on the dirt bottom of a
dried-up lake. The term xerotic eczema is used when the cracks and
fissures are deep enough to cause visible inflammatory changes and
symptoms of burning or itching. Factors which reduce surface lipid
and thus enhance water loss include aging, excess bathing, and
excess rubbing of the skin. All of these factors are particularly
troublesome for atopic individuals since they have skin which is
drier than normal anyway. Environmental factors also adversely
influence water loss from the skin. Thus low humidity, especially
that which occurs in heated homes in the winter, shifts the
equilibrium toward increased water loss. The presence of air flow
such as occurs with wind and fan driven air for heating aggravates
the effect of low humidity.

THERAPY

The therapy of xerotic eczema depends on reducing the rate of
water loss from the skin. This is approached by attempts to reduce
the removal of natural lipid and by the addition of artificial
lipid. Lipid loss is lessened by requesting that patients bathe
less frequently, that cooler water be used, that use of soap be

sharply restricted, and finally that patients pat, rather than rub, dry. Artificial lipid is added through the process of lubrication (see also Chapter 4). Hand cream should be applied four to eight times per day on the hands and twice daily on the trunk and extremities. Lubricants are particularly helpful when applied while the skin is wet since they then trap additional moisture before evaporation occurs. Bath oils are often recommended but their overall role in skin lubrication is minor.

Inflammation, when present, must also be treated. This is accomplished through the twice daily application of mid potency steroids. In the setting of xerosis an ointment base is frequently preferable to a cream base. Rarely, short term use of systemic steroids is also necessary.

Scratching, when present, must also be controlled lest further epithelial destruction occur. This subject is covered in the therapy section on atopic dermatitis.

MISCELLANEOUS NONEXCORIATED ECZEMATOUS DISEASES

Impetigo (see also Chapter 7) often presents as a shallow, red erosion covered with crust. The presence of weeping, crusting, and pruritus allows the nonbullous form of the disease to be placed within the group of eczematous diseases. Impetigo is identified by its location around the nose and mouth, by its rapid appearance and spread, by the presence of pus underneath the crust, and by its prompt response to antibacterial therapy. Other clues include the history of contagion, the paucity of inflammation compared to the magnitude of crusting, and the recovery of streptococcal or staphylococcal bacteria on culture.

The term infectious eczematoid dermatitis was originally used for those eczematous lesions which appeared in the skin around infected, draining lesions. However, it is now apparent that this eczematization is due more to the macerating effect of the drainage than to any bacteria which it might contain. Thus the rash around an ileostomy, draining sterile fluid, is similar in appearance to that around a colostomy draining fluid with a high bacterial count. For this reason the process can be viewed as a variant of weak irritant contact dermatitis and the term "infectious eczematoid dermatitis" can be left as a historical footnote in the annals of dermatology.

The patches and plaques of perioral dermatitis are often covered with a small amount of yellow colored scale. As in seborrheic dermatitis, the yellow color is due to the exudation of small amounts of serum onto the surface of the skin. Minute pustules may stud the surface of the erythematous patches or plaques and for this reason the condition is also considered in Chapter 8. As the term "perioral" implies this condition occurs on the lower half of the face. A characteristic feature is the presence of a 1/4-inch ring

of normal skin which occurs between the lips and the beginning of
the eruption.

There are several types of <u>sunlight induced eczematous</u>
<u>diseases</u>. First, photosensitivity may be induced by internally
administered medications such as the tetracyclines, the
phenothiazines, the thiazide diuretics, the sulfonamide antibiotics,
and nalidixic acid. Second, photocontact dermatitis may occur in a
small percentage of patients applying cosmetics containing musk
ambrette; sunscreens containing PABA, PABA esters, cinnamates, or
benzophenones; and, in the past at least, soaps containing
halogenated bacteriostatic agents. Third, chronic sun exposure
occurring over years may result in the development of hundreds of
small, slightly crusted actinic keratoses superimposed on an
inflammatory background. This process can be considered
conceptually as a form of actinic dermatitis. Finally, the
photosensitivity eruption of systemic lupus erythematosus (the
"butterfly eruption") is sometimes so intense it takes on an
eczematous morphology in a sun exposed distribution pattern.

ACRAL ECZEMATOUS DISEASES (HAND AND FOOT ECZEMA)

Several of the eczematous diseases discussed in this chapter
preferentially involve the hands and feet. For this reason one
should not use the term "hand eczema" or "foot eczema" as a
diagnostic term. One must specifically attempt to identify which
process is responsible: atopic dermatitis, dyshidrotic eczema,
scabies, contact dermatitis, or secondary eczematization of a
noneczematous disease. Guidelines for the recognition of these
separate processes are covered in Chapter 17.

GENITAL AND PERIGENITAL ECZEMATOUS DISEASES

The situation for eczematous diseases of the groin is analogous
to that of acral dermatitis discussed in the paragraph above. It is
not sufficient to simply make a diagnosis of "diaper dermatitis" or
"pruritus ani." One must attempt to recognize specifically which
one of several eczematous conditions is responsible for the observed
changes. Guidelines for doing so are contained in Chapter 17.

NUMMULAR ECZEMATOUS DISEASES

The adjective "nummular" is derived from the Latin word for
coin. Thus nummular lesions are characterized by sharp margination
and by their coin-like roundness and coin-like size. This is a very
common appearance for dermatologic conditions and in fact nummular
lesions can be found in all ten disease groups. However, the term
is most commonly used for small round eczematous lesions. Nummular
patterns are most often seen in xerotic eczema and in atopic

dermatitis. Occasionally some of the lesions seen in autoeczematization (see below) are also nummular. Some clinicians use the term "nummular eczema" as if it were the name of a single disease, but in most instances such lesions can be better assigned as variations of atopic dermatitis, xerotic eczema, or autoeczematization.

AUTOECZEMATIZATION (AUTOSENSITIZATION, "ID" REACTION)

There is a marked tendency for severe eczematous disease, regardless of type, to spread spontaneously outside of its original distribution pattern. The reason for this spread is unknown but it is widely believed to occur as the result of an immunologic response mounted against antigens located at the original site of involvement. The putative antigens include proteins of external origin (bacteria and fungi) and proteins of internal origin (keratin and collagen) which have been modified in some way by the original disease process.

Conceptually autoeczematization can be considered as "metastatic" spread of an eczematous disease. Local, continguous extension could then be viewed as "lymphatic metastases" and distant, noncontiguous lesions could be viewed as "hematogenous metastases."

Autoeczematization is most often seen in association with diaper dermatitis, stasis dermatitis, external otitis, hand eczema, and foot eczema. Historically, autoeczematization was first recognized in individuals with tinea pedis who subsequently developed vesicular and eczematous disease of the hands. This process was called the "dermatophytid reaction," from which has been derived the shortened term "id" reaction.

The lesions of autoeczematization are frequently vesicular when they occur on the hands but are more typically eczematous when they occur on the face, arms, legs, and trunk. In these latter locations the lesions of autoeczematization often assume a nummular pattern.

Patients with autoeczematization usually do not respond well to simple measures such as soaks and topical steroids. In most instances a burst of systemically administered steroids will be required. When systemically administered steroids are used the autoeczematous lesions respond promptly, but the underlying, original disease clears more slowly. Failure to continue treatment until the original lesions are completely healed is usually followed by rapid recrudescence of the entire process.

SELECTED READING

Kaaman T, Torssander J: Dermatophytid -- A misdiagnosed entity?
    Acta Derm Venereol 63:404, 1983.

GENERALIZED ECZEMATOUS DISEASE (EXFOLIATIVE ERYTHRODERMATITIS)

The term exfoliative erythrodermatitis is used when eczematous disease covers 70% or more of the total body surface. Exfoliative erythrodermatitis can occur in either a primary or a secondary form. The primary form consists of the de novo development of lesions in a patient with no past history of skin disease. The secondary form arises as the result of widespread extension from an already existent skin disease.

Exfoliative erythrodermatitis of the primary type may develop as an idiopathic condition, as a medication reaction, or as a manifestation of malignant lymphoma. The two medications most often responsible for the development of exfoliative erythrodermatitis are gold and phenytoin (Dilantin). Among the lymphomas, exfoliative erythrodermatitis is most commonly seen in association with mycosis fungoides and Hodgkin's disease. When it occurs with mycosis fungoides, malignant T cell lymphocytes may be found in both the skin and bloodstream (Sezary syndrome), whereas when it occurs with Hodgkin's disease no atypical cells are found on cutaneous biopsy.

Exfoliative erythrodermatitis of the secondary type occurs most often as an extension of an eczematous disease and, in particular, as a widespread extension of atopic dermatitis. It can, however, also develop as a result of secondary eczematization of a papulosquamous disease. In this situation psoriasis, particularly in its pustular or erythrodermic form, is the most likely underlying process.

The pathogenetic mechanisms responsible for the conversion of any localized skin disease to that of exfoliative erythrodermatitis are not well understood but it is convenient to think of the process as a widespread extension of autoeczematization.

Exfoliative erythrodermatitis, regardless of cause, is often complicated by anemia, leukocytosis, hyperuricemia, hypoalbuminemia, and problems with temperature regulation. Moreover, the vasodilation which accompanies the cutaneous inflammation occasionally leads to cardiac failure of the high output type.

Therapy of exfoliative erythrodermatitis is quite difficult. Patients are terribly uncomfortable and most experience shaking, chills, and considerable malaise and toxicity. Because of this, hospitalization is usually necessary. Soaks and topical steroids are almost always desirable and any associated cutaneous infection is treated with appropriate antibiotics. Most patients will also require the use of systemically administered steroids.

SELECTED READING

Worm AM, Nielsen SL: Increased microvascular water filtration and blood flow in extensive skin disease. J Invest Dermatol 76:110, 1981.

Marks J: Erythroderma and its management. Special symposium on dermatological therapy: VII. Connective tissue and vascular disorders. Clin Exp Dermatol 7:415, 1982.

Hasan T, Jansen CT: Erythroderma: A follow-up of fifty cases. J Am Acad Dermatol 8:836, 1983.

Eczematous Diseases of the Hands, Feet and Groin

The diseases discussed in this chapter are covered more fully in Chapter 16. Only those aspects which are related to differential diagnosis are presented here.

ECZEMATOUS DISEASE OF THE HANDS (Table 17-1)

There are six conditions which must be considered in the differential diagnosis of hand eczema. These are dyshidrotic eczema, atopic dermatitis, allergic contact dermatitis, irritant contact dermatitis, scabies, and autoeczematization as a result of eczematous disease elsewhere.

The characteristic features of these diseases usually allow for identification of the specific disease responsible for the patient's problem. However, these features become less recognizable in patients with longstanding disease and in patients who happen to have two or more eczematous conditions present at the same time. In instances where the diagnosis is unclear it is sometimes helpful to clear the disease completely through the use of systemic steroids and then, when the steroids are stopped, watch for the evolution of typical features if and when the disease recurs.

Dyshidrotic eczema is characterized by a history of preceding dyshidrosis. Thus, on questioning, patients will describe the onset of their disease as consisting of pinhead sized, noninflammatory vesicles situated on the tips or sides of the fingers. Moreover, on examination, some of these minute noninflammatory vesicles can usually be found adjacent to or within the eczematous plaques. Often these vesicles are so closely set they lead to the appearance of larger, multiloculated bullae. As dyshidrosis becomes increasingly eczematized there is extension of the vesicular process from the fingers onto the palms and, through the process of autoeczematization, there may also be extension of the eczematous process onto the dorsal surface of the fingers and hands. By the time the whole hand has become involved all evidence of the original, preceding vesicular disease may have disappeared, leaving the patient's description of the original lesions as the only clue to the dyshidrotic nature of the problem.

Atopic dermatitis begins quite differently. There is no historical or visible evidence of a distinct, noninflammatory, vesicular phase. Instead, patients indicate that itching precedes all evidence of skin eruption. However, the moment scratching begins, there is the sudden appearance of a vigorous inflammatory

TABLE 17-1
DIFFERENTIAL DIAGNOSIS OF HAND ECZEMA

DISEASE	CHARACTERISTIC EARLY DISTRIBUTION	OTHER CHARACTERISTICS
Dyshidrotic eczema	Tips and sides of fingers; palms	History of preceding noninflammatory vesicles (dyshidrosis)
Atopic dermatitis	Dorsal surface of hands and fingers	Itch-scratch cycle; nummular pattern
Irritant contact dermatitis	Volar surface of fingers, palms, and knuckles	Excess of soap, water, or solvent exposure; dry shiny skin; fissuring out of proportion to inflammation
Allergic contact dermatitis	Dorsal surface of hands and fingers	Pattern corresponds to contactant such as watch bands and rings
Scabies	Web spaces	History of contagion; typical lesions elsewhere; linear vesicles (burrows)
Autoeczematization	Palms and volar fingers	Presence of significant eczematous disease on the feet or elsewhere

reaction characterized by redness, swelling, weeping, crusting, and excoriation. These initial plaques of atopic dermatitis are found on the dorsal surface of the fingers and hands. Later in the course of the disease varying degrees of autoeczematization sometimes lead to the development of eczematous lesions on the palms, wrists, and forearms. The itch-scratch cycle as defined in Chapter 16 is invariably present.

Allergic contact dermatitis, like atopic dermatitis, almost always begins on the dorsal surface of the fingers and hands. This predilection is most likely due to the protective effect of the thick keratin found on the palmar aspect of the fingers and hands. Allergic contact dermatitis differs from atopic dermatitis in that excoriations are less prominent and a visible eruption precedes the scratching. However, before a diagnosis of allergic contact dermatitis can be proven a suspected contactant must be identified, a positive result to patch testing must be obtained; and the patient must demonstrate improvement when the contactant is removed. The most readily identifiable type of allergic contact dermatitis is that of nickel allergy simply because the eruption occurs in such close promixity to the offending ring, bracelet, or watch band. Many industrial chemicals cause allergic contact dermatitis of the hands. The agents most commonly involved are chromates and epoxy resins. Cosmetics (cinnamates, lanolin, Peruvian balsam) are uncommon, although occasional, offenders. Soaps and detergents for all practical purposes cause irritant contact dermatitis rather than allergic contact dermatitis.

Irritant contact dermatitis is dominated by the presence of chapping, cracking, and fissuring. Inflammation, weeping, crusting, and excoriations are considerably less prominent. The changes of irritant contact dermatitis occur most commonly on the volar aspects of the fingers, but the palms and dorsal surface of the hands, particularly over the knuckles, may also be involved. The skin is dull red in color and often has a shiny or glistening surface. Tingling or burning pain is present; pruritus is minimal to moderate in intensity. The diagnosis is based on the clinical appearance and on the history of frequent exposure to soap, water, or other solvents. Irritant contact dermatitis is an occupational hazard for mothers, housewives, nurses, dentists, waitresses, and bartenders. A second type of irritant contact dermatitis occurs because of moisture retention and maceration under wide-band rings. Thus eczematous changes around rings may be either allergic or irritant in etiology. Patch testing to metals may be necessary to differentiate the two causes.

Scabies is an infrequent cause of hand eczema. It is characterized by the fact that the earliest lesions develop in the web spaces as solitary vesicles or inflammatory vesicopapules. From there eczematous changes sometimes spread onto the dorsal surface of the hands and fingers. The diagnosis is based on this distribution pattern, evidence of contagion, recovery of the mite, and the presence of typical lesions in other body sites.

Autoeczematization (or autosensitization) is a reaction pattern in which eczematous disease elsewhere on the skin induces "metastatic" eczematous lesions at some distant site. The hands, particularly the palms and fingers, are frequently involved in this reaction. A vesicular component that resembles dyshidrosis is often present. A diagnosis of autoeczematization should be considered if vesiculation is explosive in onset, if there is minimal grouping of the vesicles, and most importantly, when marked eczematous disease is found on the feet or elsewhere on the body.

The diagnosis and therapy of hand eczema are complicated by the fact that frequently more than a single process is involved. Thus, dyshidrotic eczema, allergic contact dermatitis, and scabies are often complicated by the concomitant presence of either the itch-scratch cycle (atopic dermatitis) or irritant contact dermatitis due to soap and water exposure. With so many things going on at once it is easy to see why many clinicians give up trying to sort out the individual processes and simply label the problem "hand eczema." Nevertheless, since the treatment varies with each of the processes, it is important to identify them individually. As mentioned above, where this cannot be done on the basis of history and examination, it may be necessary to use a short course of systemic steroids so that the initial characteristic changes can be identified as they recur.

ECZEMATOUS DISEASE OF THE FEET (Table 17-2)

Eczematous disease of the feet may be caused by any one of the following six processes: dyshidrotic eczema, atopic dermatitis, vesicular tinea pedis, allergic contact dermatitis, irritant contact dermatitis, and stasis dermatitis. The problems in differential diagnosis are quite similar to those discussed for hand eczema but recognition is further hampered by the confounding effect of shoes and stockings.

Dyshidrotic eczema of the foot is distinguished from the other eczematous diseases by the fact that the process begins as dyshidrosis. Patient history identifies the fact that minute, noninflammatory vesicles preceded the appearance of the eczematous changes. These changes begin on the tips and sides of the toes; the clinical characteristics are otherwise similar to those described for dyshidrotic eczema of the hands. Dyshidrotic eczema of the feet is a particularly common problem in children.

Atopic dermatitis of the foot is distinguished by the fact that itching precedes any evidence of skin disease. Moreover, the distribution pattern, which involves the dorsal surface of the second and third toes and the dorsal surface of the foot, is highly characteristic. Lesions may also occur around the ankle near the malleoli. The plaques of atopic dermatitis on the foot are often quite sharply marginated and are nummular in size and shape. However, in some instances autoeczematization causes the disease to cover the entire foot. The itch-scratch cycle can be identified. Excoriations are prominent; lichenification is frequently present.

Tinea pedis is an extraordinarily common condition but it is less often the cause of foot eczema than one might expect. Those patients who do develop foot eczema due to tinea pedis are rather likely to give a history of preceding, chronic fissuring of the lateral toe webs. On examination, multilocular vesicles and bullae of the instep are regularly found. The dorsal surface of the foot

TABLE 17-2
DIFFERENTIAL DIAGNOSIS OF FOOT ECZEMA

DISEASE	CHARACTERISTIC EARLY DISTRIBUTION	OTHER CHARACTERISTICS
Dyshidrotic eczema	Tips and sides of the toes; soles	History of preceding noninflammatory vesicles (dyshidrosis)
Atopic dermatitis	Dorsal surface of toes and foot; around the malleoli	Itch-scratch cycle; nummular pattern
Vesicular tinea pedis	Clustered vesicles on the instep; web space fissuring	Nail dystrophy; positive KOH or culture
Allergic contact dermatitis	Dorsal surface of toes and distal foot	Positive patch test
Irritant contact dermatitis	Plantar surface of toes and foot	Fissuring with little inflammation; hyperhidrosis
Stasis dermatitis	Ankles	History of preceding noninflammatory edema (stasis)

becomes involved late in the course of the disease through the
process of autoeczematization. Foot eczema secondary to fungal
disease rarely if ever occurs prior to puberty. The typical
distribution and course, together with the presence of onychomycosis
and positive KOH preparations, allow for definitive identification.
    Allergic contact dermatitis occurs primarily on the dorsal
surface of the toes. For this reason it is easily confused with
atopic dermatitis. However, as opposed to atopic dermatitis, a rash
is present at the time pruritus is first noted. Also,
lichenification is not usually present. Most allergic contact
dermatitis of the foot is due to the products used in the
manufacture of shoes. These include glues, chemicals used in rubber
processing, and chromates used in leather tanning. A suspected
diagnosis can be confirmed by patch testing. Such tests are most

practically carried out by removal of a small piece of the inner portion of the shoe. This material can then be bandaged directly to the patient's skin in the manner described in Chapter 5. Patch testing can also, of course, be carried out with chemicals supplied in most patch testing kits. Contrary to widespread belief, allergic contact dermatitis is not a common cause of foot eczema.

Irritant contact dermatitis of the foot has a distinctive appearance. The plantar and dorsal surfaces of the toes are dull red and shiny. Careful inspection reveals chapping and hundreds of minute cracks and fissures. Peeling of the plantar surface of the toes is usually present. The problem usually starts because of maceration secondary to sweat retention. This condition is particularly likely to occur in individuals with hyperhidrosis of the feet and in those who wear shoes which retard evaporative loss of moisture. For this reason it is an extraordinarily common problem in children who wear rubber soled tennis-type shoes all day long.

Stasis dermatitis of the foot occurs in older adults who give a history of chronic ankle swelling. It is characterized by the fact that the eruption always begins first at the ankle and only subsequently extends to the rest of the foot. Appreciable swelling of the foot and ankle is always present. The dorsal aspect becomes involved first, but plantar disease is present in persistent, severe cases.

Foot eczemas, like hand eczemas, are commonly complicated by the development of autoeczematization. This process results in local as well as distant spread of eczematous disease outside of the original distribution pattern and greatly hampers recognition of the originating process. Recognition of the various foot eczemas is also hindered by the regular presence of irritant contact dermatitis secondary to the retention of serum and sweat underneath footwear. Because of these two factors it is often necessary to use a short course of systemic steroids so that the initial changes can be identified as they recur.

ECZEMATOUS DISEASE OF THE GROIN IN ADULTS (Table 17-3)

Eczematous disease of the groin in adults may be caused by atopic dermatitis, fungal eczema, or candidiasis. Irritant factors due to sweat retention may complicate these conditions.

Atopic dermatitis of the genitalia and perianal tissue is characterized by the presence of pruritus prior to the development of an observable skin rash. However, just as soon as scratching begins, inflammation, weeping, crusting, and excoriations become apparent. Prominent lichenification frequently develops once the itch-scratch cycle becomes well established. The lesions are poorly marginated. Atopic dermatitis most commonly begins on the scrotum in men and on the labia majora in women. Perianal skin is often involved in both sexes. In chronic cases the entire groin may

become eczematized. Diagnosis depends on recognition of the
itch-scratch cycle.
    Eczematized tinea cruris always begins on the upper inner
thighs. The inguinal-genital fold itself, however, is not
prominently involved. Subsequent spread leads to involvement of the
buttocks and pubic area. The genitalia and perianal skin are
usually spared. The lesions are excoriated and are usually poorly
marginated. However, one or more areas of sharp margination and
ring-like configuration can usually be found. A history of
longstanding but intermittent "jock itch" may be elicited. The

TABLE 17-3
ECZEMATOUS DISEASE OF THE GROIN (ADULTS)

DISEASE	CHARACTERISTIC EARLY DISTRIBUTION	OTHER CHARACTERISTICS
Atopic dermatitis	Scrotum, vulva, perianal skin	Itch-scratch cycle; prominent excoriation and lichenification
Tinea cruris	Inner thighs, buttocks	Mostly men; associated tinea pedis; positive KOH or culture
Candidiasis	Vulva, inguinal-scrotal fold, scrotum, preputial fold	Vaginitis; scattered pustules; positive KOH or culture

disease is considerably more common in men than in women. A
suspected diagnosis can be confirmed with KOH preparation and fungal
cultures. Unfortunately, sampling errors due to the widespread
secondary eczematization often occur. Thus the initial KOH
preparations may be negative. In such instances topical steroids
should be used for 7 to 14 days. Subsequent examination will reveal
areas of more typical tinea cruris from which repeat testing can be
carried out.
    Candidiasis as a cause for eczematous disease
of the groin develops more abruptly than atopic dermatitis and tinea
cruris. Moreover, the disease usually begins in folded
(intertriginous) areas of skin. Thus the initial lesions most often
occur in the inguinal-scrotal fold in men and in the sulcus between
the labia in women. Extension to the scrotum and labia majora

occurs rather quickly. Perianal involvement sometimes occurs in
those who have recently taken systemic antibiotics or have had
several days of diarrhea. Candidal vaginitis is usually present in
women. The lesions of candidiasis are poorly marginated and
satellite papules or pustules are usually found on the margins of
the main plaques. KOH preparations are positive only when intact
pustules are sampled, but on the other hand, cultures are usually
positive from both pustules and the eczematized skin. Cultures are
best obtained by gently rubbing a moistened cotton tipped applicator
over the inflamed surface; the applicator is then submitted for
culture.

As was true for the eczematous diseases of the hands and feet,
autoeczematization frequently complicates all three of these
conditions. Thus extension of dermatitic lesions outside of the
distribution patterns described above is rather commonly seen.
Moreover, maceration as a result of serum and sweat retention often
obscures the original morphology. Finally, eczematized psoriasis
should be considered, particularly if more typical papulosquamous
lesions can be identified elsewhere on the body.

ECZEMATOUS DISEASE OF THE GROIN IN INFANTS (Table 17-4)

There are four conditions which must be included in the
differential diagnosis of diaper dermatitis. They include irritant
contact dermatitis, candidiasis, atopic dermatitis, and seborrheic
dermatitis. Since the development of eczematous lesions in the
groin of infants is usually preceded by the retention of moisture
(intertrigo), all causes of diaper dermatitis are seen more commonly
where plastic coated disposable diapers are used or where plastic
pants are worn over conventional diapers.

Irritant contact dermatitis is the most common cause of diaper
dermatitis. It occurs as a result of prolonged maceration such as
develops when wet diapers are left unchanged for hours at a time.
The rash is most prominent on the buttocks and pubic skin; the
creases of the skin are relatively spared. The involved areas are
dusky red and have a shiny appearance. The skin seems chapped and
on close inspection many tiny cracks and fissures are seen.
Weeping, crusting, and excoriations are usually not prominent.
Retained urine is the most common offending substance but sweat
retention is often a complicating factor. There is little evidence
that either ammonia released from urine or residual detergent from
insufficiently rinsed diapers play any important role.

Atopic dermatitis occurs in a distribution pattern which often
demonstrates sparing of creases. However, the genitalia are
frequently involved. The itch-scratch cycle is present and
excoriations are prominent. The child scratches vigorously at night
and in the office when the diapers are removed for examination.
Weeping, crusting, lichenification, and scale formation are variably

TABLE 17-4
DIAPER DERMATITIS

DISEASE	CHARACTERISTIC EARLY DISTRIBUTION	OTHER CHARACTERISTICS
Irritant contact dermatitis	Nonintertriginous	Dusky red, shiny skin
Seborrheic dermatitis	Intertriginous	Dull red color; associated scalp and axillary disease
Candidiasis	Intertriginous	Bright red color; scattered pustules; positive KOH or culture
Atopic dermatitis	Nonintertriginous	Itch-scratch cycle; prominent excoriations

present. Lesions of atopic dermatitis are frequently found outside
of the groin; the cheeks in particular may be involved.

Seborrheic dermatitis is characterized by the presence of dusky
red patches and plaques deep within the creases. Nonintertriginous
skin is relatively spared. Weeping, crusting, scale formation, and
excoriations are not prominent. Seborrheic dermatitis rarely
involves only the groin area; similar lesions will often be found in
other folded areas such as the retroauricular areas and the axillary
folds. Scalp involvement, if present, is a helpful sign. Since
signs of epithelial disruption are often minimal, seborrheic
dermatitis is often confused with papulosquamous disease such as
psoriasis.

Candidiasis is characterized by initial involvement of the
creases with relatively rapid extension onto other surfaces.
Inflammation is intense. The color is bright red and accompanying
edema is often present. Isolated satellite papules and pustules are
frequently found at the margin of the inflammatory plaques.
Excoriations are often prominent. Positive KOH preparations can be
obtained from intact pustules. Positive cultures can be obtained
both from pustules and from the eczematized skin.

As is true for the other diseases discussed in this chapter,
autoeczematization frequently leads to spread of eczematous disease
outside of the diaper area. Thus, the lower trunk and upper legs

frequently become involved. Finally, two or more of the eczematous diseases discussed above are often present concomitantly. If more than one problem is present, both conditions should be treated simultaneously.

Hair Loss (Alopecias)

Hair loss is separable into two major categories: that which occurs with associated, visible scalp disease and that which occurs in the absence of visible scalp disease. In separating these two categories one must ignore the presence of mild, noninflammatory dandruff since this condition occurs in such a large proportion of the population and is rarely associated with significant hair loss. The major causes of alopecia are listed in Table 18-1.

TABLE 18-1
DISEASES ASSOCIATED WITH HAIR LOSS

    Alopecia with visible scalp disease
        Localized loss
                Tinea capitis
                Discoid lupus erythematosus
        Diffuse loss
                Seborrheic dermatitis

    Alopecia without visible scalp disease
        Localized loss
                Alopecia areata
                Trichotillomania
                Secondary syphilis
        Diffuse loss
                Telogen effluvium
                Male and female pattern loss
                Hypothyroidism

ALOPECIA WITH SCALP DISEASE

Tinea Capitis. Most cases of tinea capitis occur in children, but adult infections, especially with Trichophyton tonsurans, are occasionally seen. Sharply localized patches of alopecia are an integral part of tinea capitis. This hair loss is characterized by the fact that the hairs are broken off at, or close to, the surface of the skin. This results in the presence of fine stubble which, if too short to palpate, is sometimes visible as a series of black dots within the patch of alopecia. The patches of alopecia in tinea capitis are also characterized by their sharp margination and their confinement precisely to the area of scalp disease. The associated scalp disease consists of one or more sharply marginated scaling

plaques with varying degrees of inflammation. Infection with
Microsporum audouinii and T. tonsurans may be relatively inapparent
and noninflammatory whereas those due to Microsporum canis and
Trichophyton mentagrophytes are usually bright red and edematous.
These inflammatory changes, known as kerion formation, may be
accompanied by pustulation around some of the follicles. Only the
Microsporum sp. infections fluoresce under Wood's lamp
illumination. Confirmation of suspected tinea capitis depends on
the performance of KOH preparations and fungal cultures. Treatment
of tinea capitis (see Chapter 15) is almost always accompanied by
complete regrowth of hair.

Lupus Erythematosus. Localized patterns of hair loss regularly
develop when lesions of discoid lupus erythematosus occur in the
scalp. Here, too, the area of hair loss is very sharply localized.
However, since the centers of such lesions are often hypopigmented,
the presence of actual scalp disease may at first go unrecognized.
In such cases careful examination of the margins will reveal the
annular, active erythematous border which is distinctive for the
disease. The scalp lesions of discoid lupus erythematosus rarely
occur alone; the presence of typical facial lesions helps to suggest
the correct diagnosis. Hair loss occasionally occurs in systemic
lupus erythematosus but it is more diffuse and is often unassociated
with visible scalp disease. Lupus erythematosus is discussed in
greater detail in Chapter 15.

Seborrheic Dermatitis. Some patients with inflammatory dandruff
(seborrheic dermatitis) complain of diffuse hair loss. Such loss
may be real, although it is probably only exaggerated normal telogen
loss and in any event is seldom visible to the examiner. When
present it occurs from all portions of the scalp and thus lacks the
patchiness found in tinea capitis and discoid lupus erythematosus.
The underlying scalp disease is that of a mild inflammatory, scaling
process. The amount of scale varies with the frequency and vigor
with which the patient shampoos. Seborrheic dermatitis of the scalp
severe enough to result in hair loss is generally accompanied by
seborrheic dermatitis of the retroauricular and nasal folds.
Alopecia associated with seborrheic dermatitis may be continuous but
it is not progressive. For this reason visible baldness should not
be ascribed to seborrheic dermatitis. A vicious cycle often occurs
in this condition: patients experience most of their hair loss
during shampooing and thus decrease the frequency of hair washing
which in turn allows the seborrheic dermatitis to worsen. Hair
regrowth occurs when seborrheic dermatitis is adequately treated.
Seborrheic dermatitis is discussed in greater detail in Chapter 16.

ALOPECIA WITHOUT SCALP DISEASE

Alopecia Areata. Alopecia areata consists of sharply localized
patches of sudden hair loss unaccompanied by any visible evidence of

scalp disease. Usually the patches are completely devoid of hairs, but sometimes a few spared, normal hairs are present. Less often "broken off" hairs are scattered throughout the bald areas. These presumably occur because of mild cyclic exacerbations of the disease which lead to hair shaft fragility but not complete cessation of protein growth. Typical lesions are 2 to 3 cm in diameter. Often only a single lesion is present but careful examination may reveal two or three additional lesions in other areas of the scalp. In less typical cases multiple, larger patches of hair loss are present and in very rare instances total hair loss (alopecia totalis) occurs. Alopecia areata typically affects the scalp but occasionally involves the eyebrows, eyelashes, beard area, axillae, and pubis. The disease can occur at any age but it is most commonly found in late childhood and the early teen years. A family history of similar hair loss is found in about 25% of cases. Women are affected more often than men. Fingernail changes, especially pitting, occur in 20% of patients.

The course and prognosis in alopecia areata are highly variable. Patients destined to undergo complete remission generally develop only a few small patches. These grow to a maximum size of 2 or 3 cm over 6 to 12 months and then remain stable in appearance for another 6 to 12 months. Thereafter new hairs, which are often initially white in color, begin to regrow. By 18 to 24 months the healing process is complete. Patients with larger or more numerous patches of alopecia have a poorer prognosis. In such patients individual patches of alopecia may expand centrifugally for many months before undergoing stabilization. An estimate of the likelihood of continued expansion can be obtained by gently tugging on the hairs at the edge of the bald spot. Several hairs will be removed with each tug in cases where expansion is actively evolving; no loose hairs will be found in cases which have reached stabilization. A few patients with numerous large patches of alopecia eventually obtain complete regrowth but most go through years of dynamic equilibrium in which new patches develop as quickly as old patches regrow. A very unfortunate few patients go on to total alopecia. The outlook for complete regrowth in these individuals is extremely poor. Patients with alopecia areata who have obtained complete remission have about a 25% chance of developing one or more subsequent episodes later in life.

Alopecia areata can be viewed as a patterned induction of telogen effluvium. That is, for unknown reasons, lymphocyte attack of growing (anagen) hair follicles causes an abrupt, synchronized switch of these follicles to the resting (telogen) phase. This switch is marked by the spontaneous loss (or easy removal) of the telogen, or club, hairs.

The actual cause of alopecia areata is unknown. Genetic factors are probably important since a considerable proportion of patients have a family history of the same disease. There is also considerable evidence pointing toward an autoimmune etiology. Patients are rather likely to have autoantibodies directed against thyroid cells, parietal cells, adrenal cortex cells, or intracellular proteins. Vitiligo and autoimmune thyroid disease are seen with increased frequency in patients with alopecia areata. Emotional factors probably also play a role, although it is often difficult to decide whether those present are a cause or a result of the disease. When stress is a prominent, early causative factor, it may act through a triggering process even as it does in autoimmune Graves's disease.

There are difficult decisions to be made regarding the treatment of alopecia areata. The lesions which respond best to therapy are the small, unobtrusive lesions which also are the most likely to resolve spontaneously. The larger, more troublesome lesions seldom resolve spontaneously and are extraordinarily resistant to therapy. Therapy, if it is to be attempted at all, should begin with the use of high potency topical steroids together with nighttime shower cap occlusion. The success of this approach is not great but it does buy time during which spontaneous remission sometimes occurs. If this approach fails, the intralesional injection of steroids (see Chapter 4) can be attempted. Such injections frequently lead to sprouts of new hair growth but tissue atrophy and eventual reloss from injected sites limit the acceptability of such treatment. In desperate cases systemic steroids administered on alternate days can be tried but the degree of response is unpredictable. Moreover, if acceptable hair growth is achieved, therapy must usually be continued indefinitely since relapse rapidly occurs when the steroids are discontinued.

Three alternative treatment programs are worth considering. First, minoxidil made up in a 1 to 3% solution can be applied several times daily. Second, the photosensitizer oxsoralen can be applied topically or may be given orally. This is followed by exposure to ultraviolet light in the UVA spectrum (PUVA therapy) which in turn induces a mild erythema. Finally, patients can be sensitized to certain chemicals such as dinitrochlorobenzene (DNCB). Reapplication of the chemical to the bald areas at a later date causes induction of a (mild) contact dermatitis. The mechanisms through which these three therapies act are unknown though the latter two are thought to be "immunostimulating." The results with all three approaches are similar. About 25% of patients experience a cosmetically satisfying response; another 25% obtain very limited regrowth; and 50% do not respond at all.

Trichotillomania. Some individuals, when under significant psychic stress or as part of a habit tic, chronically pull, twist, or rub a localized patch of hair. The configuration of these patches is often strikingly angular in shape. No scalp disease is present but invariably all of the hairs within the patch have fractured distal ends. Most of these broken hairs are about 1 cm long because broken hairs must grow out to this length before they can be once again manipulated.

Secondary Syphilis. Patients with long standing secondary syphilis often develop a peculiar pattern of patchy, "moth eaten" alopecia. The large number of patches, their small size, and their indistinct margins help to separate this condition from that of alopecia areata. The hair loss is transient; regrowth occurs following adequate antibiotic therapy. Syphilis is discussed in more detail in Chapter 15.

Telogen Effluvium. Telogen effluvium is a diffuse type of alopecia which occurs when numerous but scattered hair follicles simultaneously change from the growth (anagen) phase to the resting (telogen) phase of the hair growth cycle. This may be compared to the situation in alopecia areata where a similar switch to telogen phase occurs in a tightly localized area. This similarity has led some clinicians to view idiopathic telogen effluvium as a type of diffuse alopecia areata.

Patients who seek medical attention for diffuse hair loss of telogen effluvium type seldom have much alopecia visible to the examiner. However, proof of increased hair loss is easily obtained by gently tugging at random tufts of hair. One or more telogen hairs will be removed with each tug in patients with telogen effluvium. Only an occasional loose hair will be found in individuals with normal hair growth. Alternately, the magnitude of the hair loss can be determined by asking the patient to save and count individual hairs found on the pillow, in the hairbrush, and in the basin or bathtub. Most individuals with telogen effluvium will report the loss of approximately 400 hairs per day. This is a number which is approximately four to five times greater than would be expected from individuals with normal hair growth.

Telogen effluvium is seen more commonly in women than in men. Moreover, telogen effluvium is frequently found in the postpartum state and following the discontinuation of oral contraceptive pills. These observations suggest that hormonal factors play a role in pathogenesis. However, the process is also seen following episodes of physiologic stress (high fever, myocardial infarction, cerebral vascular accidents) and in association with psychologic stress, suggesting that other, unknown factors may also be important. In many cases no specific inciting factors can be identified.

Patients with telogen effluvium rarely if ever progress to clinically significant baldness. Most instances of telogen effluvium resolve spontaneously over a 6- to 12-month period. No effective treatment is recognized.

Male and Female Pattern Baldness. Both men and women may develop distinctively patterned hair loss as they age. In men the loss is most noticeable at the vertex and in the bitemporal regions of the scalp. In women the loss is more diffuse or is restricted to the vertex. Pattern loss may be seen as early as the third decade in men but is rarely apparent prior to the sixth decade in women.

Genetic factors are important in the pathogenesis of pattern loss. Both the degree of loss and the age at which it starts seem determined by familial patterns. Hormonal factors are likewise important since men castrated at a young age do not develop pattern loss, regardless of genetic factors, until and unless supplemental testosterone is administered. The hormonal aspect of pattern loss in women is much less clear, although the usual delay in onset until after menopause suggests the possibility that estrogens are protective.

In a general sort of way there is a correlation between the age at which onset begins and the severity of eventual loss. However, the hair loss, regardless of how early it begins, is not linear with time. Individuals may go through short periods of intense loss followed by longer plateau periods of relative stability.

No effective medical treatment is recognized. Hirsutism does occur following the systemic administration of some medications, but with the possible exception of minoxidil, these drugs do not lead to a reversal of pattern loss. Based on this last observation, several clinical trials employing topically applied 1 to 3% minoxidil solution have been initiated. Incomplete reports at this time suggest that perhaps 25% of patients obtain appreciable regrowth. Cosmetic improvement of the bald areas in male pattern loss may be obtained through the use of small hair transplants taken from the lateral margins of the scalp where hair growth remains active. Scalp reduction techniques, used in conjunction with transplants, may reduce the number of transplants needed. Aesthetic success with these surgical techniques is highly variable and depends to a great deal on the skill and experience of the operator.

Hypothyroidism. Diffuse hair loss unassociated with scalp disease is occasionally seen in women with moderate to severe hypothyroidism. The mechanism through which this occurs is unknown, but it is not likely related to serum levels of thyroid hormone since replacement, while preventing further loss, fails to reverse the process.

SELECTED READING

Dawber RPR: Common baldness in women. Int J Dermatol 20:647, 1981.
Mitchell AJ, Krull EA: Alopecia areata: Pathogenesis and treatment. J Am Acad Dermatol 11:763, 1984.
Nelson DA, Spielvogel RL: Alopecia areata. Int J Dermatol 24:26, 1985
Olsen EA, Weiner MS, DeLong ER, et al: Topical minoxidil in early male pattern baldness. J Am Acad Dermatol 13:185; 1985.
Rudolph AH: The diagnosis and treatment of tinea capitis due to trichophyton tonsurans. Int J Dermatol 24:426, 1985.

Solomon LM: Tinea capitis: Current concepts. <u>Pediatr Dermatol</u>
    <u>2</u>:224, 1985.
Villez RL: Topical minoxidil therapy in hereditary androgenetic
    alopecia. <u>Arch Dermatol</u> <u>121</u>:197, 1985.
Messenger AG, Slater DN, Bleehen SS: Alopecia areata: Alterations
    in the hair growth cycle and correlation with the follicular
    pathology. <u>Br J Dermatol</u> <u>114</u>:337, 1986.

Nail Diseases

NAIL DYSTROPHY

The formation of normal nails is discussed in Chapter 1. Damage to the nail as a result of trauma or specific disease results in nail dystrophy. Nail dystrophy is defined as the presence of misshapen or partially destroyed nail plates. Soft, yellow keratin often accumulates between the dystrophic nail plate and nail bed, resulting in elevation of the former. Various aspects of nail dystrophy are discussed below.

Trauma. Trauma to the tips of the digits occasionally results in the formation of a subungual hematoma. The severe pain which accompanies this problem can be relieved by piercing the nail plate with a heated needle or paper clip. Large subungual hematomas result in sloughing of the nail plate weeks to months later. Permanent scarring with nail plate thickening and ridging sometimes accompanies trauma. Scarred nails seem particularly predisposed to the subsequent development of onychomycosis. Unfortunately, surgical removal of the scarred nail plate is simply followed by regrowth of an equally dystrophic nail.

Onychomycosis. Fungal infection is a very common cause of toenail dystrophy. The great toenail in particular seems prone to infection. Infection of the fingernails occurs only in nails previously traumatized or when nail involvement is part of tinea manum. The likelihood of onychomycosis increases with age; children are rarely if ever involved. Nails in men are somewhat more frequently involved than are those in women.

The first sign of onychomycosis is generally the development of a small area of onycholysis (separation of the nail plate from the nail bed) at the distal tip of the nail. Shortly thereafter a buildup of soft yellow keratin occurs in the space created by the onycholysis. This is accompanied by further lifting of the more proximal nail. Eventually the process results in a partially destroyed, heaped up, misshapen, yellow nail. The entire process is asymptomatic unless a thickened toenail begins to press against the top of the shoe.

Most onychomycosis is due to infection with Trichophyton rubrum but in a few cases Epidermophyton floccosum and Trichophyton mentagrophytes may be recovered. Infection with T. mentagrophytes is particularly likely to be associated with a more mild form of onychomycosis in which portions of the nail plate whiten and become superficially dystrophic. Treatment is the same regardless of which organism causes the disease. Orally administered griseofulvin or ketoconazole (see Chapter 4) is generally required if treatment is

desired; topical therapy is for practical purposes never curative.
Most fingernail infections will clear after 3 months of continuous
therapy. Toenails, because of their slower growth rate, will
require 9 to 12 months of treatment. Nearly all fingernail
infections respond to therapy but the response rate for toenail
infections is considerably lower. Moreover, the recurrence rate,
once treatment is stopped, is extremely high. For this reason many
clinicians discourage treatment of toenail onychomycosis.

   Psoriasis. Nail dystrophy occurs in a considerable proportion
of patients with psoriasis. Most often nail changes follow the
development of cutaneous lesions, but on rare occasions, they may
precede any other clinical evidence of the disease. Several types
of nail dystrophy are recognized. The specific clinical appearance
depends on whether the pathology occurs in the nail matrix, nail
plate, or nail bed.

   Onycholysis occurs as the result of nail bed involvement. In
early lesions the normally smooth, curvilinear distal junction of
the nail plate with the nail bed becomes irregular. In more
advanced disease, soft yellow keratin accumulates between the nail
plate and nail bed in a manner clinically indistinguishable from
that which occurs in onychomycosis. Another type of psoriatic
lesion occurs in the nail plate or between the plate and bed. This
results in the appearance of sharply marginated, yellow-brown,
nonpalpable color changes in the nail plate. These changes have
been likened to "oil spots." The earliest reflection of nail matrix
disease is the development of "ice pick" stippling or pitting on the
surface of the nail plate. This type of pitting occurs only in
patients with psoriasis and alopecia areata. More advanced
involvement of the nail matrix, in concert with nail bed disease,
leads to the development of grossly misshapen nails. These more
serious nail dystrophies are often accompanied by inflammatory,
arthritic changes in the distal interphalangeal joint.

   There is no widely acceptable, effective treatment for psoriatic
nail dystrophy. Topical steroid therapy used under finger cot
occlusion can be tried but the degree of improvement is usually
disappointing. Steroids injected into the nail matrix are more
efficacious but the considerable discomfort associated with multiple
injections discourages most patients. Improvement following the
long term use of topically applied fluorouracil has been reported in
a few patients but larger trials will be necessary before this
approach can be routinely recommended. Concomitant improvement in
nail dystrophy often occurs during spontaneous or therapeutically
induced remission of the accompanying cutaneous lesions.

   Arteriosclerotic Changes of the Toenails. A decrease of blood
flow to the distal toes regularly results in the development of nail
dystrophy. The nail changes found in these circumstances are nearly
identical with those seen in onychomycosis; the two diseases can be
correctly identified only when KOH preparations and fungal cultures

are carried out. Arteriosclerotic dystrophy is seen only in the toenails; fingernails are not affected. There is no effective treatment for these changes.

Beau's Grooves. Beau's grooves are depressions about 1 mm wide in the nail plate. These grooves extend horizontally from one lateral nail groove to the other. All nails are simultaneously affected. The depression occurs as the result of decreased nail protein synthesis during an episode of significant physiologic stress. Beau's grooves most commonly develop following dramatic illnesses such as myocardial infarction and periods of high fever. Similar grooving also develops after isolated periods of severe malnutrition. These grooves develop as the nail plate is forming in the nail matrix. Because of the slowness with which the nail plate grows, the groove first becomes visible at the posterior nail fold several weeks after the original insult. The groove then remains in the nail plate, slowly moving distally during the several months it takes for the nail plate to renew itself completely.

Clubbing. Clubbing of the distal fingers is identified by the following three criteria: 1) flattening of the angle formed by the junction of the proximal nail plate and the paronychial fold, 2) rounding of the nail plate such that the distal edge curves slightly around the distal tip of the digit, and 3) widening or thickening of the digit from the distal interphalangeal joint to the tip. Clubbing is most commonly seen with chronic pulmonary or cardiopulmonary disease but also occurs with some tumors, especially those of the lung parenchyma. A somewhat similar process occurs in the thyroid acropachy of Graves's disease.

Nail Splitting. Splitting of the nail plate can occur in either of two forms: cracks which are oriented parallel to the length of the finger or through separation of the nail plate layers such that "flakes" of nail chip off the distal edge. Some instances of splitting occur as the result of scar formation within the nail matrix but most are idiopathic. Splitting generally worsens with aging. The ingestion of gelatin, calcium, or vitamins is commonly recommended for the treatment of nail splitting but proof of efficacy is lacking. Cosmetic improvement can be obtained by applying multiple layers of clear fingernail polish such that the fissures or flakes are cemented together. False fingernails can also be cemented over the underlying dystrophic nail.

Warts. Periungual warts often distort the nail plate. In most instances the dystrophy is not permanent and the nail plate returns to normal following therapeutic or spontaneous resolution of the warts. Permanent nail dystrophy occasionally occurs when warts have been present for long periods of time or when they have been aggressively treated with modalities such as electrosurgery or intralesional injection of bleomycin.

NAIL COLOR CHANGES

   White Banding. Horizontal white banding or opacification
(Terry's nails, half and half nails, Muercke's lines) occurs in a
variety of settings. Clear-cut distinction among the various types
of white nail banding is not usually possible. In most instances
these changes are seen in the presence of hypoalbuminemia
accompanying chronic hepatic or renal disease.
   Brown Banding. Brown banding occurs in either of two
directions: a vertical band running from the posterior nail fold to
the distal tip of the nail or a horizontal band running from one
lateral nail fold to the other. The former occurs as the normal
finding in black patients and can be seen secondary to the presence
of a nevus or melanoma in the nail matrix of white patients.
Because of the risk of melanoma such lesions, when newly acquired,
should be biopsied. Heme pigment, rather than melanin, can also
cause this type of banding as a post-traumatic event.
   Horizontal bands of pigment may be found in Addison's disease
and following systemic administration of various cancer
chemotherapeutic agents.
   Splinter Hemorrhages. Splinter hemorrhages occur as vertical,
thin, dark red lines 1 to 3 mm in length. They represent small
hemorrhages at the junction of the nail plate and the nail bed.
These hemorrhages are carried outward to the distal tip of the
finger as the nail grows. The presence of these hemorrhages is
believed by some to be a helpful diagnostic sign of bacterial
endocarditis and trichinosis but their frequent occurrence in
totally healthy individuals makes their significance doubtful in
most clinical settings.

ONYCHOLYSIS

   If you look at the distal tip of your fingernail you will notice
that the free edge, where it grows outward beyong the nail bed, is
white. This opacification occurs because of the second air-nail
interface which is present on the underside of the nail. In
situations where the nail plate is separated more proximally from
the nail bed, a similar white opacification occurs. This separation
and whitening is known as onycholysis. Onycholysis is a
noninflammatory, asymptomatic condition.
   Onycholysis is most commonly caused by infection with Candida
sp., especially C. albicans. These candidal infections occur with
particular frequency in individuals such as dishwashers, bartenders,
waitresses, and dentists who are regularly involved in wet work.
Onycholysis due to candidal infection is often, but not always,
accompanied by paronychial swelling and inflammation (see below).
Onycholysis also occurs in psoriasis and is somewhat less often seen
with trauma, hyperthyroidism, and as a result of photochemical

separation in patients taking tetracycline. Bacteria which may colonize this blind pocket of onycholysis add color: <u>Pseudomonas</u> sp. causes a green color and <u>Proteus</u> sp. causes a brown or black color.

A diagnosis of onycholysis due to candidiasis is generally made on a clinical basis. KOH preparations are not very helpful in confirming the diagnosis, but positive cultures can usually be obtained from pieces clipped from the overlying, separated nail. In any event overlying nail should be clipped away in order that topically applied preparations such as clotrimazole (Lotrimin) solution can be appropriately applied. Bandaging of the fingertip following such clipping should be avoided since the maceration which this induces favors further growth of the yeast.

PARONYCHIAL INFLAMMATION

<u>Candida</u> <u>Paronychia</u>. Infection with <u>Candida</u> sp. (usually <u>C.</u> <u>albicans</u>) is the most common cause of paronychial inflammation. It occurs with considerable frequency in people such as dishwashers, bartenders, and waitresses who are regularly involved in wet work. Candidal paronychia is characterized by: 1) lack of pain, 2) lack of warmth, 3) absence or paucity of pus, and 4) chronicity. Onycholysis frequently accompanies candidal paronychia. The diagnosis is usually made on a clinical basis. KOH preparations are difficult to carry out and often there is insufficient material for culture.

Candidal paronychia can be treated with the application of clotrimazole (Lotrimin) solution three times daily to the inflamed tissue. A faster response may be obtained if a topical steroid antiyeast combination cream such as Lotrisone is used. Bandaging of the finger should be avoided since resultant maceration encourages further candidal growth and may even lead to secondary bacterial infection

<u>Bacterial</u> <u>Paronychia</u>. Bacterial paronychia is an acute, painful process. It is usually preceded by an episode of trauma such as the tearing of a hangnail. It presents with all of the classical signs of a bacterial process: redness, warmth, swelling, and tenderness. Gentle pressure on the swollen tissue often results in the expression of a drop of pus which can then be picked up on an applicator for culture. From a practical standpoint, however, culture is not usually necessary. Almost all bacterial paronychia is due to staphylococcal infection and treatment appropriate for such infection (see Chapter 4) can be started at the time of first examination. Incision and drainage are rarely if ever indicated; soaks are occasionally helpful.

<u>Herpetic</u> <u>Whitlow</u>. Herpetic whitlow is the name given to paronychial infection with <u>Herpesvirus</u> <u>hominis</u> type I or type II. Like bacterial paronychia, this infection occurs acutely and is

associated with redness, swelling, warmth, exquisite tenderness, and regional lymphadenopathy. It is regularly confused with bacterial paronychia, but careful examination will reveal the presence of multiple, grouped, minute vesicles. The disease is an occupational hazard for individuals such as nurses, dentists, and dental assistants who are routinely involved in mouth care. Herpetic whitlow runs its course in approximately 10 days. No medical therapy is required but the level of discomfort usually warrants a trial of orally administered acyclovir (see Chapter 4). Soaks are usually recommended although there is no proof that they are helpful. Topically applied steroids, although theoretically contraindicated, reduce the discomfort by way of lessening the inflammation. Orally administered analgesics may be necessary if the pain is severe. Incision and drainage are contraindicated. Recurrent disease in the same location is possible but it is not a common event.

Ingrown Toenails. Ingrown toenail is the most common cause of paronychial inflammation of the great toe. It develops when the sharp edge of the great toenail pierces the surrounding fold of paronychial tissue. Ingrown toenail is likely to occur when one or more of the following are present: 1) the nail is curved to a greater degree than normal, 2) the toenail is clipped back too far allowing tissue to roll up over it, 3) athletic activities which require sudden stops ("toejamming") are undertaken, and 4) ill-fitting shoes are worn such that the toe of the shoe presses against the nail and surrounding tissue. Bacterial infection frequently develops in the paronychial tissue traumatized by the presence of an ingrown nail.

Therapy of an acute ingrown nail requires that the nail corner be lifted free of the surrounding, inflamed paronychial tissue. This is easily (although uncomfortably) carried out by the application of a mosquito forceps to the incurved edge of the nail plate. When the plate is lifted a small pledget of cotton can be wedged under the nail. Soaks and antibiotics are also started. This program leads to gratifying improvement within a week, at which time surgical correction, if necessary, can be carried out. Such surgery generally requires permanent removal of a lateral portion of the nail plate and accompanying nail matrix.

SELECTED READING

Norton LA: Nail disorders. J Am Acad Dermatol 2:451, 1980.
Achten G, Parent D: The normal and pathologic nail. Int J Dermatol 22:556, 1983.
Jeanmougin M, Civatte J: Nail dyschromia. Int J Dermatol 22:279, 1983.
Daniel CR: Symposium on the nail. Dermatol Clinics 3:37, 1985.
See also the list of monographs in Appendix C.

Chapter 20

Genital and Oral Erosions

GENITAL EROSIONS AND ULCERS

Herpes genitalis is by far the most common erosive disease of the genitalia. A rough estimate suggests that 1% of the sexually active population will have one or more episodes of herpes genitalis each year. The disease is due to infection with Herpesvirus hominis. Approximately 80% of the genital lesions are type II and 20% are type I infections. There is no clinical difference in the infections due to the two types of virus. However, patients with type II infection are considerably more likely to experience recurrent episodes.

Most initial symptomatic episodes of the disease occur as the result of direct viral transmission from an infected sexual partner. However, occasionally the initial episode occurs as the result of reactivation of a latent infection which had been asymptomatically acquired months or years earlier. The course, prognosis, pathogenesis, and therapy of herpes genitalis are covered in Chapter 7.

The clinical appearance of herpes genitalis depends on many factors. The disease is, of course, basically vesicular, but the thin roofs of the blisters are easily broken, leading to a common presentation as an erosive disease. The degree of coalescence which develops is directly related to the amount of immune responsiveness that is present. Thus individuals, especially women, experiencing their first attack of herpes may lack clustering altogether. Recurrent lesions, on the other hand, demonstrate considerable clustering; all of the vesicles occur in an area no more than 2 or 3 cm in diameter. Thus, coalescence of the closely set vesicles often leads to the formation of a large erosion recognizable because of its irregular shape and the presence of one or more 2- to 3-mm nearby satellite erosions.

The erosions of herpes genitalis are rather shallow but are quite painful. A moderate amount of inflammation accompanies the lesions but there is no undermining of the edges or pus formation. The base of the erosions lacks substance on palpation. Regional lymphadenopathy may or may not be present. The lesions of herpes genitalis can occur anywhere in the groin; both mucosal and nonmucosal surfaces can be affected.

The diagnosis of herpes genitalis depends on the history of blister formation, the presence of multiple, grouped small lesions, recurrence in the same location each time, and the absence of substance on palpation. Tzanck smears (see Chapter 5) or, more preferably, viral cultures should be carried out in previously unconfirmed cases. Some clinicians believe that a dark field examination or a serologic test for syphilis also ought to be obtained because of the occasional coexistence of syphilis and herpes.

The chancre of primary syphilis usually but not always appears as a single ulcer which is deeper and less irregularly shaped than the central coalescent erosion of herpes genitalis. Chancres are also less painful and the base has considerably more substance on palpation. Undermining of the edges and pus formation are usually not found. Only a moderate amount of erythema surrounds the ulcer Lymphadenopathy is usually present. Chancres may occur on either mucosal or nonmucosal surfaces. A dark field examination, if available, and a serologic test for syphilis (see Chapter 5) should be obtained in all instances where syphilis is even remotely likely.

Candidiasis is a frequent cause of erosive disease of the genitalia. The erosions of candidiasis are distinctive because of the magnitude of the surrounding inflammation. They are easily separated from chancres because of the shallowness, irregular shape, and painfulness of candidal erosions. Separation from herpes genitalis is more difficult but the course of candidiasis is chronic rather than intermittent. Moreover, a blistering component is never present. On the other hand, satellite papules and pustules are often present. The lesions of candidiasis occur most often where skin is folded and are particularly common under the prepuce in uncircumsized men. In women, an associated candidal vaginitis is usually present. A suspected diagnosis can be confirmed by culture. A moistened swab, rolled over the involved area several times, is put into transport media and is submitted for fungal culture. KOH preparations are not usually helpful unless material from an intact pustule can be examined.

Miscellaneous additional causes of genital ulcers include trauma, chancroid, granuloma inguinale, aphthous ulcers, Behcet's disease, and ulcerating carcinoma. All of these diseases are too rare to warrant discussion here.

ORAL EROSIONS AND ULCERS

Aphthous ulcers (aphthous stomatitis) and herpes simplex infections (herpes labialis) account for approximately 95% of all oral ulcers. Both are often grouped together under the title of "cold sores" but separation is desirable and important.

Aphthous ulcers occur entirely within the mouth. Often only a single ulcer is present, but even when multiple, there is little tendency for the clustering which occurs with herpes. The individual lesions are true ulcers. That is, they are approximately as deep as they are wide. The smallest ulcers are only 1 or 2 mm in diameter but lesions up to 1 cm in size are occasionally found. The central crater is often filled with a white coagulum and a thin violaceous rim often encircles each ulcer. The lesions are usually quite painful. Aphthous ulcers may be located anywhere within the mouth but they are most commonly seen on the buccal surfaces, the gingival margins, the gingival sulci, and on the floor of the mouth, particularly around the frenulum of the tongue. Tender lymphadenopathy is often present.

Individual aphthous ulcers appear suddenly and then remain stable in size and symptoms for 7 to 10 days before resolving spontaneously. Multiple lesions may develop either simultaneously or sequentially. In the more severe cases new lesions appear before old lesions have healed.

Aphthous ulcers are intermittently recurrent over many years but there is no particular tendency for reappearance in exactly the same sites as were involved originally. In most instances aphthous ulcers are not associated with disease elsewhere in the body. They are, however, occasionally seen in association with chronic inflammatory bowel disease and Behcet's syndrome. An infectious etiology is suspected but no single causative organism has been repeatedly or convincingly demonstrated. Immune mechanisms are important in pathogenesis. Mucosal cells from patients stimulate blast transformation of their own lymphocytes and patients' lymphocytes may be cytotoxic for their own mucosal cells.

The discomfort associated with aphthous ulcers may be treated with oral analgesic solutions (elixir of Benadryl, Xylocaine Viscous, or Dyclone) which are swirled in the mouth for several minutes. Unfortunately, the duration of analgesia obtained is rather short. Some clinicians apply the tip of a silver nitrate stick to the base of each ulcer to necrotize the exposed nerve endings but it is difficult to justify using such a destructive approach. Tetracycline and other antibiotic suspensions have been demonstrated in controlled studies to reduce the duration and discomfort of the disease. They are held and swirled in the mouth for several minutes before being spit out or swallowed. Their effectiveness is presumably related to their anti-inflammatory properties rather than to their antibiotic effect. Sometimes topically applied steroids (Kenalog in Orabase, Vanceril aerosol), intralesionally injected steroids, or even systemically administered steroids will be required.

Herpes simplex viral infections, on the other hand, occur as shallow erosions rather than ulcers. Actually the lesions begin as vesicles but trauma quickly leads to breakdown of the vesicle roofs. Individual vesicles and erosions are 1 to 3 mm in diameter, but they are usually clustered such that three to eight individual erosions coalesce, forming a single, large erosion with a distinctly irregular configuration. The erosions are surprisingly uncomfortable considering how shallow they are. The base of the erosion is red but there is little perilesional inflammation. Tender lymphadenopathy is sometimes present.

Herpetic lesions are found almost exclusively on the lips at or near the vermillion border; less than 1% of patients have lesions contained entirely within the mouth. Individual herpetic erosions heal spontaneously in 5 to 10 days without scarring. Most patients with herpes labialis experience recurrent episodes intermittently throughout their lives. Recurrent episodes are triggered by psychologic stress and by physiologic stress such as sunburn, coryza, and fever.

Herpes labialis is caused by Herpesvirus hominis. Approximately 80% of the time labial herpes is due to type I infection; in the remainder it is due to type II infection. These two types of infection cannot be distinguished clinically. Further discussion on diagnosis, therapy, and pathogenesis of herpes labialis can be found in Chapter 7.

Miscellaneous causes of oral erosion include erythema multiforme bullosum (Stevens-Johnson syndrome), pemphigus, and cicatricial pemphigoid. These diseases are discussed in Chapter 7. Erosive degeneration occasionally develops in the white, oral plaques of several additional diseases as discussed in Chapter 21. Finally, painless, single ulcers occur in primary syphilis and squamous cell carcinoma of the mucous membranes.

SELECTED READING

Bell GF, Rogers RS: Observations on the diagnosis of recurrent aphthous stomatitis. Mayo Clin Proc 57:297, 1982.
Felman YM, Nikitas JA: Primary syphilis. Cutis 29:122, 1982.
Odds FC: Genital candidosis. Clin Exp Dermatol 7:345, 1982.
Felman YM, Nikitas JA: Genital candidiasis. Cutis 31:369, 1983.
Chapel TA: Primary and secondary syphilis. Cutis 33:47, 1984.
Dreizen S: Oral candidiasis. Am J Med 77(4D):28, 1984.
Manzella JP, McConville JH, Valenti W, et al: An outbreak of herpes simplex virus type I gingivostomatitis in a dental hygiene practice. JAMA 252:2019, 1984.
Mertz G, Corey L: Genital herpes simplex virus infections in adults. Urol Clin North Am 11:103, 1984.
Wong RC, Ellis CN, Diaz LA: Behcet's disease. Int J Dermatol 23:25, 1984.
Marlowe SI: Medical management of genital herpes. Arch Dermatol 121:467, 1985.
Jorizzo JL, Taylor RS, Schmalstieg FC, et al: Complex aphthosis: A forme fruste of Behcet's syndrome? J Am Acad Dermatol 13:80, 1985.

White Plaques
in the Mouth

The most common and important causes of white lesions in the mouth include the normal bite line, lichen planus, lupus erythematosus, secondary syphilis (lues), leukoplakia, candidiasis, and human papilloma virus infection. All of these diseases except candidiasis occur because of the development of a hyperkeratotic surface in an area normally lacking cornification. This cornified layer is white while wet, just as one's fingertips become white after prolonged exposure to water. The whiteness in candidiasis represents the actual yeast organisms present in a thick mycelial plaque.

The bite line is the most common white lesion in the mouth. This lesion is characterized by its linearity and by its location at the dental occlusion line. Often the bite line has several irregular extensions which correspond to grooves between the teeth. It is asymptomatic. The bite line probably arises as a type of "callus" formation secondary to presence of chronic trauma. The condition has no pathologic significance and requires no treatment.

Lichen planus is the most common pathologic explanation for white plaques on the oral mucous membranes. In milder lesions the plaques are made up of a network of criss-crossed, gray-white lines, whereas in more severe cases the plaques are thicker and are less reticulate. The mucosal lesions of lichen planus are most commonly located on the buccal surfaces, but involvement of the gingivae, lips, and tongue is occasionally seen. The buccal plaques occasionally become deeply eroded. Patients with mild oral lichen planus are asymptomatic but in more severe cases the lesions can be very painful. The diagnosis is easily made when typical cutaneous lesions are found elsewhere on the body. However, lichen planus does sometimes exist solely within the mouth and in such instances biopsy will be necessary to confirm the diagnosis. The mucosal lesions of lichen planus are chronic in nature; buccal plaques in particular may remain for years. Very rarely squamous cell carcinoma has arisen in older lesions of lichen planus. Asymptomatic plaques require no treatment. Painful, eroded lesions are partially responsive to topically applied steroids (Kenalog in Orabase, Vanceril aerosol spray) and to topically applied Vitamin A acid (Retin-A). In some cases orally administered retinoids or intralesionally injected triamcinolone will be required.

Both discoid and acute systemic lupus erythematosus may be accompanied by mucosal lesions in about 20% of cases. The gray-white plaques caused by lupus erythematosus are clinically rather similar to those found in lichen planus though they do tend to be less reticulate. They most often occur on the buccal surface, lips, and palate. Erosions may be present but such lesions are less symptomatic than those found in lichen planus. Diagnosis depends on the presence of typical lesions of lupus erythematosus elsewhere on the skin. Biopsy is distinctive but not pathognomonic. Treatment of the mucosal lesions is generally not necessary.

Secondary syphilis (lues) is frequently accompanied by the presence of white plaques in the mouth. These plaques are whiter, thicker, and more sharply marginated than the otherwise similar plaques of lupus erythematosus and lichen planus. They are generally asymptomatic. The mucosal lesions of syphilis are teeming with treponemes and are thus very contagious. Since these lesions occur during the secondary stage of syphilis serologic tests will always be positive. Dark field examinations may be helpful but care must be taken in differentiating T. pallidum from the Borrelia treponemes which are normal inhabitants of the mouth. Typical cutaneous lesions of secondary syphilis will nearly always be found. Treatment of the patient with penicillin as described in Chapter 15 results in resolution of mucosal lesions.

Leukoplakia is derived from the Greek word for "white plaque." By dermatologic convention use of the word is restricted to lesions which show evidence of dysplasia on biopsy. Intraoral lesions are particularly likely to be seen in patients who have chronically used intraoral tobacco products whereas lip lesions are usually due to chronic sunlight exposure. Diagnosis is established by way of biopsy. Most often only mild atypia is present but in more chronic cases the picture may be that of carcinoma in situ. Such lesions should be treated with excision, electrosurgical destruction, or, on the lip, topical application of fluorouracil.

Candidiasis (moniliasis, thrush) represents infection with Candida sp., most often C. albicans. The white plaques formed as the result of such yeast infection are thick and soft. They are loosely adherent and one can dislodge pieces of the plaque with the edge of a scalpel blade. Material removed in this manner will reveal dense mats of hyphae on KOH examination. Lesions of candidiasis can occur anywhere in the mouth but are particularly common on the buccal surfaces. Oral candidiasis may be found in infants and in immunosuppressed or debilitated adults. Patients with acquired immunodeficiency syndrome (AIDS) are almost universally affected. Treatment is carried out by the application of an oral solution of nystatin (Mycostatin oral suspension) or through the use of clotrimazole (Mycelex) troches. Extemporaneous solutions can also be prepared using the intravenous forms of amphotericin B and miconazole.

Human papilloma virus infection may result either in the appearance of flattopped individual or coalescent warts (Heck's disease) or, in patients with AIDS, shaggy white plaques known as oral hairy leukoplakia. In the latter situation concomitant infection with Epstein-Barr virus may also be present. Treatment usually requires local destruction with electrosurgery or the use of cytotoxic agents.

SELECTED READING

Brightman VJ: Red and white lesions of the oral mucosa. In Lynch MA, Brightman VJ, Greenberg MD (eds): Oral Medicine, 8th edition. J.B. Lippincott Co., Philadelphia, 1984, pp 209-292.

Greenspan D, Greenspan JS, Conant M, et al: Oral "hairy" leukoplakia in male homosexuals: Evidence of association with both papillomavirus and a herpes-group virus. Lancet 2:831, 1984.

Giustina TA, Stewart JCB, Ellis CN, et al: Topical application of isotretinoin gel improves oral lichen planus. Arch Dermatol 122:534, 1986.

Chapter 2

Keratotic Papules
Actinic Keratoses, Seborrhei
Keratoses and Wart

Similarity in names, overlap in distribution, and concomitant occurrence in older adults sometimes lead to confusion in the identification of seborrheic and actinic keratoses. Appropriate recognition, however, is important because actinic keratoses are premalignant and seborrheic keratoses are totally benign. The two conditions are discussed in detail in Chapters 9 and 11 but clinical attributes helpful in their recognition are reviewed below.

Distribution. Actinic keratoses are found on chronically sun exposed skin. The face and dorsal surface of the hands and arms are most often involved. Occasional lesions are seen on the chest and shoulders. Seborrheic keratoses occur predominantly on the chest, back, shoulders, and, occasionally, the face. In the areas of overlap (the face and the shoulders) consideration should be given to the appearance of the skin adjacent to the lesions. Actinic keratoses do not develop unless there is clinical evidence of chronic sun damage such as pigmentary change, mild inflammation, telangiectasia, and atrophy.

Color. Seborrheic keratoses are primarily brown but range considerably in hue from light tan to a dark brown-black. Actinic keratoses are generally white or gray although some crusted lesions have a yellow color. Occasionally large, well established seborrheic keratoses are covered with a small amount of dirty gray scale.

Surface Texture. Actinic keratoses demonstrate visible scale and are rough surfaced on palpation. Seborrheic keratoses generally lack visible scale and are more smooth surfaced when palpated. However, as mentioned above, larger, well developed seborrheic keratoses may develop a small amount of palpable scale. Most seborrheic keratoses have a somewhat pitted or dimpled surface; this feature is not seen in actinic keratoses.

Margination. Seborrheic keratoses are very sharply marginated. In cross section they appear square shouldered. Actinic keratoses are less sharply marginated and in fact sometimes it is difficult to say just exactly where the lesion starts and stops. However, an occasional dysplastic actinic keratosis will be surmounted by sharply marginated yellow crust.

Superficiality. Seborrheic keratoses often have a slight "rolling under" of their margins. This gives them a "stuck on" appearance which has often been likened to drops of dirty candle wax lying on the skin. On the other hand, actinic keratoses, while also superficial in location, look like they are growing from within the skin rather than having been "dropped" onto the surface.

Size. While there is overlap in size, actinic keratoses average 2 to 10 mm in diameter whereas seborrheic keratoses average 7 to 20 mm in diameter.

Biopsy. Biopsy should be carried out in any instance where clinical diagnosis is uncertain. Superficial shave biopsy (see Chapter 5) is all that is necessary for microscopic recognition. Such a procedure heals rapidly without significant scarring and is usually curative as well.

Warts. Most warts occur in children and are distributed in locations different from those listed for actinic and seborrheic keratoses. However, warts in older adults are sometimes encountered on the face, trunk, and dorsal surface of the arms and hands. In such instances differentiation may be difficult. Generally warts are skin colored without any of the pigment changes described above. Moreover, their rough surface usually has a distinctive digitate or filiform appearance. Finally, these sharply marginated lesions, which average 2 to 7 mm in diameter, tend to be as tall, or taller, than they are wide. Nevertheless, in spite of these differences, clinical separation of warts from those actinic keratoses known as cutaneous horns is sometimes impossible without the aid of biopsy.

Pigmented Lesions and the Recognition of Melanomas

In most instances the failure to recognize a given skin disease correctly does not have life or death consequences. One exception to this rule occurs in the case of melanoma. The prognosis in melanoma corresponds most directly with the depth of invasion and this in turn relates at least in part to the age of the lesion. Correct identification and early removal of superficial melanomas are associated with gratifyingly high cure rates, whereas failure to recognize a melanoma might well lead to a disasterous outcome. Any clinician would have great moral (and possibly legal) difficulty living with a misdiagnosis and yet evaluation of most pigmented lesions is carried out in a hurried and superficial manner. Biopsy of all pigmented lesions is not the answer. The cost in time and money is far too great when one considers that each of us has an average of about 15 pigmented nevi. The only practical approach is to develop our clinical skills to as great a degree as possible. A remarkably high degree of accuracy can be obtained when systematic criteria are used for evaluation. The most important of these criteria are discussed below. General discussion of melanomas is found in Chapter 11.

OBJECTIVE CRITERIA

Lesional Configuration. Most benign pigmented lesions are perfectly round. Melanomas, on the other hand, are often somewhat irregular in shape. The earliest irregularity is often the appearance of a small area of pigment spread (pigment "bleeding") onto the flat skin surrounding the lesion. More advanced change consists of one or more areas of irregular, peninsular growth of the elevated portion of the lesion. Some individuals, especially those of Celtic origin, will demonstrate some irregularity of configuration in almost all of their nevi. When multiple nevi are irregularly shaped one should consider the possibility of the dysplastic nevus syndrome.

Surface Smoothness. Benign lesions generally have a smooth surface. Melanomas, on the other hand, sometimes show some irregularity of surface growth. The development of one or more "bumps" on the surface of a pigmented lesion suggests that clusters of the underlying cells may be growing at different rates. Thus, the presence of surface irregularity is analogous to the presence of configurational irregularity as described above. However, it should be noted that superficial melanomas may be essentially flat, smooth, and nonelevated.

Pigment Homogeneity. Most benign lesions are evenly colored throughout. Most melanomas show some variation in pigment density throughout the lesion. For example, one or more dark colored speckles might be present against a lighter brown background. Some benign nevi, especially those of the dysplastic nevus syndrome, do show speckling of pigmentation but a single speckled nevus when all others are more normal in appearance should arouse concern about the presence of a melanoma. It should be emphasized that only irregularity in density of pigment is important. Absolute density of pigmentation does not correlate with malignancy. Benign lesions can be very black in color and melanomas can be rather light.

Nonbrown Colors. Most benign pigmented lesions are brown or brown-black in color. Most superficial spreading melanomas have hues of red, white, or blue in various portions of the lesion. These lesions which fall toward the notably red end of the brown spectrum should be considered as possible dysplastic nevi. White areas are also quite important. These represent areas of pigment destruction due to immunologic attack. Since benign pigmented lesions are ordinarily not recognized as foreign by the body, no immunologic reaction is directed against them. One important exception to this rule is the presence of a white halo which completely surrounds pigmented lesions. Such "halo nevi" are rather common in childhood and are invariably benign in nature. Halo nevi are not common in adults and such lesions should be viewed with considerable suspicion. The reasons for the blue and red hues are unknown.

Presence of Inflammation. Inflammation does not spontaneously appear around benign lesions. The presence of such inflammation suggests that the body recognizes the lesion as "foreign" and is mounting an attack against it. In spite of the theoretical value of this sign it happens that most inflamed pigmented lesions turn out to be small underlying ruptured epidermoid cysts rather than melanomas.

Firmness on Palpation. Benign pigmented lesions feel quite soft when they are picked up between the thumb and forefinger. Firm lesions suggest that cellular proliferation is occurring at a rather rapid rate -- a finding often associated with malignancy of rather advanced stages.

Epithelial Disruption. Benign lesions never show evidence of spontaneous epithelial disruption. Thus the presence of weeping, crusting, or ulcer formation in any pigmented lesion is a highly suspicious sign. Here again, however, on biopsy many eroded pigmented lesions turn out to be benign nevi which have been scratched or otherwise traumatized.

Miscellaneous Objective Criteria. Pigmented lesions occurring against a background of chronic sun damaged skin are more suspect than those occurring on covered skin. Darkly pigmented (black) lesions in light skinned individuals are more suspect than black

lesions occurring in dark skinned individuals. Large lesions are
more suspect than small lesions; melanomas are almost always larger
in diameter than a lead pencil eraser (7 mm), whereas benign nevi,
other than those which are congenital, are usually less than 7 mm in
diameter.

SUBJECTIVE CRITERIA

     Criteria which depend on patient history are inherently less
accurate than the objective criteria described above. Nevertheless,
several aspects of history may be helpful. The first aspect has to
do with the timing of appearance. Pigmented lesions which have been
present from birth (congenital nevi) are more likely to undergo
melanomatous degeneration than are nevi acquired in childhood.
Likewise, newly acquired pigmented lesions after age 30 in adults
are more suspect than those acquired in childhood. The second
aspect has to do with the history of change in a single lesion. A
single lesion described voluntarily and spontaneously by the patient
as having changed in size, configuration, or pigment density should
be viewed with considerable suspicion. The third aspect has to do
with the development of symptoms in a single pigmented lesion.
Thus, a single lesion described as pruritic or painful should be
examined with particular care. On the other hand, when patients
describe multiple lesions as symptomatic they are usually expressing
anxiety about the possibility of their having melanomas.

DYSPLASTIC NEVI

     The dysplastic nevus syndrome (see Chapter 11) causes special
problems in recognition and therapy. The nevi found in patients
with this syndrome should be viewed as premalignant, that is, as
precursors to full blown melanomas. Individual lesions which have
clinical features of dysplastic nevi (red hues, irregular shape,
speckled pigment, and diameter greater than 7 mm) should be removed
by excision or the patient should be referred to a dermatologist for
regular, careful examination. As indicated in Chapter 11 it is
almost certain that one or more of these dysplastic nevi will
undergo frankly malignant change during the lifetime of the patient.

CONCLUSIONS

     All pigmented lesions should be systematically examined with the
foregoing criteria in mind. Biopsy can be justified when even one
of these criteria is met. Nevertheless, a melanoma is not
particularly likely to be present unless two or more of the criteria
discussed above are present. In such a situation biopsy is
mandatory.

Many physicians cover their uncertainty regarding recognition of possible malignant features in a pigmented lesion by suggesting that the patient watch it on a regular basis and return for repeat examination if any evidence of change develops. Unfortunately, patients are neither emotionally nor medically prepared to carry out this advice. Thus, while it appears to relieve the physician of responsibility it transfers an undue burden onto the patient. In almost all instances when a question arises about a single lesion it is better to make a commitment one way or the other. If, after examination, question remains about a pigmented macule or papule, biopsy is warranted. If, on the other hand, you are satisfied that no criteria for suspicion are present, the patient should be so notified. When multiple suspicious lesions are present a diagnosis of dysplastic nevus syndrome should be considered. This diagnosis should be confirmed through multiple biopsies or by way of referral to a dermatologist.

Biopsy of any suspicious pigmented lesion ought to be carried out by elliptical excision. With this technique the entire specimen is available for stepped histologic examination. Moreover, the possibility of repigmentation (which often causes alarm both in the patient and in a subsequent examiner) is eliminated. Excisional biopsies with margins of only 1 or 2 mm are adequate. This approach is justifiable because even if melanoma should be present, re-excision with wider margins is usually desirable anyway. Lesions too large to be removed by simple excision should have one or more punch biopsies taken from the most suspicious areas. Re-excision with grafting can be carried out a week or so later if necessary. It is not completely clear whether such incisional biopsies influence the ultimate prognosis but when confronted with a large lesion it represents the only practical approach.

Good color photographs of the various types of melanoma can be found in the first three references listed below.

SELECTED READING

Mihm MC, Fitzpatrick TB, Lane-Brown MM, et al: Early detection of primary cutaneous melanoma. A color atlas. N Engl J Med 289:989, 1973.
Leider M, Brauer EW: A clinical atlas of pigmented lesions. J Dermatol Surg Oncol 5:705, 1979.
Sober AJ, Fitzpatrick TB, Mihm MC, et al: Early recognition of cutaneous melanoma. JAMA 242:2795, 1979.
Mackie RM, Young D: Human malignant melanoma. Int J Dermatol 23:433, 1984.
Friedman RJ, Heilman ER, Rigerl DS, et al: The dysplastic nevus. Clinical and pathologic features. Dermatol Clinics 3:239, 1985.
Friedman RJ, Rigel DS: The clinical features of malignant melanoma. Dermatol Clinics 3:271, 1985.

Greene MH, Clark WH, Tucker MA, et al: Acquired precursors of
    cutaneous malignant melanoma. The familial dysplastic nevus
    syndrome. N Engl J Med 312:91, 1985.
Greene MH, Clark WH, Tucker MA, et al: High risk of malignant
    melanoma in melanoma-prone families with dysplastic nevi. Ann
    Intern Med 102:458, 1985.
Metcalf JS, Maize JC: Melanocytic nevi and malignant melanoma.
    Dermatol Clinics 3:217, 1985.

Chapter 24

Annular (Ring Shaped) Lesions

All too often "ringworm" is the only diagnosis that occurs in one's mind when an annular lesion is found on physical examination. In fact, annularity is an extremely common configuration. It can be found in more than a dozen diseases spread out among several of the ten major diagnostic groups. Some of the diseases in which annular patterns are commonly seen are discussed below.

INFLAMMATORY PAPULES AND NODULES

Granuloma Annulare. As the name suggests, annularity is an almost constant finding in this disease. In most instances complete circles are formed but occasionally only partial circles are present. Most of the rings are 2 to 5 cm in diameter; the annulus itself is usually 3 to 5 mm wide. The rings are perfectly round except where two or more merge to form a single larger lesion with a gyrate or serpiginous border. Scale is not present. The color is usually violaceous but pink and skin colored lesions are sometimes seen. The annular border is made up of individual papules and in many instances, because of incomplete coalescence, this border appears "beaded." The lesions of granuloma annulare are most commonly found on the dorsal surface of the feet and hands; the ankles and elbows are also frequently involved. Biopsy reveals a diagnostic pattern.

VASCULAR REACTIONS

Urticaria. Urticarial lesions often fade in the center, leaving a ring-like border which advances centrifugally. In most patients with urticaria, annular lesions account for only a minority of all lesions present. Rarely, annular forms predominate. Both partial and full rings can be seen. Tremendous variation in size occurs; coalescence of two or more small rings leads to the formation of larger lesions with gyrate or serpiginous borders. No scale is present. The color varies from pink to red. Lesions may occur anywhere on the body. The rapidity with which the lesions appear, expand, and resolve is highly characteristic for urticaria. Lines drawn around lesions at any one point in time will no longer correspond to the new positions of lesions when the patient is examined several hours later. Diagnosis of urticaria is made on a clinical basis; biopsy is not particularly helpful.

Erythema Multiforme. At least a few annular lesions are regularly present in patients with erythema multiforme. Those

lesions which occur distally on the extremities are more likely to
be annular than are those on the trunk. Most annular lesions in
erythema multiforme will be formed of two concentric rings arranged
around a central bull's-eye. Such "target" lesions are
pathognomonic for the disease. The annular lesions of erythema
multiforme are small, seldom measuring more than 2 to 4 cm in
diameter. No scale is present. In questionable cases biopsy can be
helpful.

   Annular and Gyrate Erythemas. As the name implies, annular
lesions are a constant feature of these diseases. All of the
lesions present will be annular; solid papules and plaques are not
found. The number of lesions present is generally small. Sometimes
only a solitary ring is noted. The size of the annular lesions is
highly variable but most are palm sized or larger. In most
instances they begin as small lesions which then demonstrate slow
centrifugal growth over a period of several weeks. The lesions are
red but the hues vary from pink to violaceous. A small amount of
scale may be present on the active border. The center of the ringed
lesion may be darker in hue than the normal skin color. This color
change represents postinflammatory hyperpigmentation. Biopsy is
helpful in distinguishing these lesions from annular conditions
found in the papulosquamous group of diseases.

   Vasculitis. Small, annular lesions 1 or 2 cm in diameter are
occasionally found on the lower extremities in patients with
vasculitis. The active border of these lesions is purpuric; it is
violaceous in color and does not blanch on pressure. Often a
purpuric papule, hemorrhagic vesicle, or tiny infarct is found in
the center of these lesions. Scale is not present. The lesions
remain stable in size; centrifugal growth is not notable.
Individual lesions fade over a period of several weeks, but if the
process is ongoing, new annular lesions may appear while old ones
resolve. Biopsy confirms a clinical diagnosis.

PAPULOSQUAMOUS DISEASES

   Psoriasis. Annular patterns are particularly likely to be found
in psoriasis as individual lesions are undergoing resolution. In
such a situation the central portion of a plaque fades, leaving an
erythematous border at the periphery. This border is generally
wider than that found in the other annular diseases and there is a
tendency for the border to break up into individual papules. The
size of the annular lesions and their configuration depend on the
appearance of the plaque which preceded them. Since annularity
usually occurs during resolution, centrifugal growth is not commonly
seen. Typical psoriatic scale is usually present on the border but
in instances where the disease is under active treatment the
formation of scale is minimal or absent. Diagnosis is not

ordinarily difficult since more typical lesions of psoriasis can be found elsewhere on the body.

Tinea Corporis. Annular lesions are found in Microsporum sp. infections of children and in Trichophyton rubrum infections of adults. In children the lesions are solitary or are few in number. They are usually only 2 to 4 cm in diameter and are generally found on exposed surfaces. Complete circles are formed and there is relatively little tendency for coalescent growth of adjacent lesions. Scale is always present at the active border. The amount of inflammation, and thus the intensity of redness, is highly variable. KOH preparations or fungal cultures, or both, should be carried out to confirm a clinical diagnosis.

The annular lesions of tinea corporis in adults are quite different. Larger rings are noted and coalescent growth frequently results in the development of very large lesions with serpiginous borders. Complete circles are not often found and, in fact, normal appearing skin areas between active portions of the border may be large enough to interfere with recognition of the annular pattern. The active, advancing border is quite narrow (1 to 3 mm) and is usually scaling. Postinflammatory hyperpigmentation may be found within the central portion of the lesions as centrifugal growth occurs. New circles can sometimes redevelop in the cleared central area of the larger rings. Tinea corporis in the adult usually begins on the upper, inner thighs and from there extends onto the buttocks and lower trunk around the belt line. Less commonly the face or dorsal surface of the hands may be involved. The disease is pruritic and excoriations (fungal eczema) are often present. KOH preparations or fungal cultures, or both, should be used to confirm a clinical diagnosis.

Lupus Erythematosus. The lesions of discoid lupus erythematosus regularly assume an annular configuration as the central portions of otherwise solid plaques begin to undergo resolution. This resolution often results in the development of hypopigmentation and scarring in the central area. The presence of scarring is a pathognomonic feature. Some of these annular plaques are stable in size while others show evidence of very slow centrifugal growth. The active border is usually thin with some evidence of scale formation. Most lesions are 2 to 5 cm in diameter. Lesions are most often found on the face, scalp, and neck but occasionally the upper trunk and arms are involved. A clinical diagnosis can be confirmed by biopsy.

Annular lesions are also occasionally seen in subacute cutaneous and in systemic lupus erythematosus. Such lesions greatly resemble those of the gyrate erythemas (see above). They lack the central hypopigmentation and scarring found in discoid-type disease. The distribution is that of the upper trunk rather than the face and arms.

Pityriasis Rosea. The herald patch of pityriasis rosea regularly demonstrates an annular configuration. The border is brown-red in color and fine (pityriasis-type) scale is present. The lesion is usually 3 to 5 cm in diameter and, once present, does not grow in size. The herald patch when seen in the presence of full blown pityriasis rosea is not difficult to recognize, but when present before the rest of the disease develops it is easily misdiagnosed as tinea corporis. KOH preparations will, of course, distinguish between the two. The smaller lesions of pityriasis rosea are only rarely annular.

Lichen Planus. Ringed lesions are sometimes seen in lichen planus but they are generally outnumbered by more typical flattopped papules and plaques. Annular lesions when present are quite small, rarely measuring more than 2 or 3 cm in diameter. Both partial and complete circles may be formed. It is sometimes possible to distinguish within the annulus individual papules which have not completely coalesced. The color is distinctively violaceous and the surface is shiny because of the reflective properties of compacted lichenoid scale. Annular lesions are particularly likely to be found on the volar surface of the wrists and on the shaft of the penis. The presence of one or more linear lesions occurring as a result of the Koebner phenomenon is a very helpful diagnostic sign. Biopsy is pathognomonic.

Secondary Syphilis. Annular lesions are occasionally seen in secondary syphilis. As in lichen planus, the annular lesions are small, most being less than 2 or 3 cm in diameter. The color is red rather than violaceous. Linear lesions are not found. The annular lesions of secondary syphilis are particularly common on the face and genitalia. Clinical recognition is assisted by the regular presence of other symptoms and signs of secondary syphilis. The serologic test for syphilis will be positive. Biopsy of the lesions is highly distinctive.

ECZEMATOUS DISEASES

Xerotic Eczema. Annular patterns occur with some frequency in xerotic eczema. The border of such lesions is made up of a fine, red line. Actually this line is really a superficial fissure but this feature may not be recognized unless a hand lens is used for examination. Similar fissures may criss-cross throughout the patch, dividing the central area into small islands of normal appearing skin. The lesions of xerotic eczema are usually 1 to 4 cm in diameter and they are most commonly found on the thighs and lower legs. In older individuals the trunk may be involved. The diagnosis is made on the basis of clinical examination.

SELECTED READING

See "Selected Reading" lists for each of the above diseases as they are individually covered in Chapters 13-16.

Pruritus

Patients with pruritus can be divided into two major groups: those with and those without associated, readily visible skin disease. In either case, episodes of pruritus may occur spontaneously or may be precipitated by the presence of chapped, dry skin (xerosis), retained sweat, or psychologic factors such as anxiety or depression. Again, in either case, the severity of the pruritus waxes or wanes depending on the degree to which the mind is occupied with other matters. Thus, patients with pruritus of all types generally experience their worse itching during the evening and nighttime hours.

PRURITUS ASSOCIATED WITH VISIBLE SKIN DISEASE

Itching frequently occurs in association with inflammatory skin diseases (Table 25-1) and, in this setting, is probably due to the action of inflammatory mediators (such as histamine, prostaglandins, and kinins) on cutaneous nerve endings. The release of proteinases during the process of inflammation may also play an important role. The same lightly myelinated (or nonmyelinated) nerves responsible for the transmission of light pain appear to carry these itch impulses to the brain. Conventional wisdom suggests that all itching is qualitatively the same but empirical observations suggest that this might not be so. For instance, patients with urticaria often complain of extremely severe itching but only rarely does this pruritus lead to excoriation. On the other hand, patients with dermatitis herpetiformis regularly scratch their lesions even when the pruritus is perceived as only moderately severe in intensity. Moreover, those individuals who are genetically atopic (see Chapter 16) seem predisposed to vigorous excoriation at the slightest provocation whereas nonatopics rarely scratch uncontrollably. From a practical standpoint pruritus then appears to depend on four major factors: 1) the type of disease (some conditions are inherently more pruritic than others); 2) the environmental condition of the skin (xerotic and sweaty skin favors itching); 3) genetic factors (atopics have a lower threshold for itching than do nonatopics); and 4) the psychologic set of the patient (itching is more severe in anxious and depressed individuals). Those diseases which are to a greater or lesser degree inherently pruritic are listed in Table 25-1. But, based on the discussion above, the severity of pruritus experienced will be at the least partially dependent on other factors.

TABLE 25-1
DERMATOLOGIC DISEASES OFTEN ASSOCIATED WITH PRURITUS

Vesiculobullous diseases
    Herpes simplex (recurrent nonlabial, nongenital lesions)
    Vesicular tinea pedis
    Dyshidrosis
    Poison-ivy-type contact dermatitis
    Pemphigoid
    Dermatitis herpetiformis
    Scabies

Erythematous papules and nodules
    Insect bites

Vascular reactions
    Urticaria
    Fixed erythemas -- erythema multiforme

Papulosquamous diseases
    Psoriasis (primarily in intertriginous areas)
    Tinea corporis (primarily in groin and lower trunk)
    Parapsoriasis/mycosis fungoides
    Pityriasis rosea
    Lichen planus

Eczematous diseases -- all eczematous diseases

PRURITUS OCCURRING IN THE ABSENCE OF READILY APPARENT SKIN DISEASE

Pruritus occurring in the absence of visible skin disease is
termed essential pruritus. Excoriations may or may not be present
but, if present, will always occur without associated primary
lesions. Thus, patients will indicate that, at the time they began
scratching, there was no visible skin disease. Essential pruritus
can be divided into three subgroups: pruritus occurring as a result
of underlying systemic disease, pruritus associated with
"nondetectable" skin disease, and pruritus of purely psychologic
origin.

Pruritus Associated with Systemic Disease. Generalized itching
may be an early presenting sign (and thus a diagnostic clue) for
polycythemia vera, Hodgkin's disease, and some types of hepatic
disease. Pruritus in polycythemia vera is said to be particularly
prominent following the ingestion of alcohol or the use of hot water
for bathing. The pruritus of Hodgkin's disease may be related to
the presence of xerosis (see below) since acquired ichthyosis is

sometimes concomitantly present. Pruritus is often a prominent, early indicator of biliary cirrhosis but in most other forms of hepatic dysfunction itching occurs late in the course of the disease. Itching may thus accompany the jaundice of obstructive hepatic disease and is occasionally seen with hepatitis B virus infection. The itching in hepatic disease was originally believed to be related to increased tissue levels of bile salts but this explanation has recently been questioned. Ultraviolet light therapy and the ingestion of cholestyramine may be helpful in the treatment of pruritus associated with hepatic disease.

Generalized pruritus occurs late in the course of pregnancy and in end stage chronic renal disease. The itching in pregnancy is probably related to the mild cholestatic hepatic changes which are present as a normal part of late pregnancy. Hormonal factors and simple stretching of the skin may also play a role. The pruritus associated with chronic renal failure is often extremely severe. The cause of this pruritus is unknown but reported improvement following parathyroidectomy suggests that imbalances in calcium and phosphorus metabolism may play a role. Dialysis alone does not always lead to relief of the pruritus but the ingestion of activated charcoal and the use of ultraviolet light therapy have been reported as helpful.

Textbooks state that itching also occurs with diabetes mellitus, iron deficiency, and both hyper- and hypothyroidism. I cannot confirm these observations on the basis of my own experience.

Pruritus Associated with "Nondetectable" Skin Disease. Excess dryness (xerosis) of the skin is an extraordinarily common cause of generalized pruritus. Xerosis sufficient to cause itching is seen in a variety of circumstances. People who bathe or shower more than once a day often complain of itching. This is particularly likely to occur when hot water and soap are liberally used. Xerosis also occurs in very dry environments even without the addition of excess bathing. Thus it can be a problem in the low humidity of desert climates and in cold winter climates where dry, forced air heating is used. Xerosis also is a component of atopy and aging. In both situations inadequate cutaneous lipid production enhances moisture evaporation and leads to a drier than normal stratum corneum. Pruritus associated with xerosis is treated by reducing lipid loss from the skin (less soap and water) and by the application of skin lubricants (see Chapter 4).

Sweat retention and other forms of mechanical irritation such as occur during contact with wool clothing, fiberglass spicules, and some plants may also be followed by itching. These mechanical factors seem to cause more problems for atopic individuals than for individuals with "normal" skin.

Patients with pediculosis pubis (pubic lice) frequently report itching in the absence of visible skin lesions. Close observation reveals the presence of lice and adherent small white larvae (nits)

on the hair shafts. Treatment is easily accomplished through use of
lindane (Kwell) or synergized pyrethrins such as R.I.D. The latter
has the advantage of being a nonprescription product.

Patients with mastocytosis may have episodes of generalized
itching. This itching is usually accompanied by the presence of
flushing or urticaria. Careful examination of the skin often
reveals minute brown papules which are barely elevated above the
surface of the surrounding skin. Such lesions are routinely missed
unless they are carefully looked for. The use of standard H1
blockers, cimetidine, disodium cromoglycate, or PUVA therapy may be
helpful in the symptomatic treatment of this disease.

Pruritus of Psychologic Origin. A considerable portion of
patients with essential pruritus fall into this category. Some of
these individuals have easily detectable and rather severe
psychiatric disorders. For instance, some patients insist that
their itching is due to the presence of "bugs" or "worms" which are
crawling about in the skin. Careful examination of their skin and
of material that they have removed from their skin invariably fails
to reveal any such organisms. These patients resist rational
explanation and also refuse to accept psychiatric consultation.
They instead seek out yet one more physician in an attempt to get
someone to support their belief. It is appropriate to treat the
pruritus symptomatically and appropriate to offer psychotropic
medication but I believe it is inadvisable to offer medications
designed "to kill the bugs" since, after a brief period of placebo
effect, the problem will return, now reinforced by the belief that
the physician had indeed found something worth treating.

Most of the other patients with psychogenic pruritus have
considerably less psychic disability. A rough judgment regarding
the degree of psychic disability present can be made on the basis of
how severely the skin is damaged by scratching. Thus those with
many "neurotic" excoriations and those with multiple scratch papules
(prurigo nodularis) seem more troubled than those with no visible
sign of scratching. Anxiety or depression, or both, may be
present. A program of counseling or behavior modification, together
with appropriate psychotropic medications (see Chapter 4), will
often be helpful. Symptomatic relief is sometimes possible with
soaks, lubrication, and topical antipruritic agents (see Chapter
4). Orally administered antihistamines, except insofar as they have
psychotropic effects, are usually not very helpful.

SELECTED READING

Summerfield JA: Pain, itch and endorphins. Br J Dermatol 105:725,
    1981.
Camp R: Generalized pruritus and its management. Clin Exp
    Dermatol 7:557, 1982.
Kantor GR, Lookingbill DP: Generalized pruritus and systemic
    disease. J Am Acad Dermatol 9:375, 1983.

Jorizzo JL: The itchy patient. A practical approach. Dermatol
    Clinics 2:141, 1984.
Tuckett RP, Denman ST, Chapman CR, et al: Pruritus, cutaneous
    pain, and eccrine gland and sweating disorders. J Am Acad
    Dermatol 11:1000, 1984.
Martin J: Pruritus. Int J Dermatol 24:634, 1985.
Denman ST: A review of pruritus. J Am Acad Dermatol 14:375, 1986.

General Signs of Systemic Disease

HYPERPIGMENTATION

Increased pigmentation of the skin is seen in a number of systemic diseases. In porphyria cutanea tarda hyperpigmentation occurs on the face and arms presumably because of the photosensitizing effect of porphyrins. It is accompanied by hirsutism of the face (see below) together with skin fragility or blistering of the dorsal hands. There often is laboratory evidence of liver disease. Elevated urine levels of uro- and corpoporphyrin are diagnostic. When skin lesions suggestive of porphyria cutanea tarda are accompanied by gastrointestinal symptoms, neurologic problems, or psychiatric changes, stool porphyrins should be obtained in order to evaluate for the possible presence of variegate porphyria.

In Addison's disease hyperpigmentation occurs over the entire body but there is accentuation of the brown color in old scars and in skin creases. The nail beds and the oral mucosa may also become hyperpigmented. Hyperpigmentation in Addison's disease is due to increased output of pituitary hormones such as MSH and ACTH, both of which are capable of stimulating pigment production. Low serum cortisol levels are present and the diagnosis is established by the failure of cortisol levels to rise following appropriate adrenal stimulation. Vitiligo is sometimes also present in patients whose Addison's disease occurs as part of a multiglandular deficiency syndrome.

In scleroderma, hyperpigmentation is generalized, but there is accentuation of the brown color on the dorsal surface of the arms and hands. Occasionally vitiligo-like macules of hypopigmentation will be interspersed with areas of darkened skin. The mechanism for the pigmentation is unknown. Diagnosis is supported by the concomitant presence of Raynaud's phenomenon, sclerodactyly, decreased esophageal motility, and, in advanced cases, by the presence of pulmonary, cardiac, and renal disease. Skin biopsy, to determine the degree of sclerosis, helps to confirm a clinical diagnosis.

The generalized hyperpigmentation of hemochromatosis is somewhat more slate colored or bronze than it is brown. Jaundice may also be present. The mucous membranes become hyperpigmented in 20% of patients. The pathogenesis of the pigmentation is unknown. Glucose abnormalities are present and the diagnosis is confirmed by liver biopsy, which on appropriate staining demonstrates elevated levels of hepatic iron.

Hyperpigmentation associated with malignancy is most classically found with carcinoma of the lung. The pigmentation occurs because of the MSH-like activity of polypeptides elaborated by such tumors. Generalized melanosis is also sometimes seen with advanced, widespread melanoma, in which case the color is due to the direct production of pigmented compounds by the malignant cells.

The pigmentation in acanthosis nigricans, although generalized, is most notable in intertriginous areas where it is accompanied by the presence of densely pigmented, soft velvety ridges. These changes are particularly notable on the side of the neck, in the axillae, and in the groin. Increased pigmentation of mucosal surfaces is also often present. The mechanism responsible for the pigmentation is unknown but increased MSH output is suspected. Acanthosis nigricans is most commonly found as an unimportant aspect of obesity but its occurrence in children and adults of normal weight should raise a question of associated malignancy. Central nervous system tumors are most often the cause in children whereas gastrointestinal tumors are usually found in adults.

Most patients with severe neurofibromatosis show some evidence of generalized hyperpigmentation in addition to the presence of cafe-au-lait patches (see also Chapters 11 and 27).

Diffuse hyperpigmentation sometimes occurs as a result of chemotherapeutic agents administered to patients with varying types of malignancy. In such situations pigmented bands on the nails may also be noted.

SELECTED READING

Rigel DS, Jacobs MI: Malignant acanthosis nigricans: A review. J Dermatol Surg Oncol 6:923, 1980.

Tsega E, Damtew B, Landells JW, et al: Hyperpigmentation without blisters: Porphyria cutanea tarda. Br J Dermatol 103:137, 1980.

Tsuji T: Experimental hemosiderosis: Relationship between skin pigmentation and hemosiderin. Acta Derm Venereol 60:109, 1980.

Nordlund JJ, Sober AJ, Hansen TW: Periodic synopsis on pigmentation. J Am Acad Dermatol 12:359, 1985.

FLUSHING SYNDROMES

Sudden reddening of the upper torso most commonly occurs with anger and embarrassment. It may also be found in the presence of pheochromocytoma, where events which trigger catecholamine release from the tumor are followed by a marked rise in blood pressure as well as by facial reddening. Diagnosis of pheochromocytoma is confirmed by the presence of increased urinary catecholamines.

Patients with mastocytosis develop cutaneous flushing due to histaminemia under two circumstances. Mastocytomas in internal organs can, following appropriate stimulation, release enough histamine to cause a sudden generalized redness. Secondly, in patients with mastocytosis of the skin (urticaria pigmentosa) direct trauma to the skin may result in sufficient histamine release to result in localized or even generalized reddening. Urticarial lesions commonly accompany flushing episodes in mastocytosis.

Those patients who have carcinoid hepatic metastases or certain primary carcinoid tumors may develop flushing as a result of serotonin and bradykinin release from their tumors. These episodes are often triggered by food or alcohol ingestion. The face is primarily involved and, with the passage of time, a permanent cyanotic blue-red color persists between flushing episodes. Gastrointestinal and pulmonary symptoms usually accompany the cutaneous changes. Diagnosis is obtained when elevated levels of serotonin metabolites (5-hydroxyindole acetic acid and 5-hydroxytryptamine) are found in the urine.

SELECTED READING

Kendall MR, Fields JP, King LE Jr: Cutaneous mastocytosis without clinically obvious skin lesions. J Am Acad Dermatol 10:903, 1984.

Travis WD, Chin-Yang LI, Su WPD: Adult onset urticaria pigmentosa and systemic mast cell disease. Am J Clin Pathol 84:710, 1985.

HIRSUTISM

Several medical syndromes are associated with increased hair growth. Patients with porphyria cutanea tarda may develop facial hirsutism which is most marked between the lateral eyebrows and the normal sideburns. The mechanism for this hair growth is not known.

Patients with Cushing's disease or syndrome develop an accentuated male hair growth pattern as part of the excess stimulation of glucocorticoid hormones. The facial redness, acne, edema, and fat deposition in the cheeks and upper back lead to a clinical diagnosis. Laboratory confirmation of this diagnosis can be obtained through determination of serum cortisol levels.

Patients with acromegaly often develop hirsutism, but it is rarely a prominent finding in comparison to the voice changes and increased size of the hands, feet, and jaw. The process appears to be due to the increased levels of growth hormone which characterize the disease.

The virilizing syndromes due to ovarian tumors, adrenal tumors, and adrenal hyperplasia lead to male pattern hair growth as well as other forms of masculinization. Diagnosis depends on the presence of increased levels of testosterone in the serum and 17-hydroxy ketosteroids in the urine.

In polycystic ovarian disease (Stein-Leventhal syndrome) the long term presence of anovulatory cycles leads to persistent stimulation of ovarian stroma by estrogenic hormones. This in turn causes increased production of ovarian androgenic hormones and

hirsutism. Virilization, however, is not usually seen. Diagnosis
is suggested by the presence of elevated levels of serum
testosterone. A somewhat similar syndrome occurs as a result of 21
hydroxylase deficiency.

Young women who, through vigorous restriction of foot intake,
maintain themselves at grossly underweight levels (anorexia nervosa)
become amenorrheic and may develop hirsutism. The mechanism for
this is unknown. The diagnosis is made on a clinical basis.

Hirsutism can develop during long term administration of
phenytoin (Dilantin) and minoxidil (Loniten). The mechanism for
development of hair growth with these two medications is unknown.
Hirsutism also occurs with administration of various hormonal agents
and has been occasionally reported with the use of a few other
medications such as the phenothiazines. A familial pattern of
hirsutism sometimes occurs as a normal finding in some women of
Mediterranean descent.

SELECTED READING

Kredar JC, Gibson M, Krusinski PA: Hirsutism: Evaluation and
    treatment. J Am Acad Dermatol 12:215, 1985.
Kuttenn F, Couillin P, Girard F, et al: Late onset adrenal
    hyperplasia in hirsutism. N Engl J Med 313:224, 1985.

CUTANEOUS ULCERS

One or more deep, undermined ulcers known as pyoderma
gangrenosum may develop on the lower extremities of patients with
inflammatory bowel disease due to ulcerative colitis, granulomatous
colitis, or regional enteritis. These ulcers are generally filled
with healthy granulation tissue and they are surprisingly free of
pus and crust. The undermined margin of skin around the ulcer is
usually deeply violaceous. A variety of bacterial organisms
colonizes these ulcers but treatment with ordinary antibiotic agents
does not lead to clinical improvement. The pathogenesis of the
ulcers is not known but both immunologic and vasculitic factors may
be important. The ulcers of pyoderma gangrenosum do not respond to
topical therapy but often resolve if the associated inflammatory
bowel disease can be successfully treated. Systemic administration
of steroids leads to direct improvement of the cutaneous ulcers as
well as to improvement of the gastrointestinal disease. The oral
administration of dapsone may enhance the effect of steroids.

Ulcers similar in appearance to those described above are
occasionally seen in patients with rheumatoid arthritis. Such
ulcers are particularly likely to occur in those patients who have
markedly elevated titers of rheumatoid factor. This observation
suggests that circulating immune complexes may play a role in the
pathogenesis. Unfortunately, the response of these ulcers even to

high dose steroids is not as good as that obtained in patients with inflammatory bowel disease.

Patients with <u>myeloma</u>, especially when the paraprotein is IgA in type, may also develop cutaneous ulcers which simulate the lesions of pyoderma gangrenosum. These individuals often have scattered purpuric and pustular lesions as well.

A small number of patients have been reported with a variant of pyoderma gangrenosum in which hemorrhagic bullae precede the breakdown and ulceration of the skin. Most of these patients have <u>leukemia</u> or preleukemia of the myelocytic type.

Ulcers due to vasculitic processes may be found in patients with nodular vasculitis (erythema induratum), polyarteritis nodosa, giant cell arteritis, and Wegener's granulomatosis. Ulcers due to vascular occlusion may develop in patients with arteriosclerosis, hypertension, and diabetes. Ulcers due to traumatic damage are sometimes seen in patients with neuropathic complications of diabetes or leprosy.

Patients with advanced <u>mycosis fungoides</u> often develop deep ulcers of the skin due to destructive infiltration with malignant T-cell lymphocytes. The presence of such ulcers signals the terminal phase of the disease. The diagnosis is ordinarily not difficult since typical plaques of mycosis fungoides usually accompany the ulcers. A clinical diagnosis can be confirmed by biopsy from the edge of the ulcers. Partial, temporary improvement of these ulcers is usually obtainable with high dose radiation therapy.

Several <u>deep fungal diseases</u> are associated with cutaneous ulceration. In the United States the most common infections responsible for ulcer formation are sporotrichosis, coccidioidomycosis, histoplasmosis, and North American blastomycosis. The diagnosis is best confirmed by culture but organisms are also sometimes visible in biopsies taken from the edge of the ulcers. The cutaneous lesions of deep fungal infection are particularly likely to be found in patients who are immunocompromised.

Several of the atypical <u>mycobacterial infections</u> also result in cutaneous ulcers. The most common of these infections is that due to <u>Mycobacterium marinum</u>. This infection is acquired among those who swim in infected swimming pools or who work with infected aquariums. Rarely, systemic atypical mycobacterial infections lead to ulceration as a result of disseminated disease. Response of the cutaneous atypical mycobacterial ulcers to conventional antituberculous drugs is not particularly good.

<u>Stasis ulcers</u> are covered in the section on stasis dermatitis.

VASCULAR REACTIONS

Urticaria, erythema multiforme, erythema nodosum, and vasculitis are all occasionally seen as markers of internal disease. They are particularly likely to occur in patients with collagen vascular disease, dysproteinemias, and tumors. These conditions are discussed individually in Chapter 14.

PRURITUS

Pruritus in the absence of skin disease is occasionally a marker for underlying renal disease, hepatic disease, lymphoma, and polycythemia vera. This subject is covered more fully in Chapter 25.

SELECTED READING

Beyt BE, Ortbals DW, Santa Cruz DJ, et al: Cutaneous mycobacteriosis: Analysis of 34 cases with a new classification of the disease. Medicine 60:95, 1980.

Hickman JG, Lazarus GS: Pyoderma gangrenosum: A reappraisal of associated systemic diseases. Br J Dermatol 102:235, 1980.

Holt PJA, Davies MG, Saunders KC, et al: Pyoderma gangrenosum. Medicine 59:114, 1980.

Kerking TM, Duma RG, Shadomy S: The evolution of pulmonary cryptococcosis. Ann Intern Med 94:611, 1981.

Wheat LJ, Slama TG, Eitzen HE: A large urban outbreak of histoplasmosis: Clinical features. Ann Intern Med 94:331, 1981.

Grange JM: Mycobacteria and the skin. Int J Dermatol 21:497, 1982.

Kane J, Righter J, Krajden S, et al: Blastomycosis: A new endemic focus in Canada. Can Med Assoc J 129:728, 1983.

Powell FC, Schroeter AL, Su WPD, et al: Pyoderma gangrenosum and monoclonal gammopathy. Arch Dermatol 119:468, 1983.

Bradsher RW, Rice DC, Abernathy RS: Ketoconazole therapy for endemic blastomycosis. Ann Intern Med 103:872, 1985.

Gibson LE, Dicken CH, Flach DB: Neutrophilic dermatoses and myeloproliferative disease: Report of two cases. Mayo Clin Proc 60:735, 1985.

Specific Signs of Systemic Disease

The diseases discussed in this chapter are for the most part uncommon diseases. They are listed here because the cutaneous manifestations are distinctive enough to be of diagnostic help or because the cutaneous involvement is an important contribution to the morbidity of the disease.

Dermatomyositis. Approximately 50% of the patients with polymyositis (inflammatory muscle disease of the autoimmune type) develop the cutaneous changes of dermatomyositis. The most common finding is a violaceous edema of the upper eyelids. This is sometimes accompanied by redness and swelling of the entire face. In contrast to the facial lesions of lupus erythematosus, the red patches of dermatomyositis are more generalized and are less distinctly marginated. Patients with dermatomyositis also may have red to violaceous patches and plaques over the elbows, knees, and dorsal surface of the knuckles. The changes on the hands are similar to those found in lupus erythematosus but those of dermatomyositis are usually located directly over the joints, whereas in lupus erythematosus they are found over the phalanges between the joints. Violaceous patches may develop over the volar tips of the fingers and on the thenar and hypothenar eminences. These are similar to palmar changes found in other collagen vascular diseases. The severity of the cutaneous involvement does not correlate particularly well with the severity of the associated myositis. A clinical diagnosis of dermatomyositis can be confirmed by the presence of elevated muscle enzymes in the serum and by recognition of the typical inflammatory changes on muscle biopsy. Systemic malignancies of various types are found with unexpected frequency in patients with dermatomyositis who are over the age of 40.

Scleroderma. Scleroderma is not ordinarily a difficult disease to recognize. It is characterized by sclerodactyly, which is defined as thickening and tightening of the skin over the fingers and hands. Other typical changes on the hand include the presence of pitted scarring on the fingertips, tapering of the fingers with fingertip soft tissue loss, telangiectasia of the posterior nail fold, and curvature of the nail over the fingertip. Palmar violaceous color changes similar to those described for dermatomyositis and lupus erythematosus may also be present. Hyperpigmentation, often interspersed with vitiligo-like hypopigmented patches, sometimes develops on the anterior chest and dorsal surface of the hands and arms. In a few patients, telangiectatic mats similar to those of the Osler-Weber-Rendu

syndrome are found on the face, upper chest, and arms. Calcinosis
of the skin and subcutaneous tissue is a late finding in
scleroderma. Skin biopsy which demonstrates an increased thickness
of the dermis and collagen entrapment of the sweat glands is helpful
in confirming a clinical diagnosis.

Lupus Erythematosus. The lesions of lupus erythematosus are
described in Chapter 15.

Hyperthyroidism. Autoimmune thyroid disease of the
hypermetabolic type (Graves's disease) is reflected by several
visible changes. The skin is soft and moist. Scalp hair is thin in
diameter and evidence of diffuse alopecia may be present. Vitiligo
occurs in 5 to 10% of the patients. Alopecia areata occurs in a
considerably smaller proportion of patients. Onycholysis of the
fingernails is sometimes seen. Late in the course of the disease a
few patients develop a peculiar form of clubbing (thyroid acropachy)
or pretibial mixedema. The latter consists of thickened,
irregularly surfaced, skin colored plaques over the lower anterior
shins. These plaques are usually symptomatic.

Diabetes Mellitus. Patients with diabetes mellitus may develop
a number of cutaneous changes. The yellow plaques of necrobiosis
lipoidica diabeticorum (see Chapter 12), most often located on the
anterior shins, are the most distinctive of these changes. Small,
hypopigmented, slightly depressed scars (diabetic dermopathy) are
also occasionally found on the anterior lower legs. These lesions
probably represent obliterative small vessel disease in an area
prone to trauma. Bullous lesions somewhat similar in appearance to
those of pemphigoid may arise from otherwise normal appearing skin
around the feet and ankles. The cause of these blisters is
unknown. Eruptive xanthomas consisting of small, smooth, pink, dome
shaped papules may appear in a sudden shower of lesions in those
whose diabetes is grossly out of control. Staphylococcal bacterial
infections and candidal yeast infections are seen with increased
frequency in diabetic individuals. Diabetes is also associated with
a variety of other cutaneous and medical conditions which are too
rare to warrant discussion here.

Neurofibromatosis. The presence of sharply marginated, light
brown patches (cafe-au-lait patches) is often the first clue to the
presence of von Recklinghausen's disease (see also Chapter 11). In
late childhood or during the teen years axillary freckling and
cutaneous neurofibromas begin to develop. The latter are soft,
smooth surfaced, pedunculated papules 0.5 to 2 cm in diameter. They
vary in number from several to several hundred and are distributed
randomly over the trunk and extremities. Patients with the most
severe forms of neurofibromatosis may develop large, grotesque,
sack-like plexiform neuromas. A small proportion of these latter
lesions undergo sarcomatous degeneration.

Tuberous Sclerosis. The earliest sign of tuberous sclerosis is
generally the presence of small, faint white, oval shaped patches

(ash leaf spots) scattered randomly on the trunk and extremities (see also Chapter 10). These lesions may be present at birth or may develop in early childhood. One or more elevated, thickened, skin colored plaques (shagreen plaques) may appear on the lower back in late childhood. Also, during late childhood, pinhead sized, smooth, red, dome shaped papules (adenoma sebaceum) begin to emerge on the central portion of the face. The upper lip is spared. Such lesions are easily mistaken for acne papules. Finally, in adult life, small, firm, skin colored, subungual or periungual fibromas may be noted. Similar lesions may also occur in mouth.

Peutz-Jehgers Syndrome. This dominantly inherited condition is characterized by the presence of small brown or black freckles which appear in clusters on and around the lips and on the fingertips. These pigmentary changes are accompanied by the development of intestinal polyps. Carcinomatous degeneration of these polyps is not common but does occur.

Osler-Weber-Rendu Syndrome. This dominantly inherited condition, also known as hereditary hemorrhagic telangiectasia, is characterized by the presence of small, dusky red, clustered macules on the fingertips, lips, and mucosal surfaces. These macules are composed of multiple telangiectatic vessels which blanch on pressure. Lesions similar to these may also occur in patients with the CRST variant of scleroderma. Patients with this disease have recurrent episodes of epistaxis and gastrointestinal bleeding. Arteriovenous fistulae are sometimes present in the lungs and liver.

Relapsing Polychondritis. Patients with relapsing polychondritis usually present with dramatically swollen, painful, red ears. Sometimes the nose is involved in a similar manner. These skin changes reflect the presence of massive inflammatory changes in the underlying cartilage. Such changes occurring in the larynx, trachea, and bronchi may lead to death. Ocular and articular abnormalities may also be present.

Reiter's Syndrome. This disease occurs almost entirely in men. The cutaneous lesions of Reiter's syndrome are similar to, if not identical with, those found in psoriasis. Pustular plaques on the palms and soles, together with small red scaling plaques on the glans penis, are characteristically present. Ocular inflammatory disease, sacroilitis, and arthritis of the spine and larger peripheral joints complete the syndrome. Most patients with Reiter's disease have an HLA haplotype which includes B27. Episodes of disease activity may be triggered by a variety of infectious etiologies.

Behcet's Syndrome. Behcet's syndrome is characterized by the presence of aphthous-like ulcers of the mouth and genitalia. These changes are usually accompanied by arthritis, uveitis, and a variety of neurologic changes. Thrombophlebitis, gastrointestinal involvement, erythema nodosum, and a peculiar pustular response to skin trauma (pathergy) are occasionally present.

Sarcoidosis. Sarcoidosis is characterized by the presence of noninfectious, noncaseating granulomas of many organs, including the skin. The most distinctive skin lesions consist of clusters of small, nonscaling, violaceous to skin colored, dome shaped papules. These papules are most often found on the face and neck. Coalescence of the papules to form annular plaques is frequently noted. Larger nodules and plaques are sometimes found on the trunk and extremities. Involvement of scar tissue with sarcoidal granulomas is highly characteristic. Erythema nodosum of the lower legs frequently accompanies active lesions of sarcoid occurring in the lungs. Biopsy of the skin lesions (except those of erythema nodosum) reveals the characteristic granulomas and allows confirmation of a diagnosis made on clinical examination.

Acquired Immunodeficiency Syndrome (AIDS). Several types of skin lesions are found in AIDS and, in fact, are often helpful in making this diagnosis. The lesions of Kaposi's sarcoma occur in about 50% of the patients. They consist of red to violaceous, smooth surfaced papules and nodules. Lesions may be found anywhere on the body, but the most frequent distribution includes the face, arms, trunk, and mucous membranes. The lesions of AIDS-related Kaposi's sarcoma differ from those of classical Kaposi's sarcoma in that the former are smaller in size, are violaceous rather than blue-black in color, and are distributed on the upper half of the body instead of the legs. Less characteristic findings include oral candidiasis, oral hairy leukoplakia (see Chapter 21), seborrheic dermatitis of the face, minute erythematous papules of the trunk, and various other types of cutaneous opportunistic infections.

SELECTED READING

Riccardi VM: Von Recklinghausen neurofibromatosis. N Engl J Med 305:1617, 1981.
Keat A: Reiter's syndrome and reactive arthritis in perspective. N Engl J Med 309:1606, 1983.
Callen JP: Dermatomyositis. Dermatol Clinics 1:461, 1983.
Connolly SM: Scleroderma: Therapeutic options. Cutis 34:274, 1984.
Kerdel FA, Moschella SL: Sarcoidosis. An updated review. J Am Acad Dermatol 11:1, 1984.
Lee EB, Anhalt GJ, Voorhees JJ, et al Pathogenesis of scleroderma. Int J Dermatol 23:85, 1984.
Sibbald RG, Schachter RK: The skin and diabetes mellitus. Int J Dermatol 23:567, 1984.
Wong RC, Ellis CN, Diaz LA: Behcet's disease. Int J Dermatol 23:25, 1984.
Manchul LA, et al: The frequency of malignant neoplasms in patients with polymyositis-dermatomyositis. Arch Intern Med 145:1835, 1985.
White JW Jr: Relapsing polychondritis. South Med J 78:448, 1985.

Acheson ED: AIDS: A challenge for the public health. <u>Lancet</u>,
    <u>1</u>:662, 1986.
Sorensen SA, Mulvihill JJ, Nielsen A: Long-term follow-up of Von
    Recklinghausen neurofibromatosis. Survival and malignant
    neoplasms. <u>N</u> <u>Engl</u> <u>J</u> <u>Med</u> <u>314</u>:1010, 1986.

Major Reference Textbooks in Dermatology

Demis DJ, Dobson RL, McGuire J: Clinical Dermatology. Harper &
Row, Hagerstown, MD, 1979.
        This is a most unusual textbook. It is bound loose-leaf
    style so that it can be continuously updated. Approximately 10
    to 15% of the book is rewritten each year. The black and white
    photographs are good. There are no color photographs. Because
    of the loose-leaf format, use of the index is somewhat
    cumbersome.

Fitzpatrick TB, Eisen AZ, Wolff K, et al: Dermatology in General
Medicine, 3rd edition. McGraw-Hill, New York, 1986.
        This is the major American reference textbook. It is
    particularly helpful in the areas of basic science, clinical
    pathogenesis, and etiology. The cutaneous manifestations of
    systemic disease are emphasized. It contains several sections
    of color clinical photographs. The third edition is
    considerably larger than the second with many new sections and
    an increased number of photographs. Coverage of pigmentation
    and pigmented lesions is particularly thorough. The section on
    photomedicine is unique.

Moschella SL, Hurley HJ: Dermatology, 2nd edition. WB Saunders,
Philadelphia, 1985.
        This is the easiest to read of all the major textbooks.
    The major emphasis is on the most important and common skin
    diseases, but there is also remarkably good coverage of esoteric
    subjects. An excellent job of editing has been done. The black
    and white photographs are very good; there are no color
    photographs.

Rook A, Wilkinson DS, Ebling FJG: Textbook of Dermatology, 3rd
edition. Blackwell Scientific Publications, Oxford, England, 1979.
        This is the foremost British reference textbook. It is
    extraordinarily complete even in esoteric areas. The clinical
    descriptions are particularly good but the sections on therapy
    are not always appropriate for American use. The index is
    particularly well organized. Black and white photographs are
    excellent. There are no color photographs. This edition is
    dated, but a new edition should soon be available.

Appendix B

Color Atlases of Skin Lesions

Edmond RTD: <u>Color Atlas of Infectious Diseases</u>. Year Book Medical Publishers, Chicago, 1974.

Fitzpatrick TB, Polano MK, Suurmond D: <u>Color Atlas and Synopsis of Clinical Dermatology</u>. McGraw-Hill, New York, 1983.

Fry L: <u>Dermatology. An Illustrated Guide</u>. Update Publications, London, 1978.

Habif TP: <u>Clinical Dermatology, A Color Guide to Diagnosis and Therapy</u>. CV Mosby, St. Louis, 1985.

Kimmig J, Janner M: <u>Pocket Color Atlas of Dermatology</u>, American edition, Goldschmidt H, translator. Year Book Medical Publishers, Chicago, 1975.

Levene GM, Calnan CD: <u>Color Atlas of Dermatology</u>. Year Book Medical Publishers, Chicago, 1974.

Lynch PJ, Epstein S: <u>Burckhardt's Atlas and Manual of Dermatology and Venereology</u>, 3rd American edition. Williams & Wilkins, Baltimore, 1977.

Rassner G, Kahn G: <u>Atlas of Dermatology</u>, 2nd edition. Urban & Schwarzenberg, Baltimore-Munich, 1983.

Reeves JRT, Maibach HI: <u>Clinical Dermatology Illustrated: A Regional Approach</u>. ADIS Health Science Press, Boston, 1984.

Rosen T: <u>Atlas of Black Dermatology</u>. Little, Brown and Company, Boston, 1981.

Sharvill DE: <u>Skin Diseases</u>. Williams & Wilkins, Baltimore, 1984.

Steigleder GK, Maibach HI: <u>Pocket Atlas of Dermatology</u>. Thieme-Stratton, New York, 1984.

Wisdom A: <u>Color Atlas of Venereology</u>. Year Book Medical Publishers, Chicago, 1973.

Recent Reference Monographs

REGIONAL DERMATOLOGY

Rook A, Dawber R: Diseases of the Hair and Scalp. Blackwell
    Scientific Publications, Boston, 1982.
Beaven DW, Brooks SE: Color Atlas of the Nail in Clinical Diagnosis.
    Year Book Medical Publishers, Chicago, 1985.
Baran R, Dawber RPR: Diseases of the Nails and Their Management
    Blackwell Scientific Publications, Boston, 1984.
Zaias N: The Nail in Health and Disease. SP Medical & Scientific
    Books, New York, 1980.
Senturia BH, Marcus MD, Lucente FE: Diseases of the External Ear,
    2nd edition. Grune & Stratton, New York, 1980.
Kritzinger EE, Wright BE: Color Atlas of the Eye and Systemic
    Disease. Year Book Medical Publishers, Chicago, 1984.
Friedrich, EG Jr: Vulvar Disease, 2nd edition. WB Saunders,
    Philadelphia, 1983.
Gardner HL, Kaufman RH: Benign Diseases of the Vulva and Vagina,
    2nd edition. GK Hall, Boston, 1981.
Lynch MA, Brightman VJ, Greenberg MS: Burket's Oral Medicine, 8th
    edition. JB Lippincott, Philadelphia, 1984.
Pindborg JJ: Atlas of Diseases of the Oral Mucosa, 4th edition. WB
    Saunders, Philadelphia, 1985.
McCarthy PL, Shklar G: Diseases of the Oral Mucosa, 2nd edition.
    Lea and Febiger, Philadelphia, 1980.
Jones JH, Mason DK: Oral Manifestations of Systemic Disease. WB
    Saunders, Philadelphia, 1980.
Samitz MH: Cutaneous Disorders of the Lower Extremities. JB
    Lippincott, Philadelphia, 1981.

DERMATOLOGIC ASPECTS OF SYSTEMIC DISEASE

Braverman IM: Skin Signs of Systemic Disease, 2nd edition. WB
    Saunders, Philadelphia, 1981.
Callen JP: Cutaneous Aspects of Internal Disease. Year Book Medical
    Publishers, Chicago, 1981.

THERAPEUTICS

Arndt KA: Manual of Dermatologic Therapeutics, 3rd edition.
    Little, Brown and Company, Boston, 1983.

Epstein E, Epstein E Jr: Skin Surgery, 5th edition. Charles C
    Thomas, Springfield, IL, 1982.
Stegman SJ, Tromovitch TA, Glogan RG: Basics of Dermatologic
    Surgery. Year Book Medical Publishers, Chicago, 1982.
Wright VC, Riopelle MA: Laser Physics for Surgeons. Biomedical
    Communications, Houston, 1982.
Zacarian SA: Cryosurgery for Skin Cancer and Cutaneous Disorders.
    CV Mosby, St. Louis, 1985.

PATHOPHYSIOLOGY

Goldsmith LA: Biochemistry and Physiology of the Skin. Oxford
    University Press, New York, 1983.
Soter NA, Baden HP: Pathophysiology of Dermatologic Diseases.
    McGraw-Hill Book, New York, 1984.
Thiers BH, Dobson RL: Pathogenesis of Skin Disease. Churchill
    Livingstone, New York, 1986.

IMMUNODERMATOLOGY

Dahl MV: Clinical Immunodermatology. Year Book Medical Publishers,
    Chicago, 1981.
Stone J: Dermatologic Immunology and Allergy. CV Mosby, St. Louis,
    1985.

DERMATOPATHOLOGY

Hood AF, Kwan TH, Burns DC, Mihm MC Jr: Primer of Dermatopathology.
    Little, Brown and Company, Boston, 1984.
Lever WF, Schaumburg-Lever G: Histopathology of the Skin, 6th
    edition. JB Lippincott, Philadelphia, 1983.
Pinkus H, Mehregan AH: A Guide to Dermatohistopathology, 3rd
    edition. Appleton-Century-Crofts, New York, 1981.

PHOTOBIOLOGY

Harber LC, Bickers DR: Photosensitivity Diseases. WB Saunders,
    Philadelphia, 1981.
Parrish JA, Kripke ML, Morison WL: Photoimmunology. Plenum Medical
    Book Company, New York, 1983.

INFECTIONS, INFESTATIONS, AND INSECT BITES

Alexander J O'D: Arthropods and Human Skin. Springer-Verlag, New
    York, 1984.
Holmes KK, Mardh PA, Sparling PF, Weisner PJ: Sexually Transmitted
    Diseases. McGraw-Hill, New York, 1984.

Noble WC: Microbiology of Human Skin, 2nd edition. Lloyd-Luke
     Medical Books, London, 1981.
Orkin M, Maibach HI: Cutaneous Infestations and Insect Bites.
     Marcel Dekker, New York, 1985.
Rippon JW: Medical Mycology, 2nd edition. WB Saunders,
     Philadelphia, 1982.

CONTACT DERMATITIS

Adams RM: Occupational Skin Disease. Grune & Stratton, New York,
     1983.
Cronin E: Contact Dermatitis. Churchill Livingstone, New York,
     1980.
Fisher AA: Contact Dermatitis, 3rd edition. Lea & Febiger,
     Philadelphia, 1986.

PEDIATRIC DERMATOLOGY

Hurwitz S: Clinical Pediatric Dermatology. WB Saunders,
     Philadelphia, 1981.

COSMETOLOGY

Frost P, Horwitz SN: Principles of Cosmetics for the Dermatologist.
     CV Mosby, St. Louis, 1982.

Pediatric Dosages of Commonly used Medications

Diphenhydramine (Benadryl)	5 mg/kg/day, divided doses
Erythromycin	30 to 50 mg/kg/day, divided doses
Griseofulvin	15 mg/kg/day, single or divided doses
Hydroxyzine (Atarax)	2 mg/kg/day, divided doses
Oxacillin, dicloxacillin, cloxacillin	50 to 100 mg/kg/day, divided doses
Penicillin, benzathine	300,000 to 900,000 units in single injection
Penicillin, phenoxymethyl	50 mg/kg/day, divided doses
Prednisone	1 to 2 mg/kg/day, single dose

These dosages and others used throughout the text are believed to be accurate. However, before prescribing, physicians should check for the manufacturer's latest recommendations. One convenient source for this infomation is the current annual edition of the Physician's Desk Reference (Medical Economics Company, Oradell, NJ).

Index

Underlined page numbers represent the page on which the most major discussion of that topic may be found.

333

Bayes' theorem, 50
Beau's grooves, 287
Bed bug bites, 179
Bee sting, 179, 187
Behcet's disease, 292
Behcet's syndrome, 293, 323
Benzocaine, 260
Benzodiazepines, 37, 196, 230
Benzoin, Tincture of, 133
Benzophenones, 30
Benzoyl peroxide, 111, 133
Betamethasone diproprionate, 25
Betamethasone valerate, 25
Bible tumor, 144
Bile salts, 312
Biliary cirrhosis, 230, 312
Biofeedback, 241
Biopsies, immunofluorescent, 219
Biopsy, punch, 56
Biopsy, skin, 57
Biopsy techniques,
 immunofluorescent, 53
Birth control pills, 113, 172,
 190, 282
Birthmark, 170, 171
Bite line, 295
Bites, bed bug, 179
Bites, chigger, 179
Bites, flea, 179
Bites, insect, 95, 184
Bites, spider, 179
Bites, tick, 201
Black dots, 124, 216, 278
Black light, 49
Blackheads, 108
Blastomycosis, 319
Bleaches, quinone type, 150
Bleaching, hydroquinone, 156
Bleeding, 56
Bleomycin, 127
Blepharitis, 115
Blistering, 315
Blisters, friction, 106
Blisters, traumatic, 106
Blood vessels, 7
Boot, Unna, 246
Borrelia treponemes, 296
Bowen's disease, 135, 226

Bowenoid papulosis, 132
Bradykinin, 317
Breasts, 247
Breslow technique, 164
Brown patches, 155
Brown plaques, 155
Brown-black lesions, 74, 155
Brown-black macules, 155
Brown-black nodules, 155
Brown-black papules, 155
Bulla, 17
Bullous, erythema multiforme,
 98, 100
Bullous diseases, 79
Bullous impetigo, 104
Burns, acid, 255
Burns, alkali, 255
Burns, thermal, 106, 152, 255
Burow's solution, 20
Burrows, 247
Burst of steroids, 35
Buschke-Lowenstein tumors, 132
Butterfly eruption, 220
Buttocks, 81, 153, 222, 247

C1 esterase inhibitor, 196
C3, 54, 98, 99
Cafe-au-lait patches, 170, 171,
 322
Calamine lotion, 21
Calcification, cerebral, 135
Calcinosis cutis, 322
Calluses, 124, 130, 177
Campbell de Morgan spots, 180
Camphor, 28
Candida albicans, 119, 288,
 289, 296
Candida paronychia, 119, 289
Candida sp., 119, 288, 289, 296
Candida vaginitis, 119
Candidiasis, 118, 251, 274, 276,
 292, 296, 324
Candidiasis, chronic
 mucocutaneous, 119
Cantharidin, 126, 143
Carbon dioxide lasers, 65
Carbon dioxide slush, 112
Carbuncle, 184